Molecular Cytogenetics

Molecular Cytogenetics

Edited by

Barbara Ann Hamkalo

and

John Papaconstantinou

Biology Division
Oak Ridge National Laboratory
Oak Ridge, Tennessee

Plenum Press • New York–London

Library of Congress Cataloging in Publication Data

Main entry under title:

Molecular cytogenetics

"Proceedings of the twenty-sixth annual Biology Division research con-
ference held April 9-12, 1973 in Gatlinburg, Tennessee; . . . sponsored by
the Biology Division of the Oak Ridge National Laboratory."
Includes bibliographies.
1. Molecular genetics—Congresses. 2. Cytogenetics—Congress. I. Hamkalo,
Barbara Ann, ed. II. Papaconstantinou, John, ed. III. United States. National
Laboratory, Oak Ridge, Tenn. Biology Division. [DNLM: 1. Cytogenetics—
Congresses. QH605 011m 1973]

| QH426.M64 | 575.2'1 | 73-18008 |

ISBN 0-306-30765-0

*Proceedings of the Twenty-Sixth Annual Biology Division Research Conference,
held April 9-12,1973, in Gatlinburg, Tennessee.*

*Dr. Hamkalo's present address is the Department of Molecular
Biology and Biochemistry, University of California at Irvine,
Irvine, California 92664.*

*© 1973 Plenum Press, New York
A Division of Plenum Publishing Corporation
227 West 17th Street, New York, N.Y. 10011*

*United Kingdom edition published by Plenum Press, London
A Division of Plenum Publishing Company, Ltd.
Davis House (4th Floor), 8 Scrubs Lane, Harlesden, London, NW10 6SE, England*

FOREWORD

This volume represents the Proceedings of the Twenty-Sixth
Annual Biology Division Research Conference held April 9-12, 1973
in Gatlinburg, Tennessee. The subject of the symposium was
Molecular Cytogenetics and the aim of the meeting was to bring
together researchers interested in problems of chromosome organization, activity and regulation in prokaryotes and eukaryotes.
Cytological, biochemical and genetic approaches to these questions
were included since the collective information gained from these
disciplines provides an integrated approach to genome structure
and function.

The meeting was sponsored by the Biology Division of the Oak
Ridge National Laboratory*. It would not have been possible without the interest and cooperation of the organizing committee under
the chairmanship of O. L. Miller, Jr. Special thanks are due to
the chairmen and speakers for making this volume possible and to
Dr. Waldo Cohn for his assistance in editing. Preparation of the
completed volume was due in large part to the efforts of Sandra
Vaughan of the Biology Division.

The Editors

Barbara Ann Hamkalo
John Papaconstantinou

August, 1973

---

  * Operated by the Union Carbide Corporation for the U.S.
Atomic Energy Commission.

CONTRIBUTORS

ALBERTS, B., Department of Biochemical Sciences, Princeton University, Princeton, New Jersey

AMENSON, C. S., Division of Biology, California Institute of Technology, Pasadena, California

BAKKEN, A. H., Department of Biology, Yale University, New Haven, Connecticut

BALSAMO, J., Laboratório de Oncologia Experimental, Faculdade de Medicina, Universidade de São Paulo, São Paulo, Brasil

BERNARDI, G., Laboratoire de Génétique Moléculaire, Institut de Biologie Moléculaire, Paris, France

BIRD, A. P., Department of Biology, Yale University, New Haven, Connecticut

BIRNSTIEL, M. L., Institute for Molecular Biology, University of Zurich, Zurich, Switzerland

BLATTNER, F. R., McArdle Laboratory for Cancer Research, University of Wisconsin, Madison, Wisconsin

BRENTANI, R., Laboratório de Oncologia Experimental, Faculdade de Medicina, Universidade de São Paulo, São Paulo, Brasil

BRESCHKIN, A., Department of Molecular Biology, Vanderbilt University, Nashville, Tennessee

BRITTEN, R. J., Division of Biology, California Institute of Technology, Pasadena, California and Kerckhoff Marine Laboratory, Corona del Mar, California

BRZEZINSKA, M., Departments of Genetics and Biochemistry, University of Washington, Seattle, Washington

BUTTERWORTH, P. H. W., Department of Biochemistry, University College, London, U.K.

CALLAN, H. G., Zoology Department, The University, St. Andrews, Scotland

CASE, M. E., Department of Zoology, University of Georgia, Athens, Georgia

CASHEL, M., Laboratory of Molecular Genetics, National Institute of Child Health and Human Development, National Institutes of Health, Bethesda, Maryland

CHESTERTON, C. J., Biochemistry Department, University College London and King's College London, U.K.

DANEHOLT, B., Department of Histology, Karolinska Institutet, Stockholm, Sweden

DAVIDSON, E. H., Division of Biology, California Institute of Technology, Pasadena, California

DE POMERAI, D. I., Biochemistry Department, University College London and King's College London, U.K.

EHRLICH, S. D., Laboratoire de Génétique Moléculaire, Institut de Biologie Moléculaire, Paris, France

FLINT, S. J., Biochemistry Department, University College London and King's College London, U.K.

GALAU, G. A., Division of Biology, California Institute of Technology, Pasadena, California

GALL, J. G., Department of Biology, Yale University, New Haven, Connecticut

GEORGIEV, G. P., Institute of Molecular Biology, Academy of Sciences of the U.S.S.R., Moscow

GILES, N., Department of Zoology, University of Georgia, Athens, Georgia

GOLDBERG, R. B., Division of Biology, California Institute of Technology, Pasadena, California

GRAESSMANN, A., Institut für Molekularbiologie und Biochemie, Freie Universität, Berlin

GRAESSMANN, M., Institut für Molekularbiologie und Biochemie, Freie Universität, Berlin

GRAHAM, D. E., Division of Biology, California Institute of
    Technology, Pasadena, California and Kerckhoff Marine
    Laboratory, Corona del Mar, California

GRUNSTEIN, M., Department of Medicine, Stanford University School
    of Medicine and Veterans Administration Hospital, Palo Alto,
    California

HALL, B. D., Department of Genetics, University of Washington,
    Seattle, Washington

HALLICK, R. B., Departments of Biochemistry and Biophysics,
    University of California Medical Center, San Francisco,
    California

HAMKALO, B. A., Biology Division, Oak Ridge National Laboratory,
    Oak Ridge, Tennessee

HAUSMANN, R., Institut für Biologie III der Universität, Freiburg,
    West Germany

HAYES, S., McArdle Laboratory for Cancer Research, University of
    Wisconsin, Madison, Wisconsin

HILL, R. J., Department of Zoology, The University, St. Andrews,
    Scotland

HOLLENBERG, C. P., Departments of Genetics and Biochemistry,
    University of Washington, Seattle, Washington

HOUGH, B. R., Division of Biology, California Institute of
    Technology, Pasadena, California

JACOBSON, J. W., Department of Zoology, University of Georgia,
    Athens, Georgia

JEANTEUR, PH., Laboratoire de Biochimie-C.R.L.C., Hoptial Saint-
    Eloi, Montpellier, France

KEDES, L., Department of Medicine, Stanford University School of
    Medicine and Veterans Administration Hospital, Palo Alto,
    California

LARA, F. J. S., Department of Biochemistry, Institute of
    Chemistry, São Paulo, Brasil

LE TALAËR, J. Y., Unité de Biochimie, Institut Gustave Roussy,
    Villejuif, France

MAHLER, H. R., Department of Chemistry, Indiana University, Bloomington, Indiana

MARQUES, N., Laboratório de Oncologia Experimental, Faculdade de Medicina, Universidade de São Paulo, São Paulo, Brasil

MAUNDRELL, K. G., Department of Zoology, The University, St. Andrews, Scotland

MILLER, O. L, JR., Biology Division, Oak Ridge National Laboratory, Oak Ridge, Tennessee

MOSIG, G., Department of Molecular Biology, Vanderbilt University, Nashville, Tennessee

MYIASHITA, M., Laboratório de Oncologia Experimental, Faculdade de Medicina, Universidade de São Paulo, São Paulo, Brasil

NEUFELD, B., Division of Biology, California Institute of Technology, Pasadena, California and Kerckhoff Marine Laboratory, Corona del Mar, California

PARDUE, M. L., Department of Biology, Massachusetts Institute of Technology, Cambridge, Massachusetts

PERRY, R. P., The Institute for Cancer Research, Fox Chase Center for Cancer and Medical Sciences, Philadelphia, Pennsylvania

REINESS, G., Department of Biological Sciences, Columbia University, New York, New York

ROCHAIX, J. D., Department of Biology, Yale University, New Haven, Connecticut

RUTTER, W. J., Department of Biochemistry and Biophysics, University of California Medical Center, San Francisco, California

SCHEDL, P., Department of Biochemistry, Stanford University School of Medicine, Palo Alto, California

SCHULTZ, L. D., Departments of Genetics and Biochemistry, University of Washington, Seattle, Washington

SMITH, M. J., Division of Biology, California Institute of Technology, Pasadena, California

STOLF, A. M. S., Laboratório de Oncologia Experimental, Faculdade de Medicine, Universidade de São Paulo, São Paulo, Brasil

SWIFT, H., Department of Biology, University of Chicago, Chicago,
    Illinois

SZYBALSKI, W., McArdle Laboratory for Cancer Research, University
    of Wisconsin, Madison, Wisconsin

THIERY, J. P., Laboratoire de Génétique Moléculaire, Institut de
    Biologie Moléculaire, Paris, France

WEINBERG, E. S., Department of Biology, Johns Hopkins University,
    Baltimore, Maryland

YANG, H. L., Department of Biological Sciences, Columbia
    University, New York, New York

ZUBAY, G., Department of Biological Sciences, Columbia University,
    New York, New York

CONTENTS

1. AS THE CONFERENCE OPENS

C. A. Thomas, Jr.

Department of Biological Chemistry, Harvard Medical School, Boston, Massachusetts

Now that we are all together at this conference on "Molecular Cytogenetics" we might consider what the subject is, or what the words mean. Everyone agrees that cytogenetics is the direct study of the hereditary apparatus of cells, as contrasted with the study of the frequency of progeny genotypes. Since most genes reside on (in or around) chromosomes, cytogenetics has been preoccupied, historically, with the study of the structure and segregational mechanics of chromosomes. The word "molecular" has a more debatable meaning, but everyone agrees that it must be *modern*, and since cytogenetics dates back to Balbiani and Carnoy in the last century, it's a welcome addition to freshen up a musty subject.

It also makes some sense to think that *molecular cytogenetics* is an effort to continue the studies of cytogenetics to a lower level of organization that lies between the chromosome and the double helix. Somewhere among the molecular organizations of this size range is the material representation of the eukaryotic gene. Some of you, who are now accustomed to think of genes as segments of a DNA molecule that contain the coding sequences for a protein will be surprised to learn that we do not yet know how genes are physically represented in higher chromosomes. The various speakers over the next few days will be revealing just how great our ignorance really is.

Those of you who are familiar with the well-developed *E. coli* and phage genetics may find it a shock to learn that it has not yet been shown in any higher system that genetically-recognized mutations affect amino acid sequences. No peptide sequences have been done on mutant proteins in *Drosophila*. Indeed point mutations, which are easy to identify by their revertability in phage or bacteria, *cannot* be so identified in flies. The best one can do is a

1

recombinational test -- and that is quite another thing. No intra-
cistronic deletions are known in any higher system. There is no
known deletion that can be shown, by genetic tests, to reside entirely within a single functional unit. There are other important areas
of ignorance that will surprise anyone who is changing his attention
from molecular genetics to molecular cytogenetics.

In a real way, the successes of molecular genetics of prokaryotes has inhibited the development of the molecular biology of eukaryotes. If point mutations can be demonstrated to cause amino-
acid substitutions in bacteria or phage, then why do it in *Drosophila,* where it is so much more difficult? There are other more serious
examples of how cytogeneticists have been swayed or perhaps even
intimidated by the successful molecular biologists. This has been
unfortunate because they may have obscured some of the very important contributions that this classical subject has made.

THE CHROMOMERE

Perhaps the most important contribution of classical cytogenetics is the identification of the *chromomere.* Unfortunately, chromomeres can only be visualized under two rather bizarre situations:
in the polytene chromosomes -- most clearly displayed in *Dipteran*
larvae, and in the meiotic chromosomes -- particularly in the spec-
tacular lampbrush chromosomes generally found in oocytes. Under
both those situations the normal mitotic chromosomes are extended
200-fold or more in length. Apparently, when chromosomes are extended to this degree, the underlying chromomeric organization is
revealed. It is the working hypothesis of many investigators that
all chromosomes are organized into chromomeres, even though they
don't reveal them and have not yet been coaxed to do so. This hypothesis contains the tacit assumption that all chromosomes share
a common structural plan, both within a given species, and between
species. At this conference you will meet those who think all
chromosomes are built on more or less the same plan and those who
think each one is an individual case.

I prefer to think that the structures of all chromosomes are
based on a common organizational plan, but there always are the
exceptions.

THE CHROMOMERE AS A UNIT OF GENETIC FUNCTION

The polytene chromosomes were first recorded in the last century, but they were not recognized as being chromosomes until their
simultaneous "rediscovery" by Heitz and by Painter in the 1930's.
The work of Muller, although far from conclusive, suggested that

individual bands might be the "dwelling place" of individual genes.
This idea gained wide currency, and it will amuse the modern reader
to see reference to the "gene bands*" in such volumes as Darlington's
little book on chromosome techniques. Here the molecular biologists
collided with the cytogeneticists -- and as usual the cytogeneticists
retreated -- or at least remained silent.

Perhaps the major contribution of a generation of molecular
biology has been the establishment of the genetic code, and its
generality. From the coding ratio one knows that a relatively small
number of nucleotides (1000 or so) would be required to code for an
average or even large peptide chain. Yet it was evident that there
is 10 or even 100-times *more* DNA per chromomere than is required to
code for an average peptide. The numbers for *Drosophila* go something like this: there are 1.5×10^8 nucleotide pairs (ntp) (sub-
stracting satellite-DNA) in a *Drosophila* sperm cell, and Bridges
counted 5149 bands in *D. melanogaster* salivary chromosomes. Therefore there are ∿30,000 nucleotides per band. Since some bands have
10 times the average there is enough DNA for 30 or even 300 coding
sequences in these bands.

Thus it has been a matter of intense interest to watch the
development of the studies of Burke Judd and his collaborators over
the past dozen years. This group has been localizing hundreds of
mutations, some of which must be point mutations, in a limited interval on the X chromosome. By strictly genetic tests, they have
put all of these mutations into 12 complementation groups. There
are exactly 12 bands that are to be seen in this interval. Deficiencies that extend into this region remove bands *and* complementation groups in serial order. Thus bands seem to correspond to individual functional genetic units. This work is corroborated by
others in several portions of the genome. The unanswered question
is: What's all that DNA doing there? Why do some chromomeres have
10 times as much DNA as the average? This is a microscopic mani-
festation of a problem that can be recognized at the level of the
whole cell. It has been found that very similar "sibling" species
can differ significantly in C-value, the total chromosomal DNA content. Is DNA content truly unrelated to information content. This
is true of course, if the information were represented more than

---

    * This corruption of words and ideas is little worse than the
lab jargon that has invaded the literature, and can be found in such
statements as "titrating the number of 5S RNA genes," or "the number
of hemoglobin genes." Clearly what is being talked about is the
number of sequences that are complementary to a given RNA. A *gene*
is an informational concept, and as such is non-material. It can
have its material representation, of course. The current confusion
in molecular cytogenetics regarding "the nature of the eukaryotic
gene" is due, in part, to semantics.

once. So one of the crucial questions that underlies much of what you will hear during the next few days is *whether coding sequences that represent individual genes are represented ONCE or more than once*. Irrespective of what the chromomere is, this question is begging for an answer.

THE CHROMOMERE AS A UNIT OF REPLICATION

We know from the work initiated by Taylor that the entire chromosome is replicated semiconservatively, so the chromomeres along it must be semiconservatively replicated. This doesn't mean that all portions of the chromosome are replicated at all times; as Joe Gall will tell you this afternoon, chromosomes can be differentially replicated to different degrees under certain circumstances. In the extreme case, an individual chromomere can be replicated free of the chromosome, as Hourcade and Bird will explain this morning. However, as Taylor demonstrated in his original work, chromosomes and parts of chromosomes are replicated according to a specific schedule of their own. This idea received strong support from the work of Pelling and of Plaut who presented evidence that the bands of the polytene chromosomes incorporate label according to a special sequence. The autoradiography of Huberman and Riggs supports the idea that the units of replication might be the size of chromomeres (since no one knows what the size of the chromomere might be in a mammalian cell). However, this idea is challenged by the experiments that Callan will tell you about this morning, and Hagness will add support to the same conclusion. If their interpretation is right, we will have to accept the idea that replication *can* be initiated at multiple points *within* individual chromomeres. Of great interest here is the *maximum* number of initiation sites, and this can only be resolved by the electron microscope.

THE CHROMOMERE AS A UNIT OF TRANSCRIPTION

As a result of careful studies, primarily by Beermann, we know that puffs and even the spectaculer Balbiani rings are the result of transcriptional activity involving a single band, or at most a few neighboring bands. We are fortunate to have Bertil Daneholt here from Sweden to tell us about his experiments that suggest a single chromomere, Balbiani ring 2, is transcribed as a single unit into one long RNA molecule. This idea is so shocking that one's first reaction is to disbelieve it. Further, this RNA is likely to contain a repeating sequence, and somewhere along its length there must be the coding sequence (or multiple copies of the coding sequence) for a protein that has already been identified.

This story can be compared with those of Darnell and Brown who will be telling us about the transcription of chromomeres that can't

be seen or isolated. Finally, near the end of the conference we
will hear talks by Hausmann and Chamberlin dealing with the transcription of a DNA molecule that is about the length of a *Drosophila*
chromomere, namely T7 DNA, which is known to contain about 30 coding
sequences for 30 different proteins (or about 1200 nucleotides per
coding sequence). Finally, we will be seeing the electron micrographs of transcription from Barbara Hamkalo and Oscar Miller that
have become justly famous.

THE ORGANIZATION OF SEQUENCES IN CHROMOMERES

But irrespective of their function or coding ability, what is
the organization of sequences in the chromomere? Dave Hogness will
have something to say about this in the afternoon. Eric Davidson
will present his picture based on a unique annealing experiment this
morning. Charles Laird and I will present our contrasting views
this afternoon. In order to keep all of these contrasting views of
the chromosome in mind, I would like to present a little diagram
that points up the various issues. Each of the subsequent speakers
who will be dealing with chromomeric organization should be able to
tell us in rather quantitative terms just what their views are.

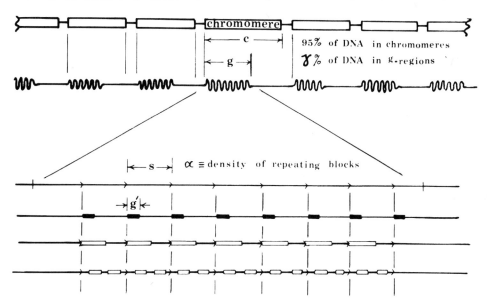

Fig. 1. POSSIBLE ORGANIZATIONS OF CHROMOSOMAL DNA SEQUENCES. This
representation assumes that most (>95%) of the mononemic chromatid
is organized into chromomeres. A certain fraction, γ, of the chromomeric DNA is in g-regions. These are regions within which clustered repetitions occur. The clustered repetitions could be either
purely tandem with repeat length s (the model preferred by us), or

intermittently spaced repetitive blocks whose length is $\underline{g}'$. These
repetitive blocks could be either internally repetitious, filled
blocks, or non-internally repetitious, open blocks. These models
are preferred by Davidson or Laird. The intermittent repetitions
are drawn with an equal spacing, $\underline{s}$, but his need not be so. They
could be located irregularly, or at random; in which case $\underline{s}$ has
less meaning, and $\underline{\alpha}$, the density of repetitious blocks, becomes a
more useful parameter.

Some of the specific questions might be:
1. How many chromomeres are thought to be in your beast. n = ?
    n = 5149 for *Drosophila*.
2. What portion of the DNA is composed in the fashion described
    γ = ?
3. What is the length in nucleotides of the regions containing the
    clustered repetitions?   g = ?
4. What is the spacing of the repetitions?   s = ?
5. What is the density of the repetitious blocks?   α = ?
6. What is the length of the repeating block or blocks, are they
    of the same or different sequence, are they internally repeti-
    tious or non-repetitious?   g' = ?

        Now one might ask whether all this is really necessary to de-
scribe the chromosome. The short answer is *yes*. It's also very
important to sharpen the definitions of what the various workers
are talking about. I will supply our own answers to these questions
this afternoon, and I'm sure that Hogness, Pardue and Laird will add
their answers as well.

        Are the Clustered Repetitions Perfect Repeats, and if So What
                    Keeps Them So Nearly the Same?

        Irrespective of the details of these models, we would like to
know whether the repetitious sequences are the same, or nearly the
same; or is there quite a lot of heterogeneity from repetition to
repetition?

        If they are nearly identical, then how is this managed. Clear-
ly, if they are replicated from a common template (the mother template) -- this perhaps by a rolling ring model -- then there is no
problem. The rolling ring will generate a series of exact tandem
repeats. In essence, this idea was introduced by Goldschmidt in
the 1930's. However, such a model is not really compatible with a
stable DNA that replicates semiconservatively. There is room for
debate here, because not all the facts are really known. The second
alternative is that repetitions are brought into agreement by a
process that has been called "rectification." Rectification would
have to occur in the germ line, but may occur in somatic cells as well.

Models for the hypothetical process of rectification all involve the reshuffling of single polynucleotide chains, the formation of mismatched nucleotides, and the operation of an excision and repair system like that found in *E. coli*. It is this collection of ideas that is generally represented by the words "masters and slaves, etc." This is presently an underground idea that may come out in the open before this conference closes.

2. SEQUENCE ORGANIZATION IN ANIMAL DNA'S

Eric H. Davidson, Barbara R. Hough, Christopher S. Amenson, Roy J. Britten[†], Dale E. Graham, Berney R. Neufeld, Michael J. Smith, Robert B. Goldberg and Glenn A. Galau

Division of Biology, California Institute of Technology, Pasadena, California and Kerckhoff Marine Laboratory, Corona Del Mar, California

Recent efforts in our laboratory have been focused on the organization of repetitive and nonrepetitive sequences in animal DNA, and the representation of these sequences in RNA. A new chapter in these studies began recently with observations that lead to the conclusion that middle-repetitive DNA sequences are interspersed in an orderly way amongst nonrepetitive sequence elements. I will begin by summarizing some of these recent experiments on sequence organization in the DNA's of *Xenopus* and the sea urchin, and then proceed to describe some new findings on the sequence constitution of sea urchin messenger RNA.

INTERSPERSION OF MODERATELY REPETITIVE DNA SEQUENCES

The mode of arrangement of middle-repetitive sequence elements appears to represent an essential key to the function of these sequences. Several previous studies by Britten and his associates indicated that, at least in the genomes of certain animals, there are middle-repetitive sequence elements that are extensively interspersed among nonrepetitive sequences. For example, it was found that for both calf and sea urchin DNA, almost 80% of labeled fragments averaging 4000 nucleotides (NT) in length would bind to hydroxyapatite after reassocation to relatively low C_ot's (<10) with

---

[†] Carnegie Institution of Washington and California Institute of Technology.

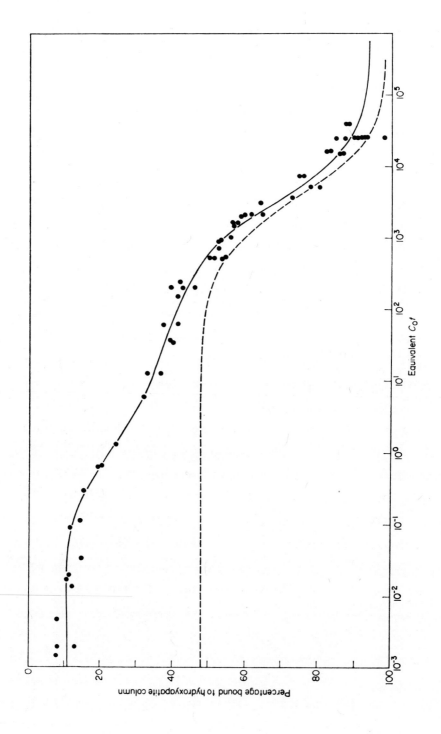

400 nucleotide long whole DNA present in excess (Britten and Smith, 1970; Britten, 1972). These experiments suggest that 80% of fragments about 4000 nucleotides must contain both repetitive and nonrepetitive sequence elements. The experiments which I will now describe began with the application of the same basic experimental procedure, *viz*. reassociation to low C_ot of long labeled DNA fragments with short carrier DNA present in large excess. The fraction of the long fragments containing repetitive sequence elements is then measured by binding to hydroxyapatite. One difference from the earlier work was than in the present study we used a series of carefully sized labeled DNA fragments. When combined with other data summarized later in this paper these hydroxyapatite binding experiments permit the construction of a quantitative model of sequence spacing in the DNA.

The choice of *Xenopus* DNA for this exploration of sequence organization is a fortuitous one. Fig. 1 shows the hydroxyapatite C_ot curve of *Xenopus* DNA, obtained with 450 nucleotide DNA fragments (Davidson and Hough, 1971). At this length about 55% of the fragments appear to contain only nonrepetitive sequence. The ideal reassociation kinetics of the nonrepetitive sequence are indicated by the dotted line. Though other frequency components may exist in small quantities, most of the repetitive DNA of the *Xenopus* genome is present in one major frequency class (Hough and Davidson, 1972). About 32% of the 450 nucleotide fragments carry recognizable seuqence elements belonging to this repetitive family, each sequence of which appears 1-2 X 10^3 times per genome.

When radioactive DNA fragments of various lengths are reassociated with a 5-10 X 10^3-fold excess of 450 nucleotide carrier DNA and passed over hydroxyapatite the results shown in Fig. 2 are obtained (Davidson *et al.*, 1973). These fragments were prepared by shearing in a Virtis homogenizer, after which fragment sizes were

---

Figure 1. Hydroxyapatite C_ot curve of sheared *Xenopus* DNA, based on data obtained from the reassociation of 13 DNA concentrations, each at one of 6 salt concentrations ranging from 0.12 to 0.32M phosphate buffer (Davidson and Hough, 1971). For details of the solutions see Davidson and Hough (1969). The C_ot values plotted are corrected for the effect on rate of salt concentrations (Equivalent C_ot). The curve is fitted to the points by a computer operating according to a least-squares method (Britten and Kohne, 1968; Britten *et al.*, 1973). The dotted line represents the computer's prediction of the reassociation reaction of the nonrepetitive component along; the nonrepetitive fraction accounts for 55% of the total DNA at the 60°C criterion applied in these experiments.

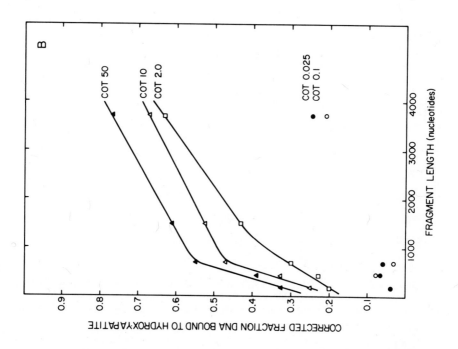

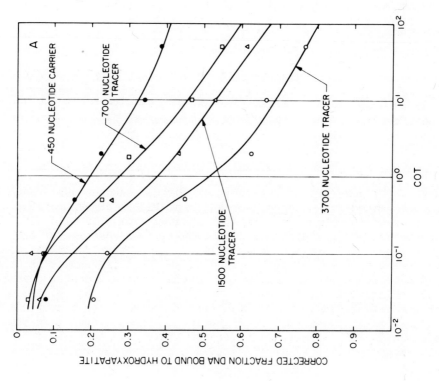

carefully measured in alkaline sucrose gradients. The experiments
of Fig. 2 show that sequence elements of the major repetitive family
must be closely interspersed with nonrepetitive sequence. This
follows from the fact that the fraction of the labeled DNA binding
to hydroxyapatite after reassociation to C_ot 50 is so large that
nonrepetitive sequence (>55% of the genome) as well as repetitive
sequence must be present on the same fragments. In fact the 3700
nucleotide fragments bearing repetitive elements evidently include
a major fraction of the nonrepetitive DNA sequence in the genome.
Since 80% of the 3700 nucleotide fragments evidently contain
repetitive elements, these must be distributed very widely in the
genome. Fig. 2 shows that the binding occurs over that range of
C_ot's expected if the duplexes are formed by reassociation of the
major repetitive sequence family, a point demonstrated directly
below.

     The presence of both repetitive and nonrepetitive sequence on
the same DNA strands can also be demonstrated directly by fractionation and shearing of long fragments. 3700 nucleotide long labeled
DNA fragments are reassociated with short carrier DNA to C_ot as in
Fig. 2, and the DNA bound to hydroxyapatite is eluted. It is then
sheared to 450 nucleotides, and more carrier DNA is added. When
reincubated to C_ot 40 hydroxyapatite binding is restricted to about
40% of the previously bound DNA, while over half the remaining labeled DNA reassociates with the carrier by C_ot 4250. This experiment
shows that by shearing, nonrepetitive sequence is released from
fragments which also contain repetitive sequence elements.

     It will be noted that the ordinates of Fig. 2 are labeled
"corrected fraction of DNA bound." This is the best estimate of
the actual fraction of fragments containing repeated sequence elements. As indicated in the caption, this correction refers to the
capacity of a small amount of single-stranded DNA to form intrastrand
structures which can bind to hydroxyapatite. These are probably

---

Figure 2. Binding of radioactive DNA of various fragment lengths
to hydroxyapatite due to reassociation with 450 nucleotide carrier
DNA (Davidson *et al.*, 1973). Radioactive DNA of various fragment
lengths was incubated with 450 nucleotide DNA present in 7000-fold
excess. Annealing mixtures were passed over hydroxyapatite operated
under standard conditions (60°C, 0.12M phosphate buffer) in the
presence of 0.06% sodium dodecyl sulfate. The data were corrected
for zero-time binding as described in text. (A) Corrected binding
as a function of carrier DNA C_ot; solid circles, averaged corrected
carrier DNA binding; open symbols, averaged tracer DNA binding.
(B) Corrected binding of DNA fragments as a function of fragment
length.

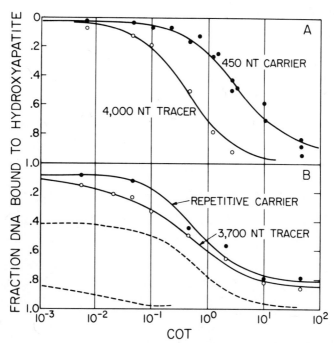

Figure 3. Test for clustering of repetitive sequences by measurement of the rate of reassociation of long fragments with short fragments (Davidson *et al.*, 1973). (A) The effect of fragment length
with bacterial DNA. A 5000-fold excess of 450 nucleotide *E. coli*
DNA carrier was mixed with 4000 nucleotide labeled *E. coli* DNA fragments. After denaturation and incubation under standard conditions
(60°C, 0.12M phosphate buffer) the samples were fractionated on hydroxyapatite: solid circles, binding of carrier DNA; open circles,
binding of labeled 4000 nucleotide fragments. Least-squares analysis yielded a second-order rate constant of 0.25 for the carrier and
2.0 for the long tracer, almost exactly in proportion to their
lengths. (B) Reassociation of 3700 nucleotide fragments of *Xenopus*
DNA bearing repetitive sequences (tracer) with 450 nucleotide repetitive DNA (repetitive carrier). Repetitive carrier was prepared as
follows: DNA was incubated to $C_o t$ 50 and passed overy hydroxyapatite;
the *bound* fraction was harvested, denatured, reincubated to $C_o t$
0.005 and the *unbound* fraction was used for the experiment; final
yield was 32% of the starting DNA in accordance with expectation.
Solid circles, reassociation of this carrier DNA; the curve drawn
through them is the least squares solution for a single second-order
component (k = 2.3 corrected to 100% purity, exactly the rate expected for the major repetitive component of the *Xenopus* genome). Tracer
was prepared from 3700 nucleotide labeled DNA, after removal of the
zero-time binding fraction, by adding a 125-fold excess of repetitive
carrier, denaturing and incubating to $C_o t$ 50. The fraction that
bound to hydroxyapatite (70%) was the tracer 3700 nucleotide DNA

"foldbacks" or "hairpins" composed of self-complementary regions. We have shown that such regions are themselves interspersed without bias with respect to the sequence families observed by reassociation kinetics for 4000 NT long fragments (Davidson *et al.*, 1973). To perform the experiments of Fig. 2, single-stranded fragments containing zero-time binding elements were either physically removed with hydroxyapatite prior to reaction (3700 nucleotide long fragments), or an appropriate numerical correction for this binding was applied at each fragment length.

MOST MIDDLE-REPETITIVE SEQUENCE ELEMENTS ARE NOT CLUSTERED

The data described above show that middle-repetitive sequence elements are widely interspersed among nonrepetitive sequence. However, these data alone do not exclude the possibility that most of the repetitive DNA could exist in arrays of clustered repetitive sequence elements with only a minor fraction of the repetitions interspersed throughout the genome. The experiment of Fig. 3 eliminates this possibility, and shows that the fraction of middle-repetitive sequence which could actually be clustered is small.

The approach used here is based on the knowledge that in a reassociation reaction between long tracer fragments and short carrier DNA fragments the rate of reassociation of the long fragments is proportional to the number of nucleation sites they contain. For a nonrepetitive DNA one expects that the number of nucleation sites is proportional to the fragment length. Fig. 3A describes an experiment which tests this expectation. Labeled *E. coli* DNA fragments sheared to an average length of 4000 nucleotides were reassociated with a great excess of *E. coli* DNA sheared to 450 nucleotides, and the reassociation kinetics measured. As shown, the long tracer DNA reassociated at about eight times the rate of the carrier DNA or in

---

containing repetitive sequence elements: open circles, reassociation of this tracer in the presence of a 9600-fold excess of repetitive carrier. The curve fitted to the tracer binding data represents a particular least-squares solution of the many possible using two second-order components. For this solution the rate constant for the slower componenet was set to that of the carrier DNA (k = 2.3). The dashed lines show the magnitude and rate of the resulting components. The data are consistent with the existence of a small (15%) rapid component whose rate constant cannot be determined from these data; the component shown has a rate constant of 90. There is no indication of the rapid reassociation of the tracer as a whole that would result if the long fragments consisted of many repetitive sequences clustered together.

proportion to their respective fragment length. On the same principle, a long DNA fragment containing many repetitive sequence elements
would also reassociate faster than the short carrier present in the
same reassociation mixture.

The kinetics of reassociation of 3700 nucleotide *Xenopus* DNA
with repetitive carrier DNA present in great excess are shown in
Fig. 3B. It is immediately clear that most of the long tracer reassociates at a rate comparable to that of the short carrier DNA
fragments. We conclude that the number of nucleation sites on the
3700 nucleotide fragments is close (within a factor of two) to the
number of such sites on the 450 nucleotide fragments. Thus there
are likely to be only one or two short repetitive sequence elements
per 3700 nucleotide fragment. Since over 80% reassociation of
tracer is obtained in this experiment, little or no strand scission
of the tracer molecules has occurred. Second order curves fit to
the data with a least-squares computer program (Fig. 3B, dashed
lines) suggest that a small (15%) rapidly binding component is present in addition to a major component reassociating at the rate of
the carrier. This small fraction represents the portion of the
fragments which *could* contain clustered arrays of middle-repetitive
sequence elements. The tracer in the experiment was preselected to
contain repetitive sequence elements (see caption for details) and
represented 79% of the total DNA. Since about 80% of it reacted,
a maximum estimate for the quantity of clustered repetitive DNA is
6-10% of the total. The experiment thus adds to the fact of middle-
repetitive sequence interspersion the additional restriction that
about 3/4ths of the middle-repetitive DNA exists in interspersed
elements. Subsequent experiments (Davidson *et al.*, 1973) in which
the long tracer bound in Fig. 3B was further fractionated, sheared
and reassociated showed a) that the interspersed repetitive sequence
elements do indeed belong to the major repetitive sequence family
in the *Xenopus* genome; b) that the clustered regions of the genome
may include a more highly repetitive reassociating class of sequence;
and c) that the best estimate for the quantity of this minor fraction
is 6-8%.

THE LENGTH OF REPETITIVE SEQUENCE ELEMENTS

The results presented in Figs. 2 and 3 imply strongly that the
middle-repetitive sequence elements must be fairly short. This expectation is confirmed in the experiments presented in Figs. 4 and
5.

Fig. 4 portrays the thermal dissociation of duplexes formed by
annealing 1400 nucleotide and 450 nucleotide long fragments to C_0t
50. The individual duplex fractions were harvested separately from
hydroxyapatite columns. The T_m's of the two samples are similar
(78.4°C and 80°C), indicating that as expected the same class(es)

of repetitive sequence are responsible for duplex formation, and that the lengths of the duplex regions are probably not greatly different. However, the 450 nucleotide duplexes display more than twice the hyperchromicity of the 1400 nucleotide duplex. This result is the expected one if the length of the average repetitive elements is less than the length of the 450 nucleotide fragments, and if these elements are interspersed with nonrepetitive DNA sequence (which of course remain unpaired in this experiment). Thus, Fig. 4 shows that, on the average, a larger fraction of the 1400 nucleotide fragments than of the 450 nucleotide fragments consists of unpaired nonrepetitive sequences contiguous to the reassociated repetitive sequence elements.

The hyperchromicity of the 450 nucleotide fragments is 17%, about two-thirds of the maximum hyperchromicity expected of perfect duplex. Since duplex formed from 450 nucleotide fragments of isolated nonrepetitive *Xenopus* DNA displays 24.6% hyperchromicity, close to that of native DNA (Davidson and Hough, 1969), it follows that some unpaired, *i.e.*, nonrepetitive sequence, must be present even on fragments as short as 450 nucleotides which also contain repetitive sequence elements. It is to be noted that C_0t 50, to which these fragments were incubated, is several times higher than is required for the complete reassociation of the major *Xenopus* repetitive DNA component, so that all available reassociable regions can be presumed to exist in the duplex form. The 17% hyperchromicity of the 450 nucleotide fragments suggests that *on the average* they contain at least two-thirds of the total fragment length as repetitive DNA duplex. A conservative interpretation of the melting curve for 450 nucleotide fragments is that the. length of the average repetitive sequence element is about 300 $\pm$ 100 nucleotides; this experiment therefore provides an estimate of the *average* repetitive sequence element length.

In order to obtain a direct measurement of repetitive sequence element length a different method is required. The principle of the approach we have taken is to use a single-strand-specific nuclease to digest away the nonrepetitive unpaired "tails" present on structures such as those melted in the upper curve of Fig. 4. The nucleotide length of the enzyme resistant duplex regions is then measured. If the conditions of enzyme digestion are set properly so that all single-strand regions are in fact digested, while little or no double-stranded structures are destroyed, such an experiment provides a precise measurement of the distribution of lengths of repetitive sequence elements as they occur in the DNA.

For the S-1 nuclease studies we have employed the *Aspergillus* single-strand-specific S-1 nuclease (Ando, 1966). Conditions were found for the enzyme digestion which appear to closely match the incubation conditions we usually use, *i.e.*, 60°C, 0.12M phosphate buffer. In these conditions (see Legend to Fig. 5) virtually all

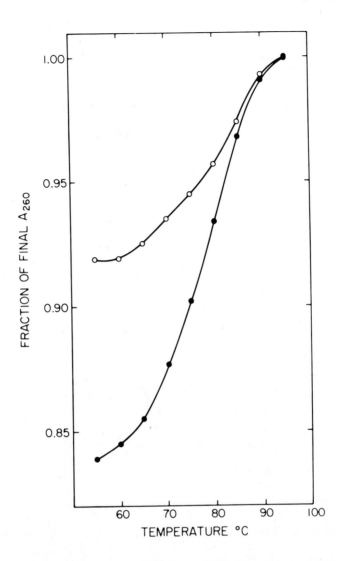

Figure 4. Optical melt of duplexes formed from long and short
fragments (Davidson *et al.*, 1973). DNA preparations averaging 1400
nucleotides and 450 nucleotides in fragment length were incubated
under standard conditions to $C_o t$ 50. Duplex fractions were eluted
from hydroxyapatite in 0.5M phosphate buffer, diluted to 0.12M
phosphate buffer and melted in water-jacketed cuvettes in a Beckman
Acta III recording spectrophotometer. Readings were made every few
seconds and the data were processed by a computer averaging program.
The plotted points represent the averages in chosen temperature-time
intervals. The accuracy of this procedure is greater than 0.2°C
error on the T_m value. T_m for the 1400 nucleotide preparation is

single-stranded "tails" are digested, since the product of the digestion has a near-native hyperchromicity of 24%. On the other hand, the amount of duplex resistant to the enzyme is about equal to the theoretical content of repetitive sequence, as shown below. Therefore it appears that no significant amount of the repetitive duplex is digested by the enzyme. The remarkable aspect of the match between the annealing conditions and the enzyme digestion conditions is that the repetitive duplex regions which are stable at the criterion conditions are also resistant to digestion even though these regions characteristically contain 10-15% base pair mismatch. Thus the T_m's of the resistant duplex regions are over $10°$ lower than can be accounted for by the measured duplex lengths. Studies of the resistant digestion products under denaturing conditions show that most of them have not been nicked by the enzyme treatment.

Xenopus DNA was sheared to about 2000 nucleotides, and reassociated to $C_o t$ 20. The annealing mixture was then treated with the S-1 nuclease under the above conditions, and the products of the digestion separated on Sephadex G-100. The annealing mixture was exposed to the enzyme for 10 times the time needed to digest half the single-stranded DNA. About 24% of the starting DNA was excluded from the Sephadex column, the remainder appearing in the nucleotide peak. Fig. 5 portrays the distribution of the excluded enzyme-resistant DNA segments on a calibrated A-50M gel filtration column. Most of the enzyme-resistant duplex chromatographs directly over a 300 nucleotide long double-stranded marker (dashed line). Thus 75-80% of the repetitive sequence elements in fact belong to a distribution of sequence lengths whose mode is 300 nucleotides. The remaining DNA is excluded from the A-50M column, and is interpreted as clustered repetitive sequence elements. It is interesting that the amount of clustered repetitive DNA recovered from this experiment is about 6% of the total starting DNA, *i.e.* just the value predicted from the experiments discussed above in connection with Fig. 3. The fact that most of the DNA falls into the 300 nucleotide distribution is powerful and independent evidence that most of the middle-repetitive sequences in the *Xenopus* genome are indeed interspersed amidst other sequences remaining single-stranded at $C_o t$ 20,

about 80°C and for the 450 nucleotide preparation is about 78.4°C. The melts were corrected for single-strand collapse. The maximum correction (at 55°C) was 0.03 for the 1400 nucleotide curve and 0.015 for the 450 nucleotide curve. Corrected hyperchromicities were 0.08 for the 1400 nucleotide preparation and 0.17 for the 450 nucleotide preparation. These represent almost exactly one and two-thirds of the hyperchromicity (0.25) observed for the melting of reassociated simple (bacterial) DNA. Open circles, 1400 nucleotide fragments; solid circles, 450 nucleotide fragments.

i.e. nonrepetitive sequence. Even more importantly, the enzyme experiments confirm the indication obtained from the experiment of Fig. 4 that the modal repetitive sequence element length is about 300 nucleotides. When measured under denaturing conditions (in alkaline sucrose, or in gel filtration columns equilibrated with 6% formaldehyde) the major fraction of the enzyme-resistant DNA fragments still correspond in size to the 300 nucleotide long marker distribution.

A QUANTITATIVE MODEL OF SEQUENCE ORGANIZATION

The data presented thus far provide the following restrictions on possible forms of sequence organization in the *Xenopus* genome: a) the largest fraction of the total DNA which can consist of clustered repetitive sequence elements is about 6%, while most of the repetitive sequence is interspersed between nonrepetitive sequence; b) the modal size of the interspersed sequence elements is 300 nucleotides. In addition we can estimate the actual amount of repetitive and nonrepetitive DNA sequence in the genome from the data of Figs. 2, 3 and 5. This knowledge permits the construction of spacing models describing the likely arrangement of repetitive and nonrepetitive sequence in the DNA. To do this we utilize the shape of the curve describing the binding of tracer DNA to hydroxyapatite after reassociation with short carrier DNA, as a function of tracer DNA fragment length.

In Fig. 6 all of the individual binding observations obtained at C_ot 50 are presented. The corrected binding of tracer of various lengths (L) due to reassociation of middle-repetitive sequences is expressed as the parameter R on the ordinate. These data are represented by the solid circles on the graph. The intercept on the R axis of the line extending through the points at 250, 450, and 700 nucleotides must represent the actual fraction of nucleotides present in repetitive sequence as measured at this criterion. The intercept value obtained should be consistent both with the hyperchromicity studies of Fig. 4 and the S-1 nuclease studies just described. It is thus gratifying that the intercept values are in fact close to 0.25, the percent of the DNA resistant to the nuclease after annealing to C_ot 20.

The data of Fig. 6 imply a sharp change in the degree of increase in binding at around 800 nucleotide fragment length. This suggests that both short and long nonrepetitive regions are found interspersed between repetitive elements. With the aid of a computer, model functions (solid lines in Fig. 6) were set up in which the shapes of the R versus L curves were determined by the lengths of repetitive and nonrepetitive sequence elements. The various model curves were compared to the data obtained at C_ot 50, and in

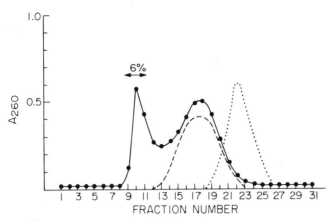

Figure 5. Size distribution of S-1 nuclease-resistant repetitive
DNA duplex. *Xenopus* DNA was sheared in a Virtis homogenizer to an
average fragment length of 2000 nucleotides, as measured in alkaline
sucrose gradients. The DNA was reassociated to an equivalent C_0t of
25 in 0.3M NaCl, 0.01M PIPES buffer, pH 6.7, at 60°C. At the end of
the incubation, an equal volume of 0.05M sodium acetate buffer, pH
4.3, containing 0.0002M Zn^{++} and 5.5mM mercaptoethanol was added.
3200 "units" of S-1 nuclease were introduced (a "unit" is the amount
of enzyme capable of digesting 40 μg of single-stranded DNA to trichloroacetic acid solubility in 10 min), and the digestion carried
out for 45 min at 37°C. The reaction was stopped by addition of 0.1
volume of 1.0M phosphate buffer and chilling. The digest was then
passed over a G-100 Sephadex column, operated in 0.12M phosphate
buffer, and the exclusion peak harvested. This represented 24% of
the starting DNA. This material was then chromatographed on an A-
50M gel filtration column, also run in 0.12M phosphate buffer (solid
circles). The exclusion peak contains about 6% of the starting DNA.
The major portion of the enzyme-resistant duplex (14% of the starting DNA) chromatographs similarly to a 300 nucleotide sheared native
marker prepared in a Virtis homogenizer (dashed line), while a small
fraction (4%) falls between the exclusion and the 300 nucleotide
peak. The size of the 300 nucleotide preparation was established
by reference to known markers in both alkaline and neutral sucrose
gradients and by electron microscopy. The hyperchromicity displayed
by all fractions of the enzyme-resistant material is in the range
24-25%, *i.e.* close to native hyperchromicity. The dotted line represents the salt peak on this A-50 column.

this way the range of nucleotide spacings consistent with the binding data obtained. Various spacing models chosen to illustrate
the extremes of the acceptable solutions, as well as median solutions, are presented in Fig. 6.

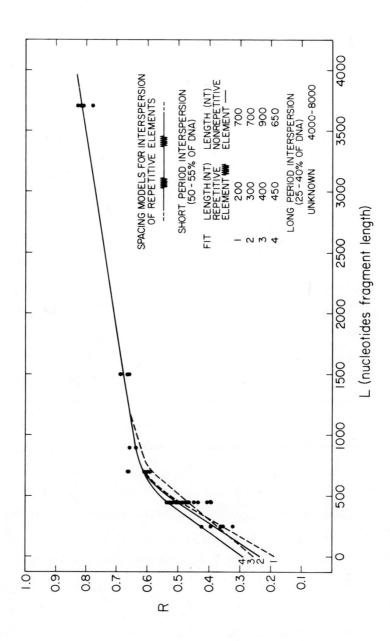

The slope of the curves in the short fragment region is almost an order of magnitude greater than the slope in the long fragment region. The higher slope at short fragment length is the result of what we term "short period sequence interspersion," while the lower slope at long fragment length results from "long period sequence interspersion." These fits assume that 6 or 8% of the DNA exists as clustered repetitive sequence. By far the largest fraction of the interspersed repetitive DNA in the genome is included in the short period interspersed class of sequence arrangements. Therefore the length of the *average* repetitive sequence elements in the Table in Fig. 6 refers to the repetitive DNA of the short period interspersed phase. The *average* length of the nonrepetitive sequence elements in the short period interspersed phase would appear to fall in the range 650 to 900 nucleotides. It is impossible to estimate the length of the infrequent repetititve sequence elements in the long period interspersed DNA from these data. Since our observations were not extended beyond 3700 nucleotides, we do not know whether the remaining 20% of the DNA also contains rare repetititve elements or no repetitive elements.

Figure 6. Plot of R versus L for C_ot 50 binding data and model interspersion spacing curves (Davidson *et al.*, 1973). Individual R values are the fractions of DNA binding to hydroxyapatite after correction for zero-time binding and for a few percent of the DNA bind-only on a second pass over hydroxyapatite. They are denoted by solid circles. The magnitude of the corrections is small and their primary utility is that they make it possible to compare the binding curves with other forms of evidence, *e.g.* hyperchromicity measurements. Scatter is somewhat greater in the optical density assays (450 nucleotide points) than in the radioactivity assays. It should be noted that three forms of reaction are included in this figure: (A) reaction of tracer fragments longer than carrier fragments with the carrier fragments (700 to 3700 nucleotide points); (B) reaction of carrier fragments with each other (450 nucleotide points); (C) reaction of tracer fragments shorter than carrier fragments with carrier fragments (250 nucleotide points). Conceivably the latter two forms of reaction could be suppressed by small factors relative to the first form of reassociation. However, we have at present no evidence that this is so. The curves fit to the data (solid and dashed lines) were generated by a computer (see text) on the basis of the spacing arrangements listed in the lower right corner of the figure opposite the respective curve designations. None of the curves can be excluded statistically. Root-mean-square values of the best fits are about 0.04. To obtain these fits standard deviations of fragment lengths equal to 0.3 of the mean fragment length were used. The ordinate intercept represents the theoretical fraction of the genome which is included in repetitive sequence elements.

In summary, the analysis summarized in Fig. 6 shows that in 50 to 55% of *Xenopus* DNA short repetitive sequence elements of *average* length 300 nucleotides alternate with longer nonrepetitive sequence elements, of *average* length 650 to 900 nucleotides. The data of Fig. 6 cannot be fit with *randomly* varying spacing intervals. We conclude that the alternating arrangement of repetitive and nonrepetitive sequence in the genome of this creature represents a high degree of order even if there is a distribution of lengths of the sequences involved. It is hard to escape the additional conclusion that the particular sequence organization we observe must be of functional significance since it has been preserved (and developed) through evolutionary selection.

GENERALIZATIONS TO OTHER ORGANISMS

An analysis similar to that illustrated in Fig. 6 has also been carried out on the DNA of the sea urchin *Strongylocentrotus purpuratus*. Space does not permit a detailed description of these results. However the overriding conclusion is that the genomes of these two virtually unrelated creatures are extremely similar in basic sequence organization. Results almost exactly similar to those shown in Fig. 5 for *Xenopus* DNA have also been obtained by application of S-1 nuclease to sea urchin DNA duplexes formed at low $C_o t$. As with *Xenopus*, middle-repetitive sequence in *Strongylocentrotus* DNA also falls predominantly into a length distribution the modal value of which is 300 nucleotides, and again there is a small class of clustered repetitive DNA. In Fig. 7 the length dependence of the hydroxyapatite binding curve for sea urchin DNA is compared to that of *Xenopus* DNA. The two curves differ at most by 10-15%. Again most of the nonrepetitive DNA of the sea urchin is interspersed with middle-repetitive sequence elements. Furthermore both long and short period interspersion is apparent in the sea urchin genome.

Analyses this extensive have not as yet been performed for other animal DNA's. However S-1 nuclease has been used to probe repetitive sequence element length in one other case, that of calf DNA. All the DNA's studied appear similar. Though it is still too early to generalize widely, a fair statement would be that at least among the deuterostomes there is widespread occurrence of the same fundamental pattern of interspersed DNA sequence organization.

SIGNIFICANCE OF INTERSPERSED SEQUENCE ORGANIZATION

A basic requirement of the Britten-Davidson theory of gene regulation is the presence of regulatory repetitive sequence elements contiguous to the structural genes (Britten and Davidson, 1969, 1971). According to the analyses presented in Figs. 6 and 7,

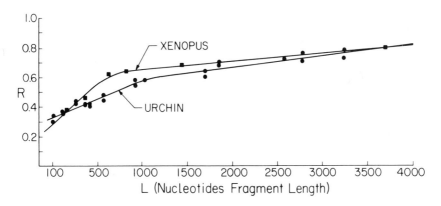

Figure 7. The relation between fragment length and hydroxyapatite binding in the DNA of the sea urchin *Strongylocentrotus purpuratus* compared to a similar curve for *Xenopus* DNA (Graham, Neufeld and Britten, in preparation). The parameter R has the same meaning as in Fig. 6. Any of a closely related set of curves can be fitted to the sea urchin data, as shown for *Xenopus* DNA in Fig. 6. The *Xenopus* curve presented here is derived from the mean R values at each point, rather than by the weighted statistical method used in Fig. 6. It is similar to one of the fits plotted in Fig. 6, assuming a 300 nucleotide repetitive sequence element length. This assumption, also used for the sea urchin curve shown, is supported for both species by the S-1 nuclease experiments discussed in the text. For the short period interspersed region of the sea urchin curve the mean nonrepetitive sequence element length is about 1100 nucleotides.

the nonrepetitive sequence lengths which separate interspersed repetitive regions are consistent with the expected lengths of structural gene regions. Apparently complete mRNA's have been isolated in the 500-1200 nucleotide range, such as for hemoglobin, immunoglobulins and ovalbumin, and many heterogeneous polysomal mRNA preparations fall within this range. On the other hand there is also evidence for mRNA's thousands of nucleotides in length, *e.g.* the message for silk fibroin (Suzuki *et al.*, 1972). Evidence was presented at this symposium (Hamkalo *et al.*) for the presence of extremely long polysomes in both HeLa and *Drosophila* cells which would also require messages thousands of nucleotides in length. These observations suggest that the nonrepetitive DNA in both long and short period interspersed arrangements could include structural genes, that is, assuming that structural genes in general belong to the nonrepetitive sequence class.

Only a few cases of animal structural genes have been examined from this point of view. Bishop and his associates, as well as

others, have demonstrated that the hemoglobin gene is probably a
nonrepetitive sequence (Bishop *et al.*, 1972; Bishop and Rosbash,
1973; Packman *et al.*, 1972; Harrison *et al.*, 1972). Suzuki and
Brown (1972) have shown that the fibroin gene is also a nonrepetitive sequence. On the other hand the work of Kedes and Birnstiel
(1971) indicates that the histone structural genes are probably
repetitive sequences. In their study a fraction of putative ">25S"
messenger RNA's was also examined, and about 90% of the hybridized
RNase-resistant labeled RNA in this fraction appears to be nonrepetitive sequence transcript. Greenberg and Perry (1971) also describe
experiments with heterogeneous-labeled mRNA's, extracted from actinomycin D-treated L-cells. Using the Nygaard-Hall (1964) filter
technique they too found that most of the labeled RNA which they
were able to hybridize reassociates with nonrepetitive DNA sequence.

This brief review indicates that little contemporary information relating to the sequence content of the total range of mRNA's
present in any given animal cells is available. Fig. 8 shows the
main results of a recent study on sea urchin mRNA's carried out in
our laboratory. The figure shows the reassociation of labeled mRNA's
from sea urchin gastrulae with DNA present in a mass ratio of 1 X
10^4 times the mRNA. The conditions of extraction ensure that the
labeled RNA in this experiment is in fact active mRNA. The polyribosomes were isolated from the >70S region of a preparative gradient, pelleted, and then treated with puromycin. The mRNP thus released appears in the form of particles sedimenting <70S. The radioactive RNA present in this area of another preparative gradient was
extracted. Contamination of these mRNA preparations with labeled
nuclear RNA has been shown to be virtually zero. At the conclusion
of all the purification procedures the modal size of the mRNA is

---

Figure 8. Reassociation of sea urchin mRNA to DNA (Goldberg *et al.*,
1973). Isotopically-labeled mRNA (50 μCi/ml [^{3}H]uridine, 3 hr, 15°
C) from 36 hr embryos was extracted as indicated in the text. The
fraction of labeled mRNA released from the resuspended polysomal
pellet was 40%. Subsequent experiments in which 90-100% of the
mRNA was recovered give substantially the same answer. Messenger
RNA was annealed to DNA (sheared at 50,000 psi to 450 nucleotides)
at 60°C in either 0.41M phosphate buffer (PB) or 0.12M PB. The
overall DNA/RNA ratio was 10,000/1. The solid circles represent
hybrids assayed by adjusting the annealing solution to 0.2M PB, 8M
urea, 1% sodium dodecyl sulfate and passing the solution over a
hydroxyapatite column equilibrated at 40°C in the same buffer. Un-
associated nucleic acids are eluted from the column at this temperature. The column temperature was then raised to 80°C in order to
elute hybrids. The percent labeled RNA in hybrids is the amount of
radioactivity eluted at 80°C divided by the total radioactivity pass-

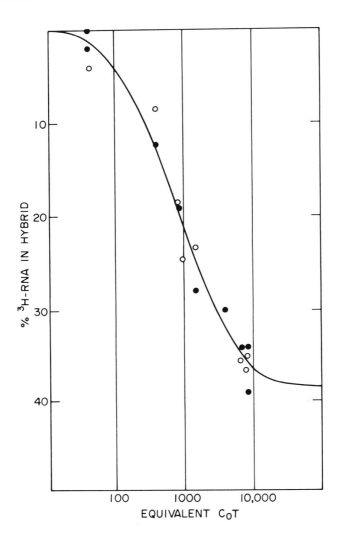

ed over the column (CPM eluted at 40°C plus 80°C). The open circles
represent hybrids which were treated with ribonuclease (10 µg/ml,
RNase A, 0.24M PB, 1 hr, room temperature) and passed over a Sephadex
G-200 column. The percent labeled RNA in hybrids is the amount of
radioactivity excluded from the G-200 column and refers to RNase-
resistant hybrids. Before assay, a fraction of each hybridization
mixture was passed over a G-100 column to check for RNA degradation.
No degradation beyond the level of G-100 exclusion occurred during
these hybridizations. The solid line describing the reassociation
of mRNA to DNA was fit to the points by a computer, using the rate
constant (0.00125) measured for nonrepetitive DNA in whole DNA
(Britten, 1972). The root-mean-square of this fit is 0.035.

about 9S, and after incubation with DNA it is still excluded by
Sephadex G-100.

The reannealing mixtures of Fig. 8 are analyzed in two ways,
as noted on the figure. For the assay of ribonuclease-resistant
hybrids the annealing mixture is treated with ribonuclease and the
RNA remaining bound to DNA is separated from nucleotides on Sephadex.
This method of assay indicates the fraction of mRNA nucleotides
transcribed from various frequency classes of DNA sequence. In the
other procedure that we have employed, the use of ribonuclease is
avoided, and the mixture is passed over hydroxyapatite directly.
Here the whole of any mRNA molecule bearing a recognizable repetitive sequence element would be trapped after annealing to a low C_ot.
In order to prevent a portion of the nonhybridized mRNA from binding
to the column, the sample is placed on the latter in 8M urea - 0.2M
phosphate buffer, at 40°C (see Legend to Fig. 8).

In the experiment of Fig. 8 both sets of data are reasonably
well fit by the same line. This line represents the measured reassociation kinetics of pure nonrepetitive sequence in whole *S.
purpuratus* DNA (Britten, 1972). Assayed either with or without
ribonuclease, less than 5% of the mRNA binds to hydroxyapatite after
annealing to C_ot 40 (all repetitive sequences in the sea urchin
genome will react by this C_ot). Thus we conclude from Fig. 8 that
almost all of the hybridizing mRNA molecules consist exclusively of
nonrepetitive sequence transcript. The failure of the mRNA hybridization reaction to exceed 40% can be shown to be due to insufficient
DNA, or in other words, to the large number of copies of each mRNA
sequence present. Increasing the DNA/RNA results in greater total
hybridization.

These experiments show that at least for one system, the sea
urchin gastrula, the active structural genes are indeed nonrepetitive sequence elements. For us the most incisive question now
becomes whether the structural gene sequences are indeed interspersed among contiguous repetitive sequence elements. Whatever the
ultimate answer, it is our belief that knowledge of the sequence
organization around the structural genes will lead to a basic understanding of regulation in the higher organism genome.

ACKNOWLEDGMENTS

Supported by grant HD-05753 from the National Institutes of
Health and grant GB-33441 from the National Science Foundation.

REFERENCES

Ando, T. 1966. A nuclease specific for heat-denatured DNA isolated from a product of *Aspergillus oryzae*. Biochim. Biophys. Acta 114: 158.

Bishop, J. O., R. Pemberton and C. Baglioni. 1972. Reiteration frequency of hemoglobin genes in the duck. Nature New Biol. 235: 231.

Bishop, J. O. and M. Roshbash. 1973. Reiteration frequency of duck haemoglobin genes. Nature New Biol. 241: 204.

Britten, R. J. 1972. DNA sequence interspersion and a speculation about evolution. In (H. H. Smith, ed.) Evolution of Genetic Systems. p. 80. Gordon and Breach, New York.

Britten, R. J. and D. E. Kohne. 1968. Repeated sequences in DNA. Science 161: 529.

Britten, R. J. and E. H. Davidson. 1969. Gene regulation for higher cells: a theory. Science 165: 349.

Britten, R. J. and J. Smith. 1970. A bovine genome. Carnegie Inst. of Wash. Year Book 68: 378.

Britten, R. J. and E. H. Davidson. 1971. Repetitive and nonrepetitive DNA sequences and a speculation on the origins of evolutionary novelty. Quart. Rev. Biol. 46: 111.

Britten, R. J., D. E. Graham and B. R. Neufeld. 1973. Analysis of repeating DNA sequences by reassociation. In (S. P. Colowick, ed.) Methods in Enzymology. In press.

Davidson, E. H. and B. R. Hough. 1971. Genetic information in oocyte RNA. J. Mol. Biol. 56: 491.

Davidson, E. H. and B. R. Hough. 1969. High sequence diversity in the RNA synthesized at the lampbrush stage of oogenesis. Proc. Nat. Acad. Sci. 63: 342.

Davidson, E. H., B. R. Hough, C. S. Amenson and R. J. Britten. 1973. General interspersion of repetitive with nonrepetitive sequence elements in the DNA of *Xenopus*. J. Mol. Biol. in press.

Goldberg, R. B., G. A. Galau and E. H. Davidson. 1973. Sequence content of messenger RNA. Proc. Nat. Acad. Sci. in press.

Greenberg, J. R. and R. P. Perry. 1971. Hybridization properties
of DNA sequences directing the synthesis of messenger RNA and heterogeneous nuclear RNA. J. Cell Biol. 50: 774.

Harrison, P. R., A. Hell, G. D. Birnie and J. Paul. 1972. Evidence
for single copies of globin genes in the mouse genome. Nature 239:
219.

Hough, B. R. and E. H. Davidson. 1972. Studies on the repetitive
seuqence transcripts of Xenopus oocytes. J. Mol. Biol. 70: 491.

Kedes, L. H. and M. L. Birnstiel. 1971. Reiteration and clustering
of DNA sequences complementary to histone messenger RNA. Nature
New Biol. 230: 165.

Nygaard, A. P. and B. D. Hall. 1964. Formation and properties of
RNA-DNA complexes. J. Mol. Biol. 9: 125.

Packman, S., H. Aviv, J. Ross and P. Leder. 1972. A comparison
of globin genes in duck reticulocytes and liver cells. Biochem.
Biophys. Res. Comm. 49: 813.

Suzuki, Y. and D. D. Brown. 1972. Isolation and identification of
the messenger RNA for silk fibroin from Bombyx mori. J. Mol. Biol.
63: 409.

Suzuki, Y., L. P. Gage and D. D. Brown. 1972. The genes for silk
fibroin in Bombyx mori. J. Mol. Biol. 70: 637.

3. DNA REPLICATION IN THE CHROMOSOMES OF EUKARYOTES

H. G. Callan

Zoology Department, The University, St. Andrews, Scotland

The first experimental evidence that the DNA of eukaryotic chromosomes replicates semi-conservatively was provided by Taylor *et al.*, 1957. Root-tip cells of the broad bean, *Vicia faba*, were allowed to incorporate tritiated thymidine during a period of DNA synthesis (S-phase), were fixed at the following mitosis, and examined by autoradiography. Each labelled chromosome showed radioactivity in both chromatids. Cells similarly labelled, but followed by a time before fixation in the absence of precursor sufficient to complete another S-phase and to reach the next mitosis (*i.e.* the second mitosis after labelling) showed radioactivity in only one chromatid at any location along each chromosome. These observations, now known to be valid for all eukaryotic chromosomes that have been studied, are evidence not only for semi-conservative replication of DNA as such, but also for the proposition of uninemy, *i.e.* that each chromatid of a eukaryote contains only one double helix of DNA.

The chromoneme of the bacterium *Escherichia coli* consists of a "naked circle" of DNA about 1.3 mm in contour length. Semi-conservative replication of this DNA proceeds in two opposite directions away from a defined initiation point (Masters and Broda, 1971; Prescott and Keumpel, 1972; Bird *et al.*, 1972) at a rate of some 20-30 μm/min one-way at 37°C, and the two replication forks can therefore converge and fuse, completing the replication of the genome, within the generation time of 30 minutes (Cairns, 1963).

Assuming the uninemy of eukaryotes' chromatids in general, for which there is compelling evidence from several other lines of investigation (reviewed by Callan, 1972), an average chromatid of the broad bean contains about 1 meter of DNA, *i.e.* is about 800 times

longer than the *E. coli* chromonema. Yet at 25°C the entire synthesis is completed within an S-phase of only 8 hours. When allowance
is made for the temperature difference, DNA replication in a broad
bean's chromatid is proceeding quantitatively about 100 times faster
than in *E. coli*. It turns out that this feat is accomplished, in
all eukaryotes so far investigated, by the presence of many initiation points, and hence many replication forks, per chromosome.

The "whole-cell" autoradiographic study of mitotic chromosomes
of various organisms, pulse-labelled with [^{3}H]dThd during the pre-
ceding S-phase, gave a decided hint that there might well be many
concurrently active sites of DNA replication, for such chromosomes
can show radioactivity throughout their lengths, not merely in the
one or two discrete and limited regions that would be expected if
there were only a single initiation point per chromosome. Furthermore in the polytene chromosomes of the larvae of dipteran flies,
exceptional not only in respect of their being multineme, but also
in that DNA replication proceeds while the chromosomes remain visible in the light microscope, hence being peculiarly amenable to
whole-cell autoradiography, short-term labelling followed immediately by fixation reveals that [^{3}H]dThd can be incorporated into DNA
concurrently at many sites along each chromosome (Keyl and Pelling,
1963; Pelling, 1966).

After studying DNA replication in the salivary gland chromosomes of a hybrid between *Chironomus thummi thummi* and *Ch. th. piger*
in this manner, this particular hybrid being chosen because the
thummi genome contains 27% more DNA than the *piger* genome (Keyl,
1965), Keyl and Pelling concluded that the units of replication are
individual chromomeres (cross-bands in these polytene chromosomes),
that replication begins simultaneously in all chromomeres, and that
replication ends in an orderly sequence, chromomeres containing
little DNA finishing early, chromomeres containing more DNA finishing late. These conclusions were supported by Mulder *et al.* (1968)
working on *Drosophila hydei,* but they have not gone unchallenged.
Howard and Plaut (1968) made an extensive analysis of labelling
patterns in salivary gland chromosomes of *Drosophila melanogaster,*
and found that they were unable to place these patterns in a single
progressive series, though the patterns could be accommodated in
two. From these observations Howard and Plaut concluded that there
must be a time-sequence of initiation as well as a time-sequence of
termination. In so far as polytene chromosomes are concerned, the
problem of whether the replicational units initiate synchronously
or in a determined sequence remains unsolved (see review by Rudkin,
1972).

A major limitation of whole-cell autoradiography results from
the fact that in general, DNA replication proceeds during interphase,
when the chromosomes cannot be resolved by the light microscope.
Thus although the incorporation of labelled precursors can be de-

tected on a gross scale, it is not possible by this method to establish precisely where replication has been in progress along any
single DNA fiber.

The limitation inherent in whole-cell autoradiography was
cleverly circumvented by a technique of DNA-fiber autoradiography
invented by Cairns (1962, 1966) and further developed by Huberman
and Riggs (1968). In this technique the cells are first labelled,
then suspended in a medium containing molar sucrose, and placed in
dialysis chambers whose walls are formed by Millipore filters. The
cells are lysed by dialysis against detergent in sucrose, the sucrose concentrations inside and outside the dialysis chamber mini-
mize shear-breakage of the DNA-fibers as these are released from
the cell nuclei. After lysis, the chambers are dialyzed against a
proteolytic enzyme, and after prolonged washing by dialysis the
chambers are punctured and drained. Some of the labelled DNA fibers
adhere to the Millipore filters and stretch out in the general
direction of drainage.

Each Millipore filter is now dried and detached from the glass
component of its chamber, stuck on to an ordinary glass microscope
slide with its former inner surface exposed, and covered with autoradiographic stripping film. After long exposure, usually several
months, the filmed slide is developed, fixed and washed, the stripping film is detached from the Millipore filter, mounted on a clean
slide, and examined by bright-field light microscopy. Tracks of
silver grains in the film mark the labelled regions of DNA fibers
trapped on the previously underlying filter, and provided the labelling regime was appropriate, the labelled fibers were sufficiently
sparse, and sufficiently devoid of shear breaks, the temporal sequence of DNA replication, its rate, and the spatial distribution
of initiation points for replication along continuous single fibers,
can be determined.

By means of this technique, and by a much simpler method introduced by Lark *et al.* (1971) whereby labelled cells are lysed and
streaked directly on to subbed slides which are later covered with
dipping emulsion, Huberman and Riggs were able to show that during
the S-phase of mammalian cells in culture, DNA replication occurs in
units that are arranged in tandem; that from any single initiation
point or origin replication progresses by two divergent forks; *i.e.*
bi-directionally, at a one-way rate of some 0.5 to 1.2 µm per minute;
that the intervals between neighboring origins vary, ranging from
some 15 to 120 µm with a mean interval of about 50 µm; and that
replication may start from neighboring origins staggered in time.
These findings have since been substantially corroborated for a
variety of mammalian cells by other investigators.

The evidence for Huberman and Riggs' discovery that replication proceeds bi-directionally from initiation points came from

"chase" experiments, and from experiments where a deliberate change
in the specific activity of radioactive precursor was introduced
at some point during the period of labelling. In chase experiments
the labelled medium is replaced, after a certain lapse of time, by
unlabelled medium, and the cells are allowed to continue growth for
a further period in this unlabelled medium before harvesting. Provided the cells have a substantial pool of DNA precursor molecules
on which to draw, the DNA which they synthesize during the chase
becomes progressively less radioactive as labelled molecules are
withdrawn from the pool. Consequently replicating units that initiated within the period of growth in labelled medium and that
continued replication during the chase, show up in autoradiographs
as heavily labelled tracks of silver grains flanked by "tails" of
diminishing grain density. An example, from cells of the South
African frog, *Xenopus laevis*, tissue-cultured at 25°C, labelled for
2 hours and chased for a further 2 hours, is shown in Fig. 2A. This
photograph should be compared with Fig. 2B which is from an autoradiograph of *Xenopus* cells labelled without any chase for 4 hours;
in the latter figure the silver grain tracks end abruptly. Replicating units that had initiated before labelling began, but that
continued replication during the period of labelling and on into a
chase period, show up in autoradiographs as heavily labelled silver
grain tracks with a tail on one side only (see Fig. 2E).

Deliberate "step-down" or "step-up" labelling regimes similarly
allow the temporal sequence of replication to be interpreted from
fluctuations in silver grain densities in the autoradiographs. The
step-down procedure is illustrated diagrammatically in Fig. 1, where
the tracks marked (i) have resulted from a labelling regime in which
the DNA synthesized during the early period of labelling had twice
the radioactivity of that synthesized during a later period. Five
stages of replication are shown, A to E, and 5 origins, O^1 to O^5;
O^2 initiated replication when the label was first supplied, and
proceeded to C without change of labelling intensity. Meantime,
but after a delay, O^3 and O^4 initiated. If harvesting were to take
place now, the autoradiograph C(i) would show one long and two
shorter tracks arranged in tandem, all of uniform grain density.
Sister strand separation is generally not apparent in autoradiographs
until 50 μm or more of DNA fiber have been replicated; that is why
these tracks are not drawn splayed apart. At the stage represented
by C, non-radioactive precursor is presumed to have been added to
the medium, thereby reducing the specific activity of labelled precursor. If harvesting were to take place at stage D, the autoradiograph D(i) would show, reading from the left, a lightly-labelled
short track representing the recent initiation of replication at O^1,
a longer track heavily labelled in the middle and flanked on both
sides by more lightly labelled regions representing the continuing
replication of O^2, and a still longer track labelled light-heavy-
light-heavy-light representing the fusion of O^3 and O^4 and continuing replication at the extremities. O^2, O^3 and O^4 may therefore be

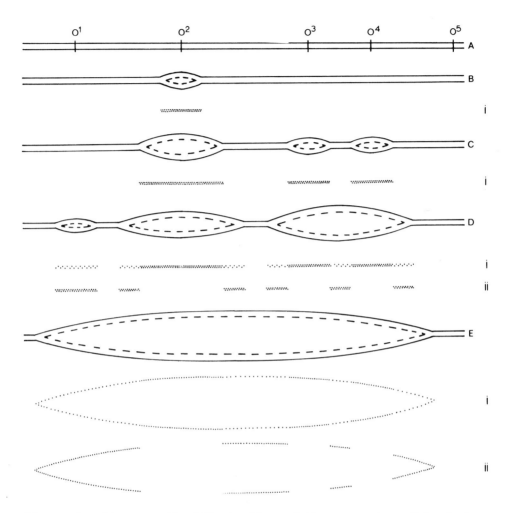

Figure 1. Diagrammatic illustration of the operation of tandemly arranged units of replication, with initiation points at O^1 to O^5. B to E represent progressive stages of replication; i and ii represent the corresponding tracks in DNA fiber autoradiographs. Further explanation in text.

located without dubiety, and O^1 tentatively. If harvesting were delayed until stage E, this would allow fusion of O^1 with O^2 with O^3/O^4, and such a long replicated section would be very likely to show up in the resulting autoradiograph as a split track, with precisely matching labelling patterns arranged in parallel. The locations of O^2, O^3 and O^4 would remain recognizable, the existence of O^1 could be inferred but its precise position not known, and the existence of O^5 would not be suspected.

There is in practice some advantage in a step-up rather than a
step-down labelling regime for the location of initiation points.
This is because an appreciable time may elapse before the specific
activity of the precursor pool inside the cell builds up to its
limit, as a consequence of which the radioactivity of DNA syntheized
at the beginning of the period of labelling increases progressively;
this effect, and it is more pronounced the bigger the intracellular
pool, can occasionally give rise to a gradient of grain density that
may be confused with a genuine tail conseqeunt upon a step-down during the labelling regime. Misreading of the spurious tail would
result in a one-way replicating section, which initiated before the
start of labelling, being taken for a two-way replicating region with
an origin at its mid-point. An autoradiograph from *Xenopus* comparable to Fig. 1 E(i) except that it results from a step-up labelling
regime (1 hour low specific activity/2 hours high at 25°C) is shown
in Fig. 2C; three origins, in the middles of the lightly labelled
regions, can be located.

Once bi-directional replication has been recognized as the
rule, it becomes possible in favorable circumstances to locate
initiation points, and hence to measure the intervals between them,
in autoradiographs from cells exposed to a radioactive medium which
remians of uniform specific activity throughout the period of labelling. This is also illustrated diagrammatically in Fig. 1. It is
here assumed that labelling began when stage C had been reached,
i.e. after replication had already been in progress from 0^2, 0^3 and
0^4. Harvesting at stage D would produce the autoradiograph shown
as D(ii), from which no information about origins could be inferred.
However if harvesting were delayed until stage E, the split track
autoradiograph shown as E(ii) would give almost indisputable evidence for origins at 0^2, 0^3 and 0^4. The only margin of uncertainty
would be that each gap in the labelling pattern might include not
just one, but more than one, origin. An example of a labelling
pattern similar to that drawn in Fig. 1 E(ii) can be seen in Fig.
2D (from chicken cells labelled for 30 minutes at 37°C).

It should then be apparent that provided cells are given labelling regimes of appropriate kind and duration and if, when interpreting the resultant autoradiographs, account be taken of the pitfalls

---

Figure 2. All are photographs of DNA fiber autoradiographs.
A. *Xenopus laevis* tissue culture at 25°C. FdUrd-treated, labelled
for 2 hours and chased for 2 hours. B. *Xenopus laevis* tissue culture at 25°C. FdUrd-treated, and labelled for 4 hours. C. *Xenopus
laevis* tissue culture at 25°C. FdUrd-treated, labelled at low specific activity for 1 hour, and at high specific activity for 2
hours. D. *Gallus domesticus* tissue culture at 37°C. FdUrd-treated,
and labelled for 30 min. E. *Gallus domesticus* tissue culture at
37°C, FdUrd-treated, labelled for 30 min and chased for 30 min.

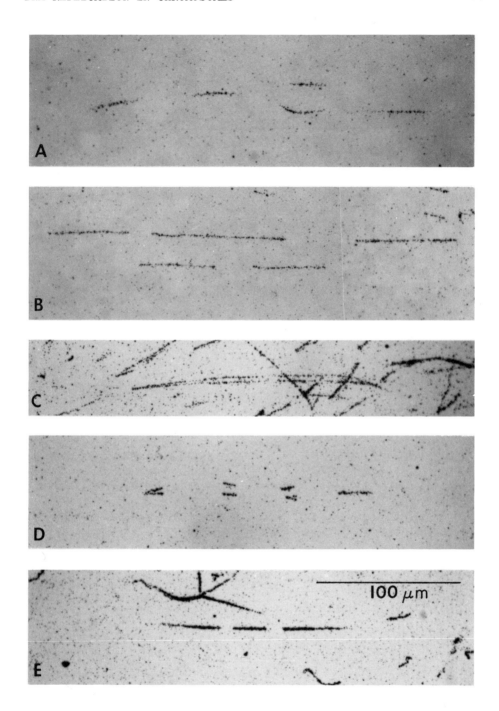

just mentioned, a measure of the frequency distribution of initiation point intervals can be obtained. Before considering some
actual examples of information that has been gained in this manner,
an additional source of bias in the data should be recognized. If
two neighboring initiation points lie far apart, they will be less
frequently identified as forming a tandem series, and further, shear
breakage will more likely occur between them, so destroying their
relationship to one another, than if they lie close together. Therefore in all frequency distributions of initiation point intervals,
longer intervals will tend to be underestimated.

When Huberman and Riggs proposed their model for the replication of DNA in the chromosomes of eukaryotes they suggested, though
not with great insistence, that termini for replication might be
disposed at symmetrical distances on both sides of initiation points.
They were led to make this proposal by the finding, in pulse-chase
experiments, of abruptly terminating heavily labelled tracks flanked
on both sides by other heavily labelled tracks each with declining
grain density tails at *both* ends. The simplest reading of such a
tandem series would be to suppose that the middle member, with its
abrupt ends, stopped replicating at the termini prior to the chase,
whilst the flanking members continued replication during the chase
period. Huberman and Riggs found very few such tandem series in
their fiber autoradiographs from mammalian cells, and that has also
been the experience of McFarlane and Callan (1973) studying chicken
material. On the other hand, in pulse-chase experiments with the
chicken cells, McFarlane and Callan have often encountered tandem
series such as the one shown in Fig. 2E, where a middle, abruptly
terminating track is flanked on both sides by tracks each showing
a well-defined tail proceeding outwards, but with an abrupt ending
towards the inside. Such tracks establish without ambiguity that
replication from an origin proceeds bi-directionally without regard
to termini, for evidently the origins lie in the midpoints of the
gaps between labelled tracks; the middle track represents the outcome of replication to fusion which occurred during the pulse,
whereas the outer tracks represent replication proceeding from the
same initiation points and continuing during pulse and chase until
the harvesting of the cells.

Estimates of the linear rate of progress of replication forks
cannot be obtained from chase experiments, because silver grain
tracks in DNA fiber autoradiographs must end abruptly if their
lengths are to be measured with accuracy. This presents a problem,
because in autoradiographs from cells labelled with radioactive DNA
precursors supplied at constant specific activity, the tracks measured are necessarily an indeterminate mixed population representing:
(1) bi-directional replication which initiated when label was first
supplied, without subsequent fusion between neighbors during the
period of labelling; (2) as 1, but with fusion; (3) as 1, but
where initiation was delayed until some time during labelling, with-

out subsequent fusion between neighbors during the period of labelling; (4) as 3, but with fusion; (5) unidirectional replication,
where initiation had occurred before labelling started, without
subsequent fusion during the period of labelling; (6) as 5, but
with fusion.

Assuming that replication rate is invariant (and remembering
that this may not be a valid assumption), only tracks of types 1
and 5 will correctly portray the full extent of replication in a
given period of time, undistorted by complications from one source
or another. However tracks of types 1 or 5 cannot in general be
distinguished from all the rest. In practice this difficulty can
be circumvented by: (a) blocking DNA synthesis in the cell culture
by an inhibitor such as 5-fluorodeoxyuridine (FdUrd), thereby ac-
cumulating cells that can only begin their S-phases when the block
is removed by supplying [^{3}H]dThd. Despite some criticisms of the
use of FdUrd, the greater the degree of synchrony in the culture
produced by this inhibitor the greater the representation of tracks
of types 1, 2 and 3 in the autoradiographs and the better the pros-
pect of accurately determining replication rate. (b) labelling for
progressively increasing periods of time, and comparing frequency
histograms of track lengths resulting from such experiments. At
least two of the labelling periods must be shorter than the time
necessary for the overwhelming majority of replicating units, that
have initiated within the labelling period to fuse with their neighbors. These periods must of course be determined empirically; they
should be unmistakably recognizable from the frequency histograms
by the absence, or virtual absence, of tracks longer than twice the
mean. Fig. 3 taken from McFarlane and Callan (1973), shows a series
of such histograms for semi-synchronized chicken cells.

Mean track lengths determined from such histograms do not give
valid estimates of replication rate, for the reasons already mentioned. But provided there is a well-defined right hand shoulder
to the histograms, its position along the abscissa will be a measure
of 2-way replication that has been in progress throughout the labelling period. Having determined replication rate in this way, the
validity of the estimate can be cross-checked against the frequency
distribution of initiation point intervals, for taken together the
two pieces of information will allow an estimate to be made of the
duration of labelling necessary to produce significant number of
long, uninterrupted tracks resulting from fusion. A frequency histo-
gram of track lengths for the appropriate labelling period and
longer should therefore include some of these long tracks.

The general impression one obtains from papers describing DNA
fiber autoradiographic studies carried out on mammalian somatic
cells in culture at 37°C is that the rate of progress of replication
forks is of the order 0.5 μm per minute; the same figure holds for
chicken cells (McFarlane and Callan, 1973). This rate, it should be

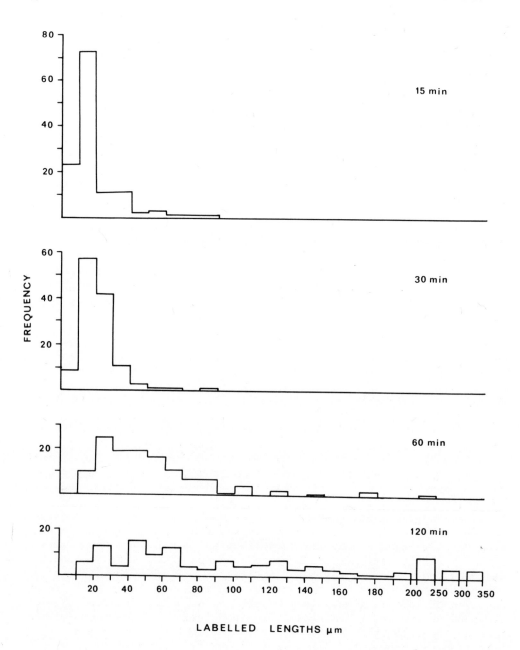

Figure 3. Frequency histograms of labelled track lengths from DNA
fiber autoradiographs derived from chick cells in culture. The cells
were FdUrd treated, and labelled with [^{3}H]dThd for 15, 30, 60 and
120 min.

noted, is about one fiftieth of the rate achieved by *Escherichia coli* growing at the same temperature. Histones have to be built into the replicating chromosomes of eukaryotes, and the manipulation of these molecules during DNA replication may well be a rate-limiting factor in higher organisms.

Huberman and Riggs have determined that the range of initiation intervals in Chinese hamster somatic cells is 15 to 120 μm, with a mean of about 50 μm. J. H. Priest (personal communication) working with rat somatic cells finds an initiation interval range of 10 to 60 μm, with a mean of about 30 μm. In chicken somatic cells McFarlane and I have found an initiation interval range of 25 to 145 μm, with a mean of about 60 μm. When cultured at 37°C these cells all have S-phases on the order of 6 to 8 hours. Assuming a one-way replication rate of 30 μm per hour, initiation intervals considerably longer than the longest recorded could evidently be bridged within S-phases of these durations. Maybe such long intervals do exist and have not been recognized, but it is more likely that extensive staggering of initiations draws out a somatic cell S-phase to a longer period of time than might otherwise be anticipated. Thus McFarlane and Callan have found evidence that in chicken somatic cells in culture some initiation points do not become effective for replication until more than two hours after neighboring units have initiated.

Amongst eukaryotes, both plant and animal, the DNA quantity per haploid genome (the C-value, Swift, 1950a,b) covers an enormous range, and remarkably enough these diverse DNA quantities are in no evident way related to organizational complexity. This is the C-value paradox (Callan, 1967, 1972). The chicken has less than half the C-value characteristic of mammals, but this lower value is not obviously reflected either in replication rate or in the initiation point intervals which operate in somatic cells. On the other hand, when replication in somatic cells of the frog *Xenopus laevis* (C-value 3 pg) is compared with that in the newt *Triturus cristatus* (C-value 29 pg), there are clear-cut differences. Rate of replication at 25°C in *Triturus* is more than twice as fast (20 μm per hour one-way) as in *Xenopus* at the same temperature (compare Figs. 2B and 4A); and whereas the initiation point intervals in *Xenopus* mostly range from 20 to 100 μm with a mean of about 60 μm, the closest intervals in *Triturus* are more than 100 μm apart, and the majority are much more widely spaced than this.

Within one and the same organism S-phase durations in cells at different developmental stages can vary enormously. S-phases are much shorter during early embryogenesis than they are in differentiated somatic cells, while the S-phase immediately prior to meiosis is exceptionally long drawn-out in all organisms so far investigated. In the newt *Triturus vulgaris* at 18°C, the S-phase in the blastula lasts for one hour, as compared with 200 hours for premeiotic S in

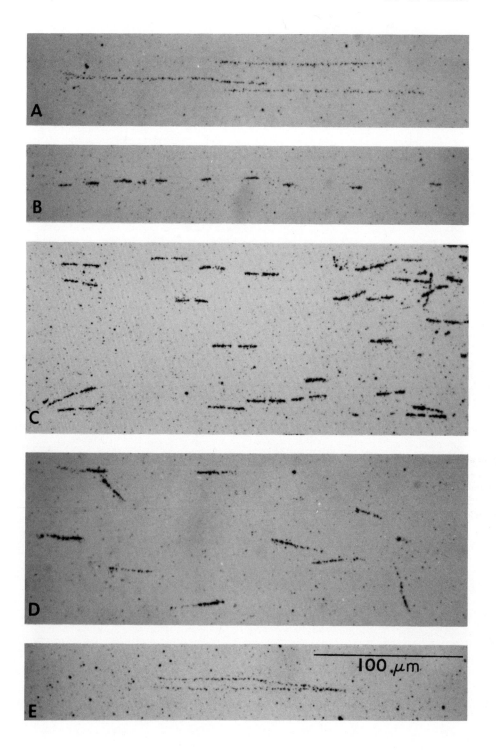

the spermatocyte (Callan and Taylor, 1968). This S-phase diversity is accommodated not by gross diversity in replication rate but rather by striking differences in the number of initiation points operative for replication. In the neurula of *Triturus*, where at 18°C the S-phase lasts some 4 hours, an order of magnitude shorter than the S-phase in newt somatic cells, most of the initiation points are about 40 μm apart. Fig. 4B shows a fiber autoradiograph from *Triturus* neurula cells labelled for one hour at 18°C. Most if not all of the tracks illustrated represent one-way replication without fusion, and the initiation points must lie at the midpoints of every alternate gap. Fig. 4B should be compared with Fig. 4A, which shows tracks from *Triturus* somatic cells in culture labelled for 4 hours at 25°C; the lengths of these tracks are such that they must represent two-way replication, with origins at the midpoints of each track - and neighboring tracks in tandem with those shown lie way beyond the limits of the photograph.

Another distinctive feature of these *Triturus* neurula cells is that replication starts in synchrony, so far as one can tell from fiber autoradiographs, at all the initiation points within one nucleus. Fig. 4C makes this point clear. The tracks shown must have originated from a single neurula cell nucleus labelled for two hours at 18°C, for the labelled cells were massively diluted with unlabelled *Xenopus* tissue culture cells just before the dialysis chambers were loaded. Essentially every track shows a small gap at its midpoint, indicating that replication had initiated just before provision of label. The one-way rate of replication can be directly assessed from Fig. 4C; it is about 6 μm/hour, surprisingly enough distinctly *slower* than in *Triturus* somatic cells in culture despite the much shorter S-phase in the cells of the embryo. If the replication rate established for the neurula also holds for the *Triturus* blastula, with an S-phase of only one hour at 18°C, no initiation points in the latter can be more than 10 μm apart.

Wolstenholme (1973) has recently been investigating DNA replication in 100 minute-old *Drosophila melanogaster* embryos by electron microscopy. In consonance with the forecast for *Triturus* blastula cells, he finds an initiation interval range of roughly 1 to 10 μm with a mean of about 4 μm. However as the S-phase in these *Drosophila* embryos lasts less than 10 minutes, replication rate must be a lot faster than any recorded for *Triturus*.

Figure 4. All are photographs of DNA fiber autoradiographs.
A. *Triturus cristatus* tissue culture at 25°C. FdUrd-treated, and labelled for 4 hours. B. *Triturus vulgaris* dissociated neurula at 18°C. Labelled for one hour. C. *Triturus vulgaris* dissociated neurula at 18°C. Labelled for 2 hours. D. *Triturus vulgaris* dissociated testis at 25°C. Labelled for 4 hours. E. *Triturus vulgaris* dissociated testis at 18°C. Labelled for 8 hours.

We have no direct information concerning the range of initiation intervals in the *Triturus* spermatocyte, but the remarkable homogeneity of track lengths in fiber autoradiographs obtained from unsynchronized spermatocytes after 2, 4 and even 8 hours of labelling at 18°C suggested that essentially all tracks represent continuing one-way replication at about 12 µm/hour, with little contribution from units which fused or initiated during the labelling period; this in turn indicates that the effective initiation points in spermatocytes must be several hundred µm apart.

Evidence for a preponderance of tracks resulting from one-way replication in fiber autoradiographs from *Triturus* spermatocytes is provided in Fig. 4D, which shows several tracks with single tails. This is the happy accidental outcome of an attempt to label spermatocytes at uniform specific activity for 4 hours at 25°C, but where evidently the [^{3}H]dThd was not properly mixed into the culture medium at the beginning of labelling! Similar evidence is provided by the many V-shaped tracks present in spermatocyte fiber autoradiographs, one of which (from 8 hours labelling at 18°C) is shown in Fig. 4E.

We are left with two clear-cut problems. One of these is how to account for the inactivity during the somatic S-phase, and still more dramatically during the premeiotic S-phase, of initiation points which are operative during embryonic S. One might postulate that there are several kinds of enzyme molecules which are responsible for the initiation of DNA synthesis and which recognize specific and different base pair sequences on the DNA, *i.e.* that there are qualitatively different initiation points, and that differences between cells arise during differentiation in regard to which initiating enzymes are available for DNA synthesis. However a more likely explanation is that while there is only one class of initiation sequence spread through the genome, any such sequence must be exposed for enzyme attachment if DNA synthesis is to begin. Occlusion of initiation sites would then presumably depend on the macromolecular packaging of DNA/histone in chromatin, a proposal supported by some rough calculations that suggest that the number of initiation points in premeiotic S equals the number of chromomeres visible in the lampbrush chromosomes at diplotene of meiosis. The chromomeres are regions of the genome where the DNA/histone fiber is densely packed; an equal number of short interchromomeric stretches, where the DNA is relatively exposed, would on this view include the only initiation sequences accessible to enzyme attachment immediately prior to meiosis. Similar considerations might be expected to apply to polytene chromosomes, and it will be recalled that already in 1963 Keyl and Pelling proposed that in such chromosomes the unit of replication is the chromomere.

The other problem concerns RNA transcription. The unit of transcription in lampbrush chromosomes of *Triturus* oocytes is generally the lateral loop projecting from a chromomere, with its single (occasionally multiple) polarized distribution of ribonucleoprotein (RNP) matrix running from "thin" to "thick" insertion. Most loops synthesize RNA throughout their lengths (Gall and Callan, 1962), and Miller and Beatty (1969) have drawn attention to the absence of any discontinuities in the distribution of RNP fibrils attached to lateral loops which might be comparable to the spacer regions of transcribing nucleolar DNA. Now the DNA being transcribed in a lateral loop of *Triturus* may be a hundred or more μm long; and even when one considers those unusual loops having multiple thin-to-thick RNP matrix distribution, *i.e.* loops that do show in the light microscope discontinuities in transcription, the transcriptional units are still exceedingly long, at least an order of magnitude longer than those of nucleolar DNA. It is a fair question what happens to the RNA transcribed across potential DNA initiation sequences, of which there may well be at least ten in a loop a hundred μm long. Such RNA sequences are probably degraded inside the nucleus, along with other sequences which have no translational meaning; this in turn raises the question as to how the "wanted" RNA sequences are protected against degradation. This problem is, however, a far cry from the topic of DNA replication. I mention it only to draw attention to the obvious: the interrelatedness of seemingly unrelated phenomena in nuclear function.

REFERENCES

Bird, R. W., J. Louarn, J. Martuscelli and L. Caro. 1972. Origin and sequence of chromosome replication in *Escherichia coli*. J. Mol. Biol. 70: 549.

Cairns, J. 1962. A minimum estimate for the length of the DNA of *Escherichia coli* obtained by autoradiography. J. Mol. Biol. 4: 407.

Cairns, J. 1963. The bacterial chromosome and its manner of replication as seen by autoradiography. J. Mol. Biol. 6: 208.

Cairns, J. 1966. Autoradiography of HeLa cell DNA. J. Mol. Biol. 15: 372.

Callan, H. G. 1967. The organization of genetic units in chromosomes. J. Cell Sci. 2: 1.

Callan, H. G. 1972. Replication of DNA in the chromosomes of eukaryotes. Proc. R. Soc. Ser. B. 181: 19.

Callan, H. G. and J. H. Taylor. 1968. A radioautographic study of the time course of male meiosis in the newt *Triturus vulgaris*. J. Cell Sci. 3: 615.

Gall, J. G. and H. G. Callan. 1962. H^3 uridine incorporation in lampbrush chromosomes. Proc. Nat. Acad. Sci. 48: 562.

Howard, E. F. and W. Plaut. 1968. Chromosomal DNA synthesis in *Drosophila melanogaster*. J. Cell Biol. 39: 415.

Huberman, J. A. and A. D. Riggs. 1968. On the mechanism of DNA replication in mammalian chromosomes. J. Mol. Biol. 32: 327.

Keyl, H.-G. 1965. Duplikationen von Untereinheiten der chromosomalen DNS während der Evolution von *Chironomus thummi*. Chromosoma 17: 139.

Keyl, H.-G. and C. Pelling. 1963. Differentielle DNS-Replikation in den Speicheldrüsen-Chromosomen von *Chironomus thummi*. Chromosoma 14: 347.

Lark, K. G., R. Consigli and A. Tolliver. 1971. DNA replication in Chinese hamster cells: evidence for a single replication fork per replicon. J. Mol. Biol. 58: 873.

McFarlane, P. W. and H. G. Callan. 1973. DNA replication in the chromosomes of the chicken, *Gallus domesticus*. J. Cell Sci. in press.

Masters, M. and P. Broda. 1971. Evidence of the bidirectional replication of the *Escherichia coli* chromosome. Nature New Biol. 232: 137.

Miller, O. L., Jr. and B. R. Beatty. 1969. Portrait of a gene. J. Cell Physiol. 74: Suppl 1, 225.

Mulder, M. P., P. van Duijn and H. J. Gloor. 1968. The replication organization of DNA in polytene chromosomes of *Drosophila hydei*. Genetica 39: 385.

Pelling, C. 1966. A replicative and synthetic chromosomal unit - the modern concept of the chromomere. Proc. R. Soc. Ser. B 164: 279.

Prescott, D. M. and P. E. Keumpel. 1972. Bidirectional replication of the chromosome in *Escherichia coli*. Proc. Nat. Acad. Sci. 69: 2842.

Rudkin, G. T. 1972. Replication in polytene chromosomes. Results and Problems in Cell Differentiation 4: 59.

Swift, H. 1950a. The desoxyribose nucleic acid content of animal nuclei. Physiol. Zool. 23: 169.

Swift, H. 1950b. The constancy of desoxyribose nucleic acid in plant nuclei. Proc. Nat. Acad. Sci. 36: 643.

Taylor, J. H., P. S. Woods and W. L. Hughes. 1957. The organization and duplication of chromosomes as revealed by autoradiographic studies using tritium-labelled thymidine. Proc. Nat. Acad. Sci. 43: 122.

Wolstenholme, D. R. 1973. Replicating DNA molecules from eggs of *Drosophila melanogaster*. Chromosoma in press.

4. THE MECHANISM OF GENE AMPLIFICATION IN *XENOPUS LAEVIS* OÖCYTES

Adrian P. Bird, Jean-David Rochaix and Aimée H. Bakken*

Department of Biology, Yale University, New Haven, Connecticut

In somatic cells the DNA coding for 28S and 18S ribosomal RNA (rRNA) is confined to the chromosomal nucleolus organizer (Birnstiel *et al.*, 1966). However, in oöcytes from a wide variety of animals, this nucleolar DNA is selectively amplified and accumulated in the nucleus free of the chromosomes (Gall, 1969). In *Xenopus laevis*, the best studied example, almost three-quarters of the nuclear DNA in a diplotene oöcyte codes exclusively for ribosomal RNA (Brown and Dawid, 1968). The extra ribosomal DNA (rDNA) is synthesized during a three-week period in early meiotic prophase (Gall, 1968; Macgregor, 1968; Bird and Birnstiel, 1971; Watson-Coggins and Gall, 1971) and during diplotene it forms hundreds of extrachromosomal nucleoli, which actively engage in rRNA synthesis (Miller and Beatty, 1969). This paper will summarize our recent studies of the amplification mechanism by autoradiography of isolated rDNA using both light and electron microscopy.

LIGHT MICROSCOPE AUTORADIOGRAPHY OF ISOLATED rDNA

To prepare DNA fiber autoradiographs of amplifying rDNA, it is first necessary to separate pulse-labelled rDNA from excess ovarian chromosomal DNA in CsCl gradients. Gentle extraction and fractionation procedures give very high molecular weight rDNA which is consistently >95% free of chromosomal radioactivity. This fraction is then dialyzed, concentrated, spread on glass slides, and exposed to autoradiographic emulsion for 3-12 weeks.

------

* Present address: Department of Zoology, University of Washington, Seattle, Washington.

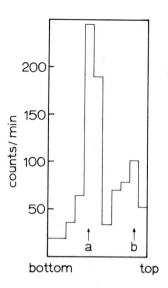

Figure 1. Fractionation of two hour pulse-labelled ovarian DNA in
a CsCl gradient. Suspended cells from a disaggregated ovary were
incubated for 2 hours at 23°C with 100 μCi/ml [^{3}H]thymidine and
100 μCi/ml [^{3}H]deoxycytidine. DNA was extracted in a centrifuge
tube using a high temperature detergent-Pronase method similar to
that of Kavenoff and Zimm (1973). Saturated CsCl solution was
carefully added, and the two layers allowed to mix by diffusion
overnight. The gradient was spun at 42,000 revs/min for 24 hours
at 18°C in a Spinco Al-50 rotor and collected by hand from the surface. Aliquots were counted to localize the peaks of incorporation.
Amplified rDNA (fraction a) and chromosomal DNA (fraction b) were
then dialyzed, concentrated and spread on slides for autoradiography.

    Typical grain tracks produced by a 2-hour-labelled rDNA prepa-
ration (Fig. 1) are shown in Fig. 2a. Only short tracks are present,
those shown corresponding in length to about 4 rDNA repeat units.
Tracks appear singly and are not obviously connected with others on
the same strand. In contrast, autoradiographs of chromosomal DNA
often contain rows of tracks that appear to be part of a single
replicating DNA molecule.

    Do rDNA grain tracks arise through semi-conservative replica-
tion at a fork in the same way as chromosomal DNA tracks (see Callan,
this volume)? Or is a non-conservative mechanism such as 'reverse
transcriptase' (Crippa and Tocchini-Valentini, 1971) operating during amplification? A semi-conservative mechanism requires that each
track is produced by two labelled arms of a replication fork lying
side by side, while in a reverse transcriptase process each track
would be formed by a single stretch of new, doubly labelled duplex.

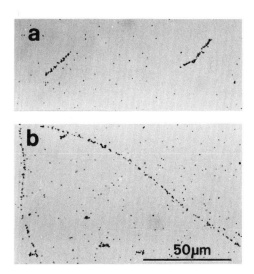

Figure 2. Grain tracks produced by amplified rDNA after (a) 2 hours
and (b) 24 hours of labelling. The rDNA fractions were prepared as
described in Fig. 1. After spreading on slides, the preparations
were air dried and treated with ice-cold 5% trichloroacetic acid
for 10 min. They were then rinsed in 95% ethanol, air-dried again
and coated with Kodak NTB-2 autoradiographic emulsion. The preparations shown were exposed for 74 days. Grain density in 2 hour
tracks is visibly higher than that of 24 hour tracks.

These possibilities can be distinguished if replication is allowed
to continue for 24 hours in the presence of label (Fig. 2b). During
this time the arms of a fork would become separated, either through
breakage in preparation, or through completion of replication, and
the grain density within tracks would drop to half its 2 hour value.
RNA-directed DNA synthesis, on the other hand, predicts a constant
grain density regardless of the labelling period.

     Chromosomal DNA synthesis is known to proceed semi-conservative-
ly, and a comparison of the tracks in 2 hour vs. 24-hour-labelled
main-peak DNA shows the expected drop in grain density (Fig. 3a).
Amplified rDNA tracks also show this halving of the grain density
(Fig. 3b), suggesting that here too, replication proceeds semi-conservatively at a fork. This conclusion is supported by occasional
observations of forked grain patterns within the amplified rDNA.

     Autoradiographs can also provide information about the direc-
tionality of synthesis during amplification. When ovaries are allowed to equilibrate gradually with labelled precursors, the grain
tracks produced display increasing density in the direction of the

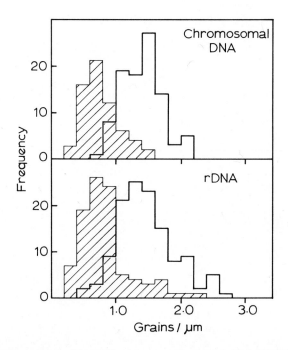

Figure 3. Frequency distributions of grain densities from chromosomal and rDNA autoradiographs. Shaded histograms represent densities in 24 hour-labelled tracks. Unshaded histograms show the distribution after 2 hours of labelling. All preparations scored were derived from one 2 hour-labelled gradient (Fig. 1), and one 24 hour-labelled gradient.

replication. Most are clearly polarized in one direction indicating unidirectional synthesis at these sites. It is also possible to estimate the rate of replication by measuring grain tracks after labelled pulses of known duration. The site of DNA synthesis travels at 10 μm/hour in both amplifying rDNA and replicating chromosomal DNA.

To summarize, DNA fiber autoradiography implies that amplification involves a fork replication mechanism. We now describe some more recent experiments, using the electron microscope, which show that this is by no means the complete story.

ELECTRON MICROSCOPY OF AMPLIFYING rDNA

Hourcade *et al.* (1973a,b) showed that electron microscope (EM) preparations of amplifying rDNA contain lariat-shaped structures. This is precisely the DNA configuration to be expected if a rolling circle mechanism is involved in amplification (Gilbert and Dressler, 1968; Buongiorno-Nardelli *et al.*, 1972). Following their example, we have prepared high molecular weight amplifying rDNA for electron microscopy by the aqueous spreading technique. In addition to lariats, (1/2-1%) (Fig. 4a), we find circles (5-11%), forked molecules 1/2-1%), and about 90% linears. Circles are occasionally super-coiled, and occur as such more frequently in higher molecular weight preparations.

As shown by Hourcade *et al.* (1973a,b), the lengths of free circles and lariat circles are not random. The smallest ones are clearly grouped at lengths corresponding to 1, 2, 3, and 4 rDNA repeat units. So far, the largest circle we have seen is part of a lariat, and corresponds to about 16 rDNA repeats. It is possible that even larger ones exist *in vivo*, but do not survive the extraction intact.

ELECTRON MICROSCOPIC AUTORADIOGRAPHY OF AMPLIFYING rDNA

In order to determine which structures actually participate in the amplification process, 6-hour-pulse-labelled rDNA was spread on grids and coated with emulsion for EM autoradiography. After 3 weeks exposure, grains were associated with some molecules. Since the background is essentially zero, the presence of one or more grains localized over a molecule is a clear indication that it was involved in DNA synthesis during the pulse. Out of 131 labelled structures on a single grid, 14 were lariats (Fig. 4 b and c), 12 were circles, and 105 were linear or, occasionally, too tangled to classify.

Thus, by scoring only labelled molecules, the proportion of lariats rises by an order of magnitude. This strongly implicates these structures in the amplification mechanism, and suggests that they are in fact rolling circles of the kind originally proposed by Gilbert and Dressler (1968).

DISCUSSION

We have described two experimental approaches to the mechanism of amplification: light microscope autoradiography, which suggests indirectly that a symmetrical fork replication mechanism is responsible; and EM autoradiography, which shows directly that rolling circle-like molecules are synthesizing DNA during amplification. Before attempting to reconcile these apparently conflicting results, it is necessary to mention some important features of the rolling circle mechanism.

A rolling circle forms when one strand of a circular DNA molecule is nicked, allowing a replication fork to travel (potentially

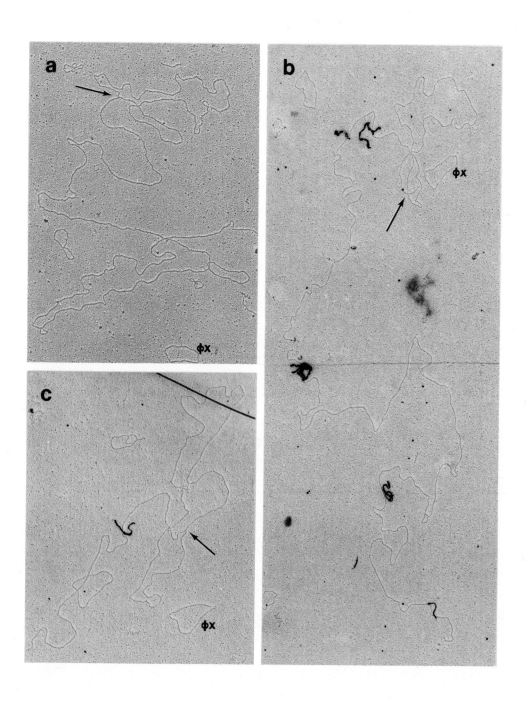

Figure 4. Rolling circle-like DNA molecules from EM spreads (a)
and autoradiographed spreads (b and c) of amplifying rDNA. Arrows
indicate the junction between 'tail' and circle. DNA of the bacteriophage φX174 (molecular weight 3.4 X 10⁶ - about 1.7 μm) was included in the spreading mixture as a size marker. Preparations were
stained by rotary shadowing with platinum-palladium. (a) The circle
on this rDNA molecule has a molecular weight of about 23 X 10⁶,
which is close to three times the size of a single rDNA repeat unit
(8.7 X 10⁶, Wensink and Brown, 1971). (b) An autoradiograph of a
rolling circle-like structure after 6 hours of labelling with [³H]-
thymidine and [³H]deoxycytidine and 3 weeks exposure. The circle
corresponds to 2 rDNA repeat units (17 X 10⁶ daltons). Four grains
are localized over the tail. (c) An autoradiograph of part of a
rolling circle-like molecule with one grain localized over the tail.
The circle corresponds to 3 rDNA repeats.

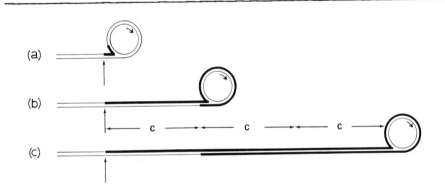

Figure 5. A diagrammatic representation of progressive stages in
the labelling of a rolling circle. Vertical arrows mark the beginning of a pulse with tritiated DNA precursors; 'c' is the circumference of the circle. (a) At this point the fork has replicated
only a small part of the circle since the beginning of the pulse.
The two labelled strands lie close together, each labelled in one
strand of the duplex. (b) The fork has now copied slightly more
than one circumference of the circle. Most DNA is labelled in one
strand. However, since the start of the second cycle, a small
region of doubly-labelled duplex has appeared. (c) The fork has
now travelled around the circle three times. Since the first cycle
was completed, all DNA appearing in the tail has been doubly labelled. The circle remains labelled in one strand, as does a section
at the distal end of the tail equal in length to 'c'.

endlessly) around the circle. The nicked strand peels off and gives
rise to a double-stranded tail which elongates as replication proceeds (Fig. 5). Thus the un-nicked strand of the original circle
is copied repeatedly by the replication fork, while the nicked

strand is copied only once before passing into the tail. It is this
asymmetrical use of template that distinguishes fork replication on
a circular DNA molecule (*i.e.* a rolling circle) from fork replication on linear DNA. The consequences of asymmetry will become clear-
er in the following example.

In the preparation of EM autoradiographs (Fig. 4), rDNA was
labelled for 6 hours. Since we know that the rate of replication
is 10 μm/hour, the fork must have travelled 60 μm during the pulse.
This means that a rolling circle 8 μm in circumference (*e.g.* Fig.
4b) has been copied 60 ÷ 8 = 7 times. DNA labelled in both strands
starts to appear in the tail as soon as the circle has been copied
more than once in the presence of label (Figs. 5 b and c). As a
result, most of the DNA synthesized by an 8 μm rolling circle should
be doubly labelled in 6 hours. Consider now a rolling circle 65 μm
in circumference - the largest we have seen so far. In 6 hours,
the fork would have completed slightly less than one cycle. Newly
synthesized DNA would therefore be labelled in only one strand, as
though symmetrical fork replication had occurred (Fig. 5a). Thus
the asymmetry of a rolling circle is not apparent until the fork
has travelled around the circle more than once in the presence of
label.

If we now refer back to the light microscope autoradiography,
it is evident that as long as a significant proportion of circles
has not rolled through more than one revolution during the 24 hour
pulse, the grain tracks predicted by a rolling circle mechanism are
indistinguishable from those predicted by a symmetrical fork mechanism. We therefore suggest that if rolling circles are the primary
source of amplified rDNA, then most will be even larger than 65 μm.
Perhaps the forked molecules seen in EM spreads of rDNA are broken
remnants of these large structures.

The ability of rolling circles to generate unlimited horizontal
repeats of whatever sequence is present in the circle may have important implications byond gene amplification. In particular, this
kind of mechanism would be capable of both creating and maintaining
uniformly repeated sequences, such as satellite DNAs and reiterated
genes (Brown *et al.*, 1972). It will be interesting to see whether
rolling circles in eukaryotes are restricted to the amplifying
oöcyte, or whether they are of more general occurrence.

ACKNOWLEDGMENTS

We are indebted to Joseph Gall for encouragement and discussions throughout this work, and to Joel Huberman for advice. Our
study would not have been possible without the personal communication of unpublished results from Dennis Hourcade, David Dressler

and John Wolfson. A.P.B. was supported by a Damon Runyon Memorial Fellowship; J.-D.R. was supported by The Swiss National Science Foundation and Hoffman La Roche; and A.H.B. was supported by U.S. P.H.S. Grant GM 12427. We thank Nigel Godson for φX174 DNA.

REFERENCES

Bird, A. P. and M. L. Birnstiel. 1971. A timing study of DNA amplification in *Xenopus laevis* oöcytes. Chromosoma 35: 300.

Birnstiel, M. L., H. Wallace, J. L. Sirlin and M. Fischberg. 1966. Localization of the ribosomal DNA complements in the nucleolar organizer region of *Xenopus laevis*. Nat. Cancer Inst. Monog. 23: 431.

Buongiorno-Nardelli, M., F. Amaldi and P. A. Lava-Sanchez. 1972. Amplification as a rectification mechanism for the redundant rRNA genes. Nature New Biol. 238: 134.

Brown, D. D. and I. B. Dawid. 1968. Specific gene amplification in oöcytes. Science 160: 272.

Brown, D. D., P. C. Wensink and E. Jordan. 1972. A comparison of the ribosomal DNAs of *Xenopus laevis* and *Xenopus mulleri*: the evolution of tandem genes. J. Mol. Biol. 63: 57.

Crippa, M. and G. P. Tocchini-Valentini. 1971. Synthesis of amplified DNA that codes for ribosomal RNA. Proc. Nat. Acad. Sci. 68: 2769.

Gall, J. G. 1968. Differential synthesis of the genes for ribosomal RNA during oögenesis. Proc. Nat. Acad. Sci. 60: 553.

Gall, J. G. 1969. The genes for ribosomal RNA during oögenesis. Genetics (Suppl.) 61: 121.

Gilbert, W. and D. Dressler. 1968. DNA replication - the rolling circle model. Cold Spr. Harb. Symp. Quant. Biol. 33: 473.

Hourcade, D., D. Dressler and J. Wolfson. 1973a. The amplification of ribosomal RNA genes involves a rolling circle intermediate. Proc. Nat. Acad. Sci. in press.

Hourcade, D., D. Dressler and J. Wolfson. 1973b. On the mechanism of ribosomal DNA amplification. Cold Spr. Harb. Symp. Quant. Biol. 38 in press.

Kavenoff, R. and B. H. Zimm. 1973. Chromosome-sized DNA molecules from *Drosophila*. Chromosoma 41: 1.

Macgregor, H. C. 1968. Nucleolar DNA in oöcytes of *Xenopus laevis*.
J. Cell Sci. <u>3</u>: 437.

Watson-Coggins, L. and J. G. Gall. 1972. The timing of meiosis
and DNA synthesis during early oögenesis in the toad, *Xenopus laevis*.
J. Cell Biol. <u>52</u>: 569.

Miller, O. L., Jr. and B. R. Beatty. 1969. Extrachromosomal nucleolar genes in amphibian oöcytes. Genetics (<u>Suppl.</u>) <u>61</u>: 133.

Wensink, P. C. and D. D. Brown. 1971. Denaturation map of the ribosomal DNA of *Xenopus laevis*. J. Mol. Biol. <u>60</u>: 235.

5. REPETITIVE DNA IN *DROSOPHILA*

Joseph G. Gall

Department of Biology, Yale University, New Haven, Connecticut

Among the higher eukaryotes, *Drosophila melanogaster* has one of the smallest reported genome sizes. According to the spectrophotometric data of Rasch *et al.* (1971) the haploid DNA content is 1.8×10^{-13} g, corresponding to 1.1×10^{11} daltons or approximately 40 times the genome size of *E. coli*. For this reason alone, analysis of the organization of DNA in *Drosophila* should be easier than in organisms with larger amounts of DNA in the haploid chromosome set. Furthermore, *D. melanogaster* has only four chromosome pairs, its formal genetics is better known than that of any other eukaryote, and cytological analysis is facilitated by the existence of the giant polytene chromosomes in larval salivary glands.

In one respect the organization of the *Drosophila* chromosome is known to be very simple. Kavenoff and Zimm (1973) have recently isolated DNA molecules long enough to contain all the DNA of a single chromosome. They have estimated the lengths of these molecules on the basis of the viscoelastic properties of the DNA solutions. They used DNA from several species and from various stocks to show that the longest molecules are obtained from the species with the largest chromosomes, and also that the molecule is continuous through the centromere region. Their experiments provide compelling direct evidence for the unineme theory of chromatid organization. Two additional features of the chromatid are reasonably clear. In all *Drosophila* species that have been adequately studied, a segment of the mitotic chromosome next to the centromere appears cytologically heterochromatic, and in those species that are well-known genetically, this segment contains very few genes. Second, the remaining portion of the chromatid, the euchromatic segment, is divided into bands (as seen in the polytene chromosomes) that in some senses correspond to genetic, transcriptional, and replicative units (reviewed in Beermann, 1972).

This paper reviews the organization of the repetitive DNA's in the chromosomes of *Drosophila*, with particular emphasis on the very highly repetitive satellite DNA's and on the genes that code for ribosomal RNA (rRNA). Some mention will be made of a few other classes of repetitive DNA.

Repetitive DNA's in *Drosophila* have been studied by essentially all of the techniques used in other systems. These methods include analysis of reassociation rates after denaturation, buoyant density profiles in CsCl, electron microscopy of molecules after various treatments (partial denaturation, cyclization), nucleic acid hybridization both *in situ* and by liquid and filter techniques, and sequencing of complementary RNA synthesized on repetitive templates. These methods have led to some fairly simple conclusions regarding the most highly repetitive fractions, but they leave considerable room for speculation about the so-called intermediate fractions, *i.e.*, those sequences present in a relatively small number of copies.

SATELLITE DNA'S

In various *Drosophila* species, as in many other organisms, the most highly repetitive DNA's often have a buoyant density in neutral CsCl different from that of the bulk of the DNA. Even when the most repetitive DNA's do not appear as "satellites" on CsCl gradients, they can frequently be separated from the main peak by centrifugation in Cs_2SO_4 gradients containing either Ag^+ or Hg^+. In other cases the "heavy" and "light" strands may be isolated from alkaline CsCl gradients because of differences in their (G + T)-content. For convenience I shall refer to all such fractions separable by centrifugation as satellite DNA's. It is now well established, on the basis of *in situ* nucleic acid hybridization experiments, that the centromeric heterochromatin in a variety of organisms is rich in satellite DNA (Pardue and Gall, 1970; Jones, 1970). This fact is particularly obvious in *D. virilis*, a species that displays prominent heterochromatic segments next to the centromeres in mitotic chromosomes, and that has approximately half of its genome devoted to three large satellite DNA's (Gall *et al.*, 1971). The various species of *Drosophila*, however, differ markedly both in the size of the centromeric heterochromatin, as seen in mitotic chromosomes, and in the amount of satellite DNA. For example, *D. melanogaster* has smaller heterochromatic segments in the mitotic chromosomes than *D. virilis*, and the total amount of highly repetitive DNA present in satellites is probably under 15% (approximately 8% in a pair of satellites at ρ = 1.689, another 3-4% in a satellite at ρ = 1.676, and a few percent in a satellite that appears as a shoulder at ρ = 1.708 on the heavy side of the main peak). In *D. melanogaster* only one of these four satellites has been shown by *in situ* hybridization to be in the centromeric heterochromatin; the other three have not been adequately investigated (Gall *et al.*, 1971). In *D. hydei* and

related species Hennig *et al.* (1970) have shown that some of the
satellites are located in the centromeric heterochromatin. It seems
probable that a reasonably good correlation will be found between
the amount of satellite DNA in a given species and the amount of
centromeric heterochromatin in the mitotic chromosomes.

   The satellite DNA's of *Drosophila* are not proportionately replicated during the formation of the giant polytene chromosomes of the
salivary glands and other organs. This fact was first shown for
D. virilis by two observations (Gall *et al.*, 1971). First, the a-
mount of satellite DNA in the total DNA isolated from larval salivary
glands is negligible, whereas the satellites constitute almost half
of the DNA from primarily diploid tissues such as the brains and
imaginal discs. Second, *in situ* hybridization experiments have been
carried out in which cRNA synthesized from satellite DNA was hybridized to diploid and polytene nuclei on the same slide. Despite the
1000-fold difference in total DNA contents, the two types of nuclei
bound comparable amounts of cRNA. The simplest interpretation of
these experiments is that the satellite DNA sequences do not replicate during polytenization, or at least do not replicate as many
times as the euchromatic sequences. These biochemical data confirm
the postulate first put forward by Heitz (1934) that the heterochromatin of the mitotic chromosome does not replicate during the formation of the salivary gland chromosomes. The same conclusion was
reached by Rudkin for *D. melanogaster* (reviewed in Rudkin 1972) and
later by Berendes and Keyl (1967) and Mulder *et al.* (1968) for *D.
hydei* on the basis of microspectrophotometric observations. All of
these authors reported an underreplication of the heterochromatin
of the diploid genome during the formation of polyploid and polytene
nuclei of the larvae.

   Dickson *et al.* (1971) have studied the reassociation of denatured DNA derived from larval salivary glands and from whole embryos
and pupae of *D. hydei*. They reported that the embryo and pupal
DNA's contain about 20% fast renaturing sequences whereas salivary
gland DNA contains less than 5%. The reduced amount of fast renaturing material in the salivary gland DNA presumably reflects the
underreplication of satellite sequences in the heterochromatin of
the polytene cells.

   It would be well to point out here a very real source of confusion in the use of the term "heterochromatin" in *Drosophila*.
Those who have worked with mitotic chromosomes refer to the proximal
region of each chromosome arm as heterochromatin or heterochromatic
on the basis of its staining properties and the tendency of the
sister chromatids to remain tightly associated at prophase. On the
other hand, cytogeneticists who work with salivary gland chromosomes
generally refer to the whole poorly banded chromocenter region as
the heterochromatin. Heitz (1934), in his original paper on the
subject, pointed out that the salivary gland heterochromatin, so

defined, consists of at least two morphologically distinct fractions. He named these α-heterochromatin and β-heterochromatin. The α-heterochromain is a relatively small, compact mass in the very center of the fused chromosome configuratin. The β-heterochromatin is the larger, loosely-textured, or poorly-banded material extending into the chromosome arms. Heitz suggested that the α-heterochromatin alone corresponds to the bulk of the mitotic heterochromatin. His suggestion was based on the simple fact that not all the chromosome arms have associated β-heterochromain in the salivary glands, where-as all do have mitotic heterochromatin. In the case of *D. virilis*, the proximal half of each mitotic chromosome is heterochromatic, but two of the five major chromosomes contain most of the β-hetero-chromatin in the salivary glands. In *D. melanogaster*, chromosome arm 3R has centromeric heterochromatin during mitosis, but as shown clearly on Bridges' map (1935) it lacks β-heterochromatin in the polytene condition. This lack of correlation between mitotic hetero-chromatin and salivary gland β-heterochromatin does not seem to be generally appreciated. That the β-heterochromatin replicates during the formation of the polytene nuclei is shown by the fact that it incorporates [^{3}H]thymidine (Plaut, 1963; Swift, 1964; Tulchin *et al.*, 1967). Also, the mass itself of the β-heterochromatin implies replication. Rudkin (1964) estimated that 3% of the DNA in the *D. melanogaster* salivary gland X chromosome is in the heterochromatin (*i.e.*, β-heterochromatin). However, 3% of one salivary gland X chromosome is the equivalent of 30 entire mitotic X chromosomes, since each polytene homologue contains approximately 1000 chromatids (Rasch, 1970). Obviously, therefore, this material must have repli-cated during formation of the giant chromosome.

I should like to emphasize, as did Heitz and later Fujii (1942), that the β-heterochromatin probably represents a relatively small part of the mitotic chromosome at the junction between the euchrom-atin and heterochromatin (Fig. 1). This conclusion implies that attempts to localize genes and the breakpoints of chromosomal re-arrangements within the salivary gland β-heterochromatin have been misleading. For instance, breakpoints known to be in the mitotic heterochromatin of the X are erroneously assigned to section 20 of the salivary gland chromosome, and conversely genes accurately as-signed to section 20 are not near the centromere of the mitotic X. A similar conclusion has been advanced on cytogenetic grounds by Lefevre (1973).

The physical properties of satellite DNA have been studied in several species of *Drosophila* (Laird and McCarthy, 1968; Rae, 1970; Hennig *et al.*, 1970; Gall *et al.*, 1971; Kram *et al.*, 1972; Tra-vaglini *et al.*, 1972a,b; Travaglini and Schultz, 1972; Laird, 1973). The three large satellites of *D. virilis* have been particularly easy to purify (Gall *et al.*, 1971; Gall and Atherton, 1973; Blumenfeld *et al.*, 1973). Each has a sharp melting curve, and reassociates rapidly after denaturation ($C_0t_{1/2}$ no greater than 0.03 and probably

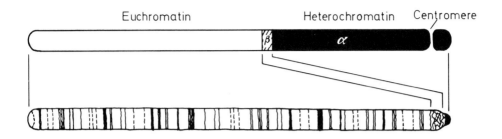

Figure 1. A comparison of a mitotic chromosome of *Drosophila* (above) with the corresponding giant polytene chromosome derived from it (below). The euchromatin of the mitotic chromosome gives rise to the regularly banded portion of the polytene chromosome. Most of the mitotic heterochromatin (α -heterochromatin) consists of highly repetitive satellite DNA which replicates little or not at all in the formation of the polytene chromosome. The β-heterochromatin represents material at the euchromatic-heterochromatic junction, and this material does replicate during the formation of the polytene chromosome.

much less). The T_m of the remelts of the reassociated satellite strands are within 0.5-1.5° of the initial T_m's, indicating little mismatching of bases and hence a high degree of sequence homogeneity. These satellites also separate into strands of differing buoyant density in alkaline CsCl, a common though not necessary characteristic of simple repeating DNA's. Similar statements can be made about the satellites of *D. melanogaster*. *D. melanogaster* possesses at least four satellites distinguishable on buoyant density gradients. Two of these have the same neutral buoyant density in CsCl (ρ = 1.689), but separate into four strands of different density in alkaline CsCl. Another satellite at ρ = 1.676 in neutral CsCl also separates into strands of different density in alkaline CsCl (ρ = 1.745 and ρ = 1.716). The fourth satellite appears as a shoulder at ρ = 1.708 on the heavy side of the main peak (Rae, Polan, personal communications) but can be separated cleanly from main peak sequences in a Ag^+-Cs_2SO_4 gradient. It likewise shows a slight strand separation in alkaline CsCl (ρ = 1.759 and ρ = 1.754 approximately). Buoyant density profiles have been examined for a number of species. The percentage of the total DNA found in density satellites is quite variable. The most extreme case that we have examined is that of *D. cyrtoloma*, in which approximately 60% of the total is satellite DNA (Craddock, personal communication). *D. virilis* runs a close second with over 40%. We have examined eleven species in the *virilis* species group (Gall and Atherton, 1973), and these range from *virilis* itself with the most satellite DNA down to *D. littoralis* and *D. lacicola*, which have only a few percent of their DNA as satellites.

These latter species could have "cryptic" satellites, *i.e.*, those of the same density as main peak sequences, that might be revealed by heavy metal binding.

We have examined DNA from salivary glands of 15 species of *Drosophila*, and in none of these were the satellites detectable when 1-2 µg of DNA was centrifuged to equilibrium in a 2° sector cell in the analytical ultracentrifuge. We conclude, therefore, that the lack of satellite DNA replication, or severe underreplication during the formation of the polytene nuclei, is a very general phenomenon. There is no theoretical reason why *all* satellite sequences should be underrepresented in the salivary gland DNA, and Hennig (1972) has suggested that some highly repetitive sequences in *D. hydei* may be replicated.

Information is now available concerning the sequences present in several satellite DNA's of *D. virilis, D. americana,* and *D. melanogaster* (Gall and Atherton, 1973). These sequences have been determined by preparing ^{32}P-labeled RNA transcripts *in vitro* from the isolated "heavy" and "light" strands of the satellites, using *E. coli* RNA polymerase. The complementary RNA's thus prepared were sequenced by standard methods (Brownlee, 1972). Several interesting facts have emerged. The three satellites of *D. virilis* are extremely simple and homogeneous in composition. They are all repeating heptanucleotides, showing little evidence of sequence heterogeneity. For example, in nearest-neighbor analyses of 12 different complementary RNA's, from 93-99% of the radioactivity was found in the nucleotides predicted from the basic seven nucleotide repeat. The sequence of the light strands of satellites I, II, and III of *D. virilis* are:

I	5' --- A-C-A-A-A-C-T --- 3'
II	5' --- A-T-A-A-A-C-T --- 3'
III	5' --- A-C-A-A-A-T-T --- 3'

It is obvious that these sequences are closely related, even though the neutral and alkaline buoyant densities of the starting materials are quite diverse. Indeed, it is the short sequence length that leads to large changes in physical properties when one base-pair is altered. Although the sequence relationships among these satellite DNA's are evident, the actual evolutionary mechanism by which one satellite could give rise to another is not clear. In a formal sense one can imagine that the basic heptanucleotide sequence is "excised" at some time and then "expanded" again into a new repeating satellite, as in the rolling-circle model of viral replication. If the basic unit used for this expansion happened to contain a base-pair change, the new satellite would incorporate the change in all of its repeats. Other schemes might involve a correction mechanism, such as postulated by Callan (1967) in his Master-Slave hypothesis. It would be particularly interesting to know in what way the three satellites are distributed among

the chromosomes, or interspersed on the same chromosome since this
information might give a clue about the history of the satellites.
It is conceivable that one or more satellite is limited to a single
chromosome. It has been shown that one satellite in another fly,
Rhynchosciara hollaenderi, is absent from one of the four chromosomes (Eckhardt and Gall, 1971).

Recently Blumenfeld *et al.* (1973) have investigated the reassociation of the satellite DNA's of *D. virilis.* They have prepared
all of the heterologous strand associations (*e.g.* IH with IIL, IH
with IIIL, etc.). Those associations with a single base-pair mismatch out of seven (I with II or I with III) have melting temperatures from 10-31° lower than those of the homologous associations.
Duplexes with two base-pairs mismatched out of seven melt approximately 40-50° lower than the homologous combination. Furthermore
the data show that a G·T mismatch is more stable than an A·C, since
the combinations involving IH with IIL or IIIL melt 13° above those
involving IL with IIH or IIIH.

D. virilis is closely related to *D. novamexicana, D. americana
americana* and *D. americana texana.* These differ in minor morphological ways from each other. The chromosome number in *D. virilis* and
D. novamexicana is 6, in *D. a. texana* 5, and in *D. a. americana* 4,
the reductions in the latter two species being due to one and two
centric fusions respectively (Robertsonian fusions). Otherwise the
chromosome banding patterns as seen in the salivary gland chromosomes are similar except for inversions. All of these species possess a large satellite whose buoyant density is 1.691 g/cm^3, identical to that of *D. virilis.* Sequencing studies show that the satellite in *D. a. americana* has the same basic heptanuclotide sequence
as satellite I in *D. virilis.* This is the first case in which
identity of satellite DNA's has been demonstrated in two closely
related species.

Some degree of homology has been demonstrated by hybridization
between the satellite DNA of the house mouse *Mus musculus* and the
DNA of three other species, M. *caroli,* M. *cervicolor,* and M. *famalus*
(Sutton and McCallum, 1972). The data from both *Drosophila* and the
mouse demonstrate that satellite DNA's can be conserved either unchanged or little changed for very long times, of the order of the
time necessary for speciation.

Sequence data are available for one other *Drosophila* satellite,
that in *D. melanogaster* having a buoyant density of 1.676 g/cm^3.
In the literature, this satellite is sometimes referred to as poly-
[d(A-T)] although the nearest neighbor analysis carried out by
Fansler *et al.* (1970) demonstrated that only 84% of the residues are
alternating A and T. As mentioned above, in alkaline CsCl the two
strands of this DNA have different buoyant densities (ρ = 1.745 and
ρ = 1.716). Therefore the material cannot be simply poly[d(A-T)]

whose strands are identical. Preliminary sequencing data show that
this DNA is $d([\text{T-A}]_n[\text{T-A-A}]_n) \cdot d([\text{T-T-A}]_n[\text{T-A}]_n)$, where $\underline{n}$ could be 1,
but where higher values have not been ruled out.

Because of their extremely short repeat lengths and the large
fraction of the genome which they represent, satellite DNA's are
present in hundreds of thousands to millions of copies of the basic
unit. For instance satellite I of *D. virilis* makes up about 25% of
the genome or roughly 5.5×10^{10} daltons. With a sequence length
of seven nucleotide pairs, there are, therefore, approximately 1.2
$\times 10^7$ copies of the basic heptanucleotide in the haploid chromosome
set.

RIBOSOMAL DNA

Several less highly repetitive sequences have been studied in
some detail in *Drosophila*. These include the genes coding for ribosomal RNA, 5S RNA, the transfer RNA's and the putative histone
messenger RNA. Of these the most thoroughly investigated are the
genes coding for ribosomal RNA, also called ribosomal DNA or simply
rDNA. Unlike the rDNA of the toad, *Xenopus*, which has been isolated
in pure form and studied by a variety of physical and chemical methods, the rDNA of *Drosophila* has not so far been purified. This is
not because it is present in unusually small amounts, since it constitutes a larger fraction of the genome than in many other organisms (at least 0.6%). However, it has a buoyant density near to
that of the main peak sequences in both *D. melanogaster* (Sinclair
and Brown, 1971) and *D. virilis*, and hence cannot be separated by
simple centrifugation. Also it fails to show any marked preferen-
tial binding of Ag^+ or Hg^+ in Cs_2SO_4 gradients, although it can be
"pulled" a few fractions to the heavy side of the main peak in both
D. melanogaster and *D. virilis* (G. Zakian, personal communication).
For these reasons we have little information on its physical characteristics. The existence of a spacer between the sequences coding
for rRNA has been inferred recently from electron microscopy of
spread nuclear contents (Hamkalo *et al.*, this Symposium).

Somewhat more is known about the cytological localization, the
replication, and the inheritance of the rDNA, and these aspects will
be briefly discussed. The association of the rDNA with the nucleolus organizer regions was first clearly demonstrated by Ritossa and
Spiegelman (1965) for *D. melanogaster* in experiments that utilized
DNA from flies having 1-4 nucleolus organizers per diploid genome.
These same experiments demonstrated that the rDNA contained 100 or
more copies of the cistrons coding for 18S and 28S rRNA. The nucleolar localization was confirmed by *in situ* hybridization of rRNA to
the nucleolar DNA in salivary gland cells of *D. hydei* (Pardue *et
al.*, 1970).

It has long been known that the nucleolus organizer in *D. melanogaster* is located in the middle of the proximal heterochromatin of the X chromosome and on the short arm of the totally heterochromatic Y (Kaufmann, 1934). This location suggests that the rDNA is probably flanked by satellite sequences, at least in the X. I say "probably" because no *in situ* hybridization experiments have been carried out on the mitotic chromosomes of *D. melanogaster*. Several studies have shown that satellite or highly repetitive sequences are located in the chromocenter of the polytene nuclei (Rae, 1970; Jones and Robertson, 1970; Botchan *et al.*, 1971; Gall *et al.*, 1971). By implication, therefore, such sequences are probably located in the centromeric heterochromatin of all the chromosomes. It has been suggested that the "poly[d(A-T)]" satellite is preferentially, though not exclusively, located in the Y chromosome (Blumenfeld and Forrest, 1971).

In any case, it is known from cytological observations that the Y chromosome is either not detectable in the polytene nucleus, or is present as only a few indistinct bands (Lindsley and Grell, 1967). Similarly the proximal part of the X is represented by very little material in the polytene chromosome. Nevertheless the nucleolus is prominent in the salivary gland. It is formed not only in normal XX and XY individuals, but also in stocks lacking the nucleolus organizer of either the Y or the X (*e.g.* XO or sc^4sc^8/Y). Thus the nucleolus forms in the salivary gland, despite the failure of adjacent chromosome regions to replicate proportionately. Various data prove that the rDNA itself replicates. The first evidence came from *in situ* hybridization experiments. If the rDNA did not replicate during the formation of the polytene nucleus, it would be present in the diploid amount, and would be too scarce to have been detected by the relatively insensitive *in situ* hybridization method. More recently, Hennig and Meer (1971) carried out filter hybridization experiments on DNA isolated from salivary glands and other tissues of *D. hydei*. They showed that the rDNA is underreplicated relative to the euchromatin, *i.e.* the saturation value for rDNA in the salivary gland averaged 0.09% compared to 0.4% found for embryonic DNA. Spear and Gall (1973) have carried out similar experiments on *D. melanogaster* and have shown that the rDNA constitutes 0.08% of the salivary gland DNA but 0.37 - 0.47% of imaginal disc DNA in two different strains.

The replicative behavior of the DNA in the salivary gland of *D. melanogaster* can be summarized as follows. Because the polytene chromosomes contain about 1024 times the DNA of a diploid nucleus, the euchromatin undergoes 10 rounds of replication ($2^{10} = 1024$). The underreplicated rDNA undergoes 7-8 replications, and the satellite sequences of the heterochromatin replicate only a few times or possibly not at all.

The replication of the rDNA during the formation of the polytene chromosomes shows other peculiar features. Spear and Gall
(1973) have shown that the percentage of rDNA in salivary gland DNA
is the same in flies of the XO and XX constitutions despite the fact
that the DNA from diploid tissues of the two genotypes shows the
expected 1:2 ratio of rDNA content. In other words the rDNA is not
only underreplicated in the polytene tissues relative to the euchromatin, but there is a disproportional underreplication such that XO
individuals "compensate" for their reduced number of X chromosomes.
The situation is somewhat comparable to the amplification of rDNA
in oocytes of the toad, *Xenopus,* where individuals with one and two
nucleolus organizers in the diploid genome produce equivalent amounts
of amplified rDNA. The disproportional replication of rDNA in polytene tissues may provide an explanation for an observation made by
Tartof (1971). Tartof showed that the rDNA content of DNA extracted
from whole, adult XO males is 0.8 times the rDNA content of DNA extracted from XX females, instead of the expected 0.5 times. It is
well known that adult *Drosophila* contain some polytene tissues, such
as the Malpighian tubules, and many other tissues have lower levels
of polyploidy. If the rDNA is disproportionately replicated in
these tissues in the XO males, as it is in the larval salivary
glands, then one would expect a ratio of the sort observed by Tartof.
There are some problems with this explanation, however, before it
can be accepted unequivocally. For instance, if the adult polyploid
tissues are as severely underreplicated as the salivary glands, then
not only should the XO:XX ratio be greater than 0.5, but the absolute saturation values for adult DNA should be considerably less
than for strictly diploid tissues. Tartof's values are not particularly low, however. It could be that the rDNA is disproportionately
replicated without being severely underreplicated in some adult
tissues, but this possibility must be examined by direct analysis
before the situation is clear.

The phenomenon described by Tartof and the disproportional
replication that we have discussed are essentially somatic phenomena.
The rDNA also behaves unexpectedly in inheritance, as shown by the
phenomenon of "magnification" described by Ritossa (1968). Magnification involves the bobbed mutants, which are known to be partial
deficiencies for the ribosomal cistrons. Under certain defined
genetic conditions, bb flies revert to the wild type, not only in
phenotype but also in the amount of rDNA in the genome. Although
there are superficial similarities between magnification and the
disproportional replication of rDNA in XO males, there is no reason
at the moment to suppose that they are related phenomenon. Since
magnification is an inherited change in rDNA content of X and Y
chromosome, it must occur in the normal mitotic chromosomes found
in the germ line. The germ cells are not polyploid or polytenic,
and so the disproportional replication seen in polytene tissue cannot be the direct explanation for magnification.

OTHER REPETITIVE DNA'S

Three other classes of repetitive DNA can be mentioned briefly: the genes coding for 5S ribosomal RNA, tRNA and histone mRNA. In addition to a single molecule of 18S and 28S RNA, ribosomes contain a molecule of a smaller RNA generally referred to as 5S RNA. Although a great deal is known about the 5S RNA in several organisms, including even its sequence, its function in the ribosome is still obscure. In *D. melanogaster*, the number of 5S genes has been estimated to be about 200 on the basis of RNA·DNA hybridization experiments (Tartof and Perry, 1970). Wimber and Steffensen (1970) carried out *in situ* hybridization of radioactive 5S RNA to the salivary gland chromosomes of *D. melanogaster* and found that hybridization is limited to a single short segment of one chromosome, comprising essentially region 56 E-F on chromosome 2R. This observation was confirmed independently by Pardue and Birnstiel using heterologous hybridization of 5S RNA from *Xenopus* tissue culture (see Pardue and Gall, 1972). It is interesting that the 5S genes are located on chromosome 2 of *D. melanogaster*, completely separate from the 18S and 28S genes on the X and Y chromosomes. Recently Prensky *et al.* (1973) utilized ^{125}I-labeling of RNA in order to improve the sensitivity of the *in situ* hybridization procedure. Using *in vitro* labeling of non-radioactive RNA, they have obtained specific activities of about 10^8 dpm/µg. This is more than an order of magnitude higher than is generally obtainable by *in vivo* labeling with ^{3}H-labeled precursors, and is comparable to the level of ^{3}H-label obtainable by *in vitro* transcription with RNA polymerase and ^{3}H-labeled nucleoside triphosphates. They have confirmed the localization of the 5S RNA genes in region 56F, but in this case their autoradiographs required only a few days' exposure, rather than a few months' as in the earlier experiments with ^{3}H-labeled 5S RNA. In principle, the specific activity of ^{125}I-labeled RNA can be increased still further. If this proves possible in practice, it should be feasible to study the *in situ* localization of unique or single-copy DNA in *Drosophila* salivary gland chromosomes. This is possible because the salivary gland chromosomes contain approximately 2000 copies of each unique gene sequence laterally apposed within a single band.

The localization of the tRNA genes was studied by Steffensen and Wimber (1971) using ^{3}H-labeled tRNA for *in situ* hybridization of salivary gland chromosomes. They obtained very few silver grains in their autoradiographs even after many weeks of exposure. By plotting the positions of all silver grains over many chromosome preparations, they defined a number of "hot spots", which they believed corresponded to the tRNA genes. There were several dozen such spots scattered widely over the genome, suggesting that the tRNA genes are not clustered in *D. melanogaster*. Similar experiments should now be possible using ^{125}I-labeled tRNA, and with the increased sensitivity the localization can be better defined.

Birnstiel *et al.* (this Symposium) have shown by hybridization of mRNA from sea urchins with *D. melanogaster* DNA that the genes coding for putative histone mRNA are reiterated in the genome of *D. melanogaster*. They also used sea urchin putative histone mRNA to demonstrate the cytological localization of the histone genes in the polytene chromosomes. They found hybridization *in situ* only to a narrowly defined region at the base of chromosome 2L, bands 39E and 39F. Whether these experiments detected all the histone genes is not clear, but they raise the interesting possibility that the genes for all the histones may be clustered at one point on one chromosome.

All the examples of *in situ* localization so far studied have involved repetitive DNA's. The reason for this is methodological, since to date the *in situ* hybridization procedure has not been sensitive enough to examine non-reiterated or unique sequences. Most of the DNA isolated from salivary glands is non-reiterated, since the major source of highly reiterated DNA, the satellites, are so drastically underrepresented. The implication is that most of the euchromatic DNA, both in the salivary glands and in the mitotic chromosomes is unique or single copy in nature. The analysis of this DNA is under active consideration in several laboratories at the moment. Hopefully, we shall soon have information on the molecular organization of the bands in the salivary gland chromosomes and their relationship to the genetic units found in them. The major amounts of repetitive DNA seem to be accounted for by the satellites, and by a few other reiterated loci, all located in special places on the chromosomes. Just how much sequence repetition occurs within the euchromatic bands remains an important question.

ACKNOWLEDGMENTS

Supported by USPHS research grant GM 12427 from the National Institute of General Medical Sciences and by American Cancer Society research grant VC 85.

REFERENCES

Beermann, W. 1972. Chromomeres and genes. Results and Problems in Cell Differentiation <u>4</u>: 1.

Berendes, H. D. and H. G. Keyl. 1967. Distribution of DNA in heterochromatin and euchromatin of polytene nuclei of *Drosophila hydei*. Genetics <u>57</u>: 1.

Blumenfeld, M. and H. S. Forrest. 1971. Is *Drosophila* dAt on the Y chromosome? Proc. Nat. Acad. Sci. <u>68</u>: 3145.

Blumenfeld, M., A. Fox and H. S. Forrest. 1973. The evolution of satellite DNA. Proc. Nat. Acad. Sci. in press.

Botchan, M., R. Kram, C. W. Schmid and J. E. Hearst. 1971. Isolation and chromosomal localization of highly repeated DNA sequences in *Drosophila melanogaster*. Proc. Nat. Acad. Sci. 68: 1125.

Bridges, C. B. 1935. Salivary chromosome maps. J. Heredity 26: 60.

Brownlee, G. G. 1972. Determination of Sequences in RNA. North Holland Publishing Co., Amsterdam.

Callan, H. G. 1967. The organization of genetic units in chromosomes. J. Cell Sci. 2: 1.

Dickson, E., J. Boyd and C. Laird. 1971. Sequence diversity of polytene chromosome DNA from *Drosophila hydei*. J. Mol. Biol. 61: 615.

Eckhardt, R. A. and J. G. Gall. 1971. Satellite DNA associated with heterochromatin in *Rhynchosciara*. Chromosoma 32: 407.

Fansler, B. S., E. C. Travaglini, L. A. Loeb and J. Schultz. 1970. Structure of *Drosophila melanogaster* dAt replicated in an *in vitro* system. Biochem. Biophys. Res. Commun. 40: 1266.

Fujii, S. 1942. Further studies on the salivary gland chromosomes of *Drosophila virilis*. Cytologia 12: 435.

Gall, J. G. and D. Atherton. 1973. Satellite DNA sequences in *Drosophila virilis*. In preparation.

Gall, J. G., E. H. Cohen and M. L. Polan. 1971. Repetitive DNA sequences in *Drosophila*. Chromosoma 33: 319.

Heitz, E. 1934. Über α- und β-Heterochromatin sowie Konstanz und Bau der Chromomeren bei *Drosophila*. Biol. Zbl. 54: 588.

Hennig, W. 1972. Highly repetitive DNA sequences in the genome of *Drosophila hydei* II Occurrence in polytene tissues. J. Mol. Biol. 71: 419.

Hennig, W., I. Hennig and H. Stein. 1970. Repeated sequences in the DNA of *Drosophila* and their localization in giant chromosomes. Chromosoma 32: 31.

Hennig, W. and B. Meer. 1971. Reduced polyteny of ribosomal RNA cistrons in giant chromosomes of *Drosophila hydei*. Nature New Biol. 233: 70.

Jones, K. W. 1970. Chromosomal and nuclear location of mouse satellite DNA in individual cells. Nature 255: 912.

Jones, K. W. and F. W. Robertson. 1970. Localization of reiterated nucleotide sequences in *Drosophila* and mouse by *in situ* hybridization of complementary RNA. Chromosoma 31: 331.

Kaufmann, B. P. 1934. Somatic mitoses of *Drosophila melanogaster*. J. Morph. 56: 125.

Kavenoff, R. and B. H. Zimm. 1973. Chromosome-sized DNA molecules from *Drosophila*. Chromosoma 41: 1.

Kram, R., M. Botchan and J. E. Hearst. 1972. Arrangement of the highly riterated DNA sequences in the centric heterochromatin of *Drosophila melanogaster*. Evidence for interspersed spacer DNA. J. Mol. Biol. 64: 103.

Laird, C. 1973. DNA of *Drosophila* chromosomes. Ann. Rev. Genetics 7. In press.

Laird, C. and B. McCarthy. 1968. Magnitude of interspecific nucleotide sequence variability in *Drosophila*. Genetics 60: 303.

Lefevre, G. 1973. The salivary gland chromosomes of *Drosophila melanogaster*. In (M. Ashburner and E. Novitski, eds.) The Genetics and Biology of *Drosophila*. In press, Academic Press, London.

Lindsley, D. and E. Grell. 1967. Genetic variations of *Drosophila melanogaster*. Carnegie Institution of Washington Publication No. 627.

Mulder, M. P., P. van Duijn and H. J. Gloor. 1968. The replicative organization of DNA in polytene chormosomes of *Drosophila hydei*. Genetica ('s-Gravenhage) 39: 385.

Pardue, M. L. and J. G. Gall. 1970. Chromosomal localization of mouse satellite DNA. Science 168: 1356.

Pardue, M. L. and J. G. Gall. 1972. Molecular Cytogenetics. In (M. Sussman, ed.) Molecular Genetics and Developmental Biology. p. 65. Prentice-Hall, Englewood Cliffs.

Pardue, M. L., S. A. Gerbi, R. A. Eckhardt and J. G. Gall. 1970. Cytological localization of DNA complementary to ribosomal RNA in polytene chromosomes of *Diptera*. Chromosoma 29: 268.

Plaut, W. 1963. On the replicative organization of DNA in the polytene chromosome of *Drosophila melanogaster*. J. Mol. Biol. 7: 632.

Prensky, W., D. M. Steffensen and W. L. Hughes. 1973. The use of iodinated RNA for gene localization. Proc. Nat. Acad. Sci. in press.

Rae, P. 1970. Chromosomal distribution of rapidly reannealing DNA in *Drosophila melanogaster*. Proc. Nat. Acad. Sci. 67: 1018.

Rasch, E. M. 1970. DNA cytophotometry of salivary gland nuclei and other tissue systems in Dipteran larvae. In (G. L. Wied and G. F. Bahr, eds.) Introduction to Quantitative Cytochemistry II. p. 357. Academic Press, New York.

Rasch, E. M., H. J. Barr and R. W. Rasch. 1971. The DNA content of sperm of *Drosophila melanogaster*. Chromosoma 33: 1.

Ritossa, F. M. 1968. Unstable redundancy of genes for ribosomal RNA. Proc. Nat. Acad. Sci. 60: 509.

Ritossa, F. and S. Spiegelman. 1965. Localization of DNA complementary to ribosomal RNA in the nucleolus organizer region of *Drosophila melanogaster*. Proc. Nat. Acad. Sci. 53: 737.

Rudkin, G. T. 1964. The structure and function of heterochromatin. In Genetics Today (Proc. XI Int. Cong. Genetics), p. 359. Pergamon Press, The Hague.

Rudkin, G. T. 1972. Replication in polytene chromosomes. Results and Problems in Cell Differentiation 4: 59.

Sinclair, J. and D. D. Brown. 1971. Retention of common nucleotide sequences in the ribosomal deoxyribonucleic acid of eukaryotes and some of their physical characteristics. Biochemistry 10: 2761.

Spear, B. B. and J. G. Gall. 1973. Independent control of ribosomal gene replication in polytene chromosomes of *Drosophila melanogaster*. Proc. Nat. Acad. Sci. 70: 1359.

Steffensen, D. M. and D. E. Wimber. 1971. Localization of tRNA genes in the salivary chromosomes of *Drosophila* by RNA:DNA hybridization. Genetics 69: 163.

Sutton, W. D. and M. McCallum. 1972. Related satellite DNA's in the genus *Mus*. J. Mol. Biol. 71: 633.

Swift, H. 1964. The histones of polytene chromosomes. In (J. Bonner and P. Ts'o, eds.) The Nucleohistones. p. 169. Holden-Day, San Francisco.

Tartof, K. D. 1971. Increasing the multiplicity of ribosomal RNA genes in *Drosophila melanogaster*. Science 171: 294.

Tartof, K. D. and R. Perry. 1970. The 5S RNA genes of *Drosophila melanogaster*. J. Mol. Biol. 51: 171.

Travaglini, E. and J. Schultz. 1972. Circular DNA molecules in the genus *Drosophila*. Genetics 72: 441.

Travaglini, E., J. Petrovic and J. Schultz. 1972a. Characterization of the DNA in *Drosophila melanogaster*. Genetics 72: 419.

Travaglini, E., J. Petrovic and J. Schultz. 1972b. Satellite DNAs in the embryos of various species of the genus *Drosophila*. Genetics 72: 431.

Tulchin, N., G. M. Mateyko and M. J. Kopac. 1967. *Drosophila* salivary glands *in vitro*. J. Cell Biol. 34: 891.

Wimber, D. E. and D. M. Steffensen. 1970. Localization of 5S RNA genes on *Drosophila* chromosomes by RNA-DNA hybridization. Science 170: 639.

6. EVOLUTION OF 9S mRNA SEQUENCES

Max L. Birnstiel*, Eric S. Weinberg** and Mary Lou Pardue[†]

*Institute for Molecular Biology, University of Zurich, Zurich, Switzerland, **Department of Biology, Johns Hopkins University, Baltimore, Maryland and [†]Department of Biology, Massachusetts Institute of Technology, Cambridge, Massachusetts

It is already clear that isolated messenger RNA's (mRNA's) are potentially very useful tools for the elucidation of gene regulation and chromosomal structure. In this paper we shall look at mRNA from a different standpoint and consider some experiments with histone mRNA which may shed some light on the evolution of protein coding DNA sequences.

Highly labelled polysomal 9S mRNA may be obtained from cells in S-phase of the cell cycle and from rapidly dividing embryonic tissues (Robbins and Borun, 1967; Gallwitz and Mueller, 1969a; Schochetman and Perry, 1972; Nemer and Infante, 1965; Kedes and Gross, 1969a,b). Four lines of evidence support the hypothesis that 9S polysomal RNA of these tissues is the messenger for histone proteins: 1) The appearance of 9S RNA is associated with DNA synthesis (Robbins and Borun, 1967; Borun et al., 1967; Gallwitz and Mueller, 1969a,b; Moav and Nemer, 1971). 2) Inhibition of DNA synthesis quickly inhibits the production of this RNA (Robbins and Borun, 1967; Borun et al., 1967; Kedes and Gross, 1969a; Gallwitz and Mueller, 1969b; Kedes et al., 1969). 3) Polysomes containing 9S mRNA synthesize histone-like peptides in vivo and in vitro (Robbins and Borun, 1967; Kedes and Gross, 1969a; Kedes et al., 1969; Gallwitz and Mueller, 1969b; Moav and Nemer, 1971). 4) Isolated 9S RNA from small polysomes of both HeLa and cleaving sea urchin cells directs the synthesis of histones (Gallwitz and Breindl, 1972; Jacobs-Lorena et al., 1972; Gross et al., 1973; Breindl and Gallwitz, 1973).

9S mRNA has certain interesting properties and some pecularities
that set it aside from most other closely investigated mRNA species.
It is derived from repetitive genes (Kedes and Birnstiel, 1971;
Weinberg *et al.*, 1972); it contains no poly(A)(Adesnik and Darnell,
1972); there is to date no conclusive evidence for the existence
of a nuclear heterogeneous high molecular weight precursor molecule;
the exit-time from the nucleus is extremely short (Schochetman and
Perry, 1972); and the half life in the cytoplasm is restricted to
a few hours at most (Borun *et al.*, 1967; Gallwitz and Mueller,
1969b; Craig *et al.*, 1971). Some of these properties, such as
gene reiteration, and some aspects of the RNA metabolism are perhaps
less astonishing if one considers that during each nuclear division
a large number of histone proteins, in vertebrates some 2×10^8
molecules, are synthesized over a short time span in each cell and
that this histone synthesis is highly coordinated with that of DNA.

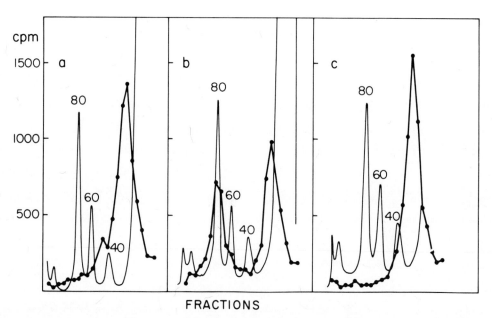

Figure 1. Addition of crude 9S RNA from sea urchin polysomes to a
rabbit reticulocyte lysate. The lysate was incubated as described
by Darnbrough *et al.* (1973) with 10^{-4} sparsomycin for 5 min before
addition of [^{3}H]uridine-labelled sea urchin RNA. After incubation
at a) 0°C, b) 30°C for 2 min, c) with 10^{-4} aurine tricarboxylic acid
at 30°C for 2 min, the samples were diluted with buffer and analyzed
on 10-30% linear sucrose gradients spun for 90 min at 45,000 rpm in
a SW50.1 rotor at 4°C. Gradients were analyzed with a recording
spectrophotometer and samples were precipitated with 1% cetyltri-
methylammonium bromide (CTAB). Solid line, A_{260}; filled circles,
radioactivity. Recovery of added radioactivity was 100%.

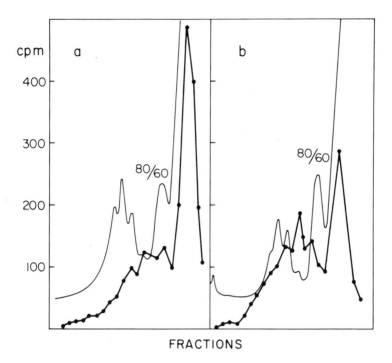

FRACTIONS

Figure 2. Binding of crude and purified sea urchin histone mRNA to polysomes. Lysate was incubated under standard conditions (Darnbrough *et al.*, 1973) for 10 min with ³H-sea urchin mRNA. No inhibitors were present. The lysate was analyzed by centrifugation in 15-30% sucrose density gradients for 30 min at 50,000 rpm in the SW50.1 rotor at 2°C. a) Sucrose gradient-purified 9S RNA; b) 9S RNA further purified by acrylamide gel electrophoresis (Weinberg *et al.*, 1972). Solid line, A_{260}; filled circles, radioactivity.

The 9S RNA of HeLa cells and sea urchins can be subfractionated into at least three major components (Gallwitz and Mueller, 1970; Weinberg *et al.*, 1972). The 9S DNA complements for each of these subfractions in two sea urchins, *Psammechinus milaris* and *Paracentrotus lividis*, are about 1000-fold repeated, as demonstrated by DNA excess hybridization. When hybridized across a CsCl density gradient containing fractionated sea urchin DNA, the 9S RNA subfractions all hybridize to DNA banding at high buoyant density (Weinberg *et al.*, 1972) and hence of high (G+C) content (Kedes and Birnstiel, 1971).

The labeled 9S RNA and one of the purified subfractions (III) used to obtain these results on gene reiteration have been shown to form 80S ribosome-mRNA complexes with good yield in a rabbit reticulocyte lysate to which sparsomycin, an inhibitor of translation, has been added. Formation of this complex is inhibited by aurine tri-

carboxylic acid. In the absence of inhibitors, the 9S RNA is to a
large extent present on light polysomes and does not accumulate on
80S ribosomes (Figs. 1 and 2; Hunt, Legon, Weinberg and Birnstiel,
unpublished experiments). Methods used in these experiments are in
press (Darnbrough et $al.$, 1973).

There is little evidence for sequence heterogeneity (disregard-
ing secondary modifications) of histones at the amino acid level
within the histone fractions. Exceptions to this are histone I
where microheterogeneity has been demonstrated (Delange and Smith,
1971), and histone V, where genetic polymorphism has been shown to
exist (Greenaway and Murray, 1971). The lack of heterogeneity in
the other histone proteins within the species is matched by a remarkable evolutionary stability of amino acid sequence, especially
of histone IV (Delange et $al.$, 1969) and probably also of III
(Panyim et $al.$, 1970); this points to exceedingly strong selective
forces acting against changes at the level of the amino acid sequence
in these proteins within and between species. King and Jukes (1969)
calculated that the minor changes observed for histone IV (Delange
et $al.$, 1969) in cows and peas amount to a rate of amino acid substitution of once every 10^{11}years per triplet, a time span 15 times
that of the age of our universe, and so one may, with some assurance,
call histone IV conservative in evolution.

Because of the degeneracy of the genetic code, one and the same
amino acid sequence may be encoded by a great number of different
DNA nucleotide sequences. It has been calculated by Kimura (1968a)
that in 23 out of 100 cases base substitutions at random along any
DNA coding sequence would be expected to lead to synonymous codons,
and therefore to an unaltered amino acid sequence. Clearly, then,
if selection acts only at the level of the protein sequence and if
consequently the DNA evolves freely within this limitation through
substitution of synonymous codons, one would expect the histone
coding genes to diverge rapidly at the level of the DNA sequence
within and between species. Conversely, if mutations to synonymous
codons are not selectively neutral, then the DNA base sequence itself would be conserved as stringently as the amino acid sequence,
both within the species and throughout the evolution of the species.
We have designed hybridization studies to test these hypotheses.

DIVERGENCE OF 9S SEQUENCES WITHIN THE SPECIES

The temperature of dissociation (melting temperature) of DNA
duplexes and RNA·DNA hybrids depends, first, on the (G+C) content
of the annealed nucleic acids. Where the (G+C) content is known,
measurement of T_m may be used as a measure of the fidelity of base
pairing, since 1% mismatching base pairs depresses the T_m by about
1.6°C (Ullman and McCarthy, 1973a,b,c).

  P^{32}-9S RNA was fractionated by gel electrophoresis, fraction A
and B isolated (Fig. 3) and base compositions determined. A (G+C)
content of 51.8 and 52.9% was obtained (Table 1; Vergin and Giudice,
unpublished). 9S RNA·DNA hybrids manufactured between purified RNA
subfractions of *Psammechinus* RNA and homologous DNA gave T$_m$'s of
75°C. The T$_m$'s of the RNA·DNA hybrids show that they are less stable, by only 1-2°C, than DNA of 53% (G+C). Thus, within the accuracy of the technique, there is no measurable sequence divergence of
the 9S sequences within the species.

Table 1. Base composition of ^{32}P-9S *Paracentrotus* RNA subfractions (H. Vergin, unpublished results). The likely base
composition for histone IV mRNA was calculated from the amino
acid sequence of the protein assuming that the choice of degenerate codons in this RNA is random.

<table>
<tr><td colspan="3" align="center">Base Composition of ^{32}P-labelled 9S RNA</td></tr>
<tr><td>Component A:</td><td>Component B:</td><td>Calculated:
(histone IV)</td></tr>
<tr><td>C   = 25.0</td><td>25.3</td><td>21.4</td></tr>
<tr><td>A   = 30.2</td><td>30.1</td><td>32.3</td></tr>
<tr><td>G   = 26.7</td><td>27.4</td><td>27.5</td></tr>
<tr><td>U   = 18.1</td><td>17.2</td><td>18.8</td></tr>
<tr><td>(G+C) = 51.7</td><td>52.7</td><td>48.9</td></tr>
</table>

  It can be easily demonstrated that the effect of degenerate
histone coding sequences would be easily detectable. For this purpose we, with A. Robertson in Edinburgh, simulated the hybridization reaction in the following way. DNA and mRNA sequences were
generated at random by a computer for histone IV amino acid sequence
making full use of the degeneracy of the genetic code. Fifty messenger sequences were matched in juxtaposition with 50 histone IV coding DNA sequences. For each matching operation a count was made of
the number of complementary runs of nucleotides in the two strands
containing 0, 1, 2....n matched base pairs. To convert the frequency distribution for each size class to the amount of the total
RNA in each size class, the number of runs were multiplied by the
number of bases in that size class, and then converted to a percent
of the total weighted sum. The percent of mismatched bases in the
50 matching operations is plotted as zero base pairs in "hybrid".
The periodicity of frequency distribution results from the fact that
base substitutions leading to synonymous codons occur mostly in the
third base position.

  Fig. 4 gives the relative proportion of RNA found in "RNA·DNA
hybrids" of various lengths after a single matching operation. Only

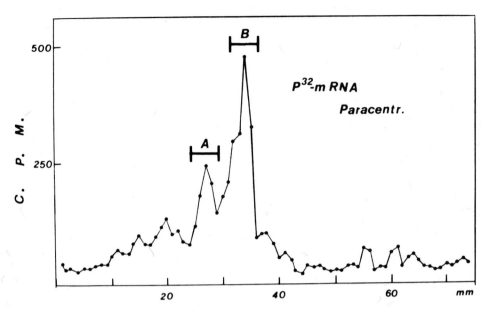

Figure 3. Electrophoresis of *Paracentrotus* ^{32}P-labelled 9S mRNA in 6% polyacrylamide gels (H. Vergin and G. Giudice, unpublished data). Fractions A and B were isolated and their base compositions determined (Table 1).

a small fraction of the matched sequences would have a length exceeding 15 nucleotide pairs, a number thought to be required for the formation of a stable hybrid. The probability of finding 10 matched base pairs is also low and that of finding two such matched regions close together connected by looped-out short RNA segments would be smaller still, although we have not considered this quantitatively. Although the simulation considers only a single matching operation, the outcome, even at completion of the reaction, can easily be foreseen. Degenerate isocoding genes and their primary products would form RNA·DNA hybrids of poor quality containing, after completion of the reaction, predominantly short matched regions attached to long unmatched tails. Furthermore, since most collisions would be unsuccessful (because they would lead to formation of hybrids shorter than that required for stabilization), the hybridization rate would be lowered. DNA specifying histones would probably behave kinetically as unique DNA (Walker, 1969; Southern, 1971). By contrast no sequence heterogeneity can be found experimentally since: 1) RNA·DNA hybrids are well matched and 2) RNA·DNA hybrids are largely insensitive to RNase and do not contain long RNA tails (Weinberg *et al.*, 1972). Obviously there is a large discrepancy between the heterogeneity which might be tolerated by the organism and that actually found in the experiment. From this one may conclude

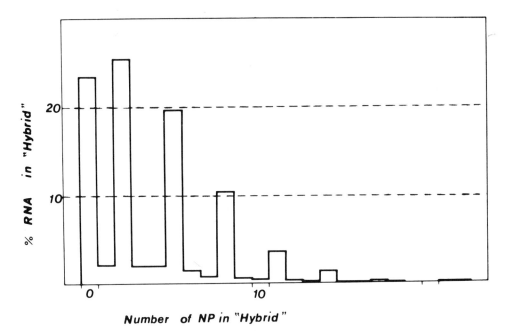

Figure 4. Distribution of RNA sequences in hybrids of increasing number of nucleotide pairs (NP) in register after a single matching operation between degenerate histone IV mRNA and its degenerate structural genes.

that the base sequences of the 9S DNA complements are themselves conserved within the species.

DIVERGENCE OF 9S SEQUENCES BETWEEN SPECIES

9S mRNA of sea urchin hybridized in excess with filter-bound DNA anneals with DNA from a variety of phyla; this could mean that mutation to synonymous codons is somehow highly restricted and that the 9S mRNA sequences are conservative in evolution (McCarthy and Farquhar, 1971).

Since the level of cross-hybridization is very low, amounting to only a few percent of the sea urchin controls, first it is necessary to show that the hybridization is by the 9S RNA itself, rather than by a minor RNA contaminant of the 9S RNA preparation. One can discriminate between these two possibilities by studying the kinetics of the RNA excess hybridization reaction. Since the rate of an RNA·DNA is proportional to the molar concentration of the reacting species (cf. Birnstiel et al., 1972), comparison of the rate of the hybridization in both homologous and heterologous systems will show

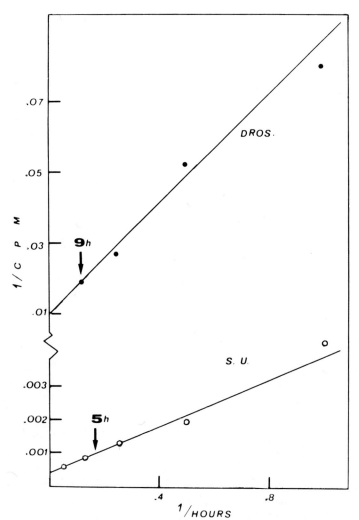

Figure 5. Kinetics of hybridization of ^{3}H-9S mRNA of *Psammechinus*
with homologous and *Drosophila* DNA (upper and lower curves, respectively). The reaction was measured according to Birnstiel *et al*.
(1972). The data is recorded in double reciprocal plots to facili-
tate determination of $t_{1/2}$. The $t_{1/2}$ for the heterologous reaction
is twice that of the homologous system. Hybridization was carried
out with 3 μg of either *Psammechinus* or *Drosophila* DNA immobilized
on a series of filters. Three filters of each DNA were averaged
for each time point; blank filters were also used for each time
point and counts hybridized to them were subtracted. Each time
point was carried out in separate vials. Hybridization conditions
were 6XSSC, 65°C, 50,000 cpm of *Psammechinus* 9S RNA in a reaction
volume of 0.3 ml.

whether the major fraction of the RNA is involved in both cases.
As seen from the double reciprocal plot in Fig. 5, for a given input
of labelled 9S mRNA the reaction half time (that is, the time taken
to saturate half of the DNA complements) is 5 hours for sea urchin
DNA, and 9 hours for *Drosophila* DNA. The reaction for *Drosophila*
is slower by a factor of about 2, but this is fully accounted for by
the effects of sequence mismatching on the rate of hybridization
(Southern, 1971). It therefore seems most probable that in both
cases we are looking at the hybridization of 9S mRNA. In addition,
the hybrids that form in heterologous systems are also locus specific
for in all cases studied the sea urchin 9S RNA reacts with DNA complements of a unique buoyant density (Kedes and Birnstiel, 1971).

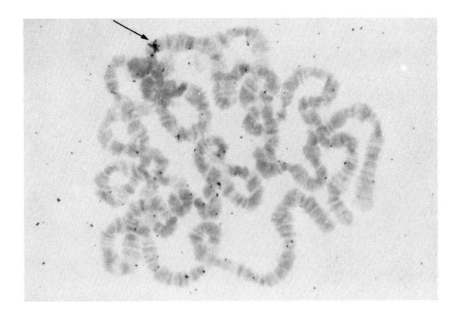

Figure 6. Autoradiograph of salivary gland chromosomes from *Drosophila melanogaster* hybridized *in situ* with ^{3}H-9S mRNA from the sea
urchin, *Psammechinus milaris*. The DNA of the chromosomes was denatured with 0.07N NaOH for 3 min and hybridized with 2 X 10^6 cpm/ml
^{3}H-9S RNA and 40 mg/ml non-radioactive *E. coli* ribosomal RNA in
6XSSC for 9 hr. The ^{3}H-9S RNA was prepared from a polysomal pellet
isolated from cleaving sea urchin embryos (Weinberg *et al.*, 1972;
Kedes and Birnstiel, 1971). Slides were stained with Giemsa. The
complete chromosome set from a polytene nucleus showing hybridization of the putative histone messenger only to region 39D-39E (arrow). Exposure 104 days (X870).

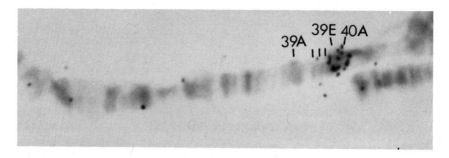

Figure 7. Autoradiograph showing the proximal end of the left arm
of chromosome 2 from a typically unstretched preparation prepared
as described in Fig. 6. Bands 39D and 39E are closely apposed and
9S hybridization is localized over the double band. Exposure 99
days (X2200).

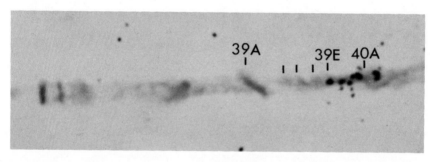

Figure 8. Autoradiograph of the proximal end of the left arm of
chromosome 2 from an extremely stretched preparation. 9S hybridization is seen to both bands and throughout the intervening region
(see Fig. 9). Exposure 99 days (X2200).

When sea urchin 9S mRNA is hybridized *in situ* to polytene chromosomes from *D. melanogaster* the RNA bands to two adjacent bands near
the centromere on the left arm of chromosome 2 (Figs. 6-8). These
two bands, which are designated 39D and 39E on the new map of G.
LeFevre, are usually closely apposed in salivary gland squash preparations. However, if the proximal part of 2L is stretched, 39D
and 39E are sometimes separated by a rather long distance and three
small bands can be seen in the newly apparent region (see Fig. 9).
Both bands 39D and 39E and the entire chromosome region between
them hybridize with sea urchin 9S mRNA. Experiments to examine the
localization of different subfractions of the sea urchin 9S mRNA
within this region are now in progress. The specific localization
of the sea urchin - *Drosophila* hybrids to a very small part of the
chromosomes is consistent with the argument that sea urchin 9S mRNA
forms heterologous hybrids with at least part of an analogous set of
repeated DNA sequences within the *Drosophila* genome.

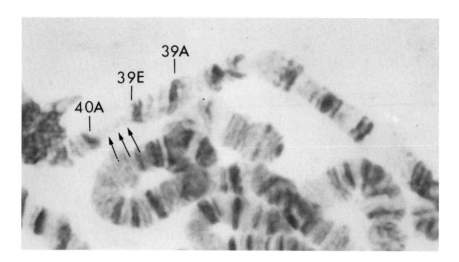

Figure 9. Salivary gland chromosomes showing the chromosome region
which becomes visible when bands 39D and 39E are spread apart.
Several very faint bands (arrows) can be seen. In most squash preparations, bands 39D and 39E form a closely united pair of bands and
no interband region is visible (Figs. 6 and 7). Acetic orcein stain
(X3200).

From RNA excess hybridization reactions (*e.g.*, Fig. 5) it remains uncertain whether the extent of heterologous hybridization is
low because 9S messenger sequences have diverged or because gene reiteration in heterologous systems is much lower. Both these points
may, in principle, be elucidated by using DNA excess hybridization
techniques. In these reactions DNA in large excess is annealed with
a trace amount of highly labelled RNA. When the concentration of
RNA·DNA hybrids is measured sequentially during the reaction and
plotted according to the convention of Britten and Kohne (1968),
a C_0t curve is obtained which is indicative of the renaturation of
the DNA complements. From the $C_0t_{1/2}$ of the trace curve, the gene
reiteration of the DNA complements may be calculated (Melli *et al.*,
1971). In homologous reactions, about 70-90% of the RNA forms RNase-
resistant hybrids. In heterologous reactions the radioactive test
RNA will trace the reiteration of the heterologous DNA complements
and, if the effect of mismatching is considered, the approximate
redundancy of the DNA complements may be determined. RNA sequences
that have diverged to the extent that they will no longer hybridize
will be hydrolyzed by the action of RNase. This will show up as a
poor yield of RNA·DNA hybrids even at very high C_0t values.

This question was first examined using different species of
sea urchins. The three main 9S mRNA subfractions were highly puri-

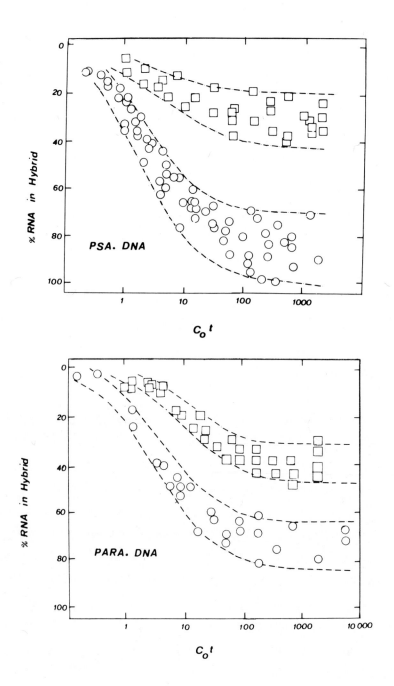

fied by gel electrophoresis from both *Psammechinus* and *Paracentrotus* embryos and reacted with both homologous and heterologous sea urchin DNA. Fig. 10 is a composite of the raw data from our experiments using pure subfractions. It may be seen that all homologous RNA fractions in both sea urchin systems trace a $C_ot_{1/2}$ of about 2 to 4 corresponding to a gene reiteration of approximately 1000. A similar redundancy is obtained for trace curves with heterologous RNA, but the reaction is clearly less complete, amounting to 40 to 50% of the control reactions.

The conclusions from these experiments are that the level of histone gene redundancy is conserved during the evolution of the two sea urchin species, but that the 9S sequences are not conserved. Since the two sea urchins are closely related to one another, it is highly unlikely that the observed sequence divergence could have arisen from amino acid substitutions in histones; it must be due to synonymous codons arising from mutations (Weinberg *et al.*, 1972).

In order to estimate the rate of evolution of the 9S sequences it would be interesting to know what percent base substitution corresponds to the disparity of hybridization between the two sea urchin species. The definition of a sequence which will no longer cross-hybridize is of course rather an arbitrary one, depending for one thing on the stringency of the hybridization reactions. For the computation of sequence divergence from a DNA excess hybridization experiment much more information is needed about the minimal stable hybrid length and also the reliability of RNase resistance as a measure of hybrid stability.

Data of a more quantitative nature is obtainable from the melting temperatures of the heterologous 9S RNA·DNA hybrids. Labelled *Psammechinus* 9S RNA or *Psammechinus* 9S RNA further purified into subfractions by electrophoresis was annealed to both *Paracentrotus* and *Psammechinus* DNA. The incubation time was sufficient to saturate at least 90% of all available DNA sites. We have used discriminating (1XSSC, 70°C) and relaxed (6XSSC, 65°C) conditions of incubation and compared the T_m's of the heterologous duplexes with those of homologous controls.

Figure 10. Hybridization of purified [3]H-9S RNA fractions I-III from *Paracentrotus* and *Psammechinus* embryos with homologous and heterologous DNA in vast excess. a) RNA fractions hybridized to *Psammechinus* DNA; b) RNA fractions hybridized to *Paracentrotus* DNA. For experimental details see Weinberg *et al.* (1972). Open circles, homologous RNA fractions; open squares, heterologous RNA fractions.

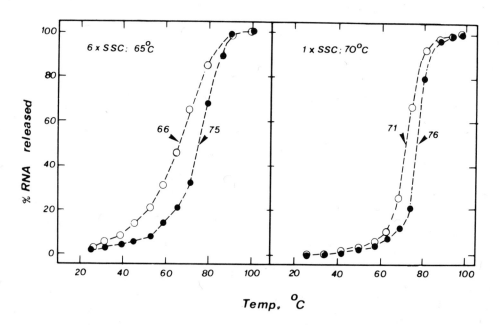

Figure 11. Melting temperature of homologous and heterologous sea
urchin 9S RNA·DNA hybrids. 9S mRNA (left panel) or electrophoretic-
ally purified 9S mRNA subfractions (right panel) from *Psammechinus*
were annealed with *Psammechinus* DNA (homologous hybrid) and *Paracentrotus* DNA (heterologous hybrid) in RNA excess under stringent
and relaxed conditions of incubation and the T_m's were determined
as described in Weinberg *et al*. (1972) and Kedes and Birnstiel
(1971). Filled circles, homologous hybrid; open circles, heterologous hybrid.

     Figure 11 shows that when *Psammechinus* 9S RNA is hybridized
under discriminating conditions to either *Paracentrotus* or homologous DNA, the heterologous hybrid melts some 5°C lower than the
homologous control. This corresponds to a sequence mismatching of
3%. Under relaxed conditions of hybridization, the difference
approximates 9°C, indicative of 6% mismatching. It should be noted,
however, that reactions in RNA excess under non-discriminating conditions would be expected to enhance hybridization of any contaminat-
ing (and perhaps less conserved), RNA species and might account for
some of the differential between the T_m's of the homologous and
heterologous hybrids. We therefore consider 3% mismatching to be
the more reliable value.

     As expected, the degree of mismatching in heterologous 9S hy-
brid for species as distantly related as sea urchins and *Drosophila*
is much greater. Here a ΔT_m of 19°C is observed corresponding to

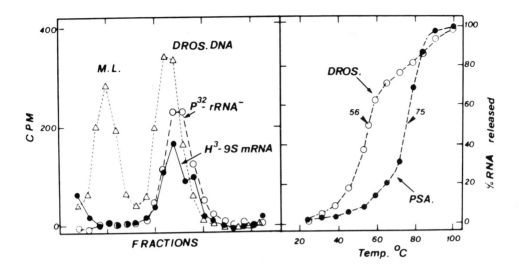

Figure 12. Properties of 9S-DNA complements in *Drosophila*. *Drosophila* DNA was fractionated on a CsCl density gradient and the fractions challenged with ^{32}P-rRNA of *Xenopus* and ^{3}H-9S mRNA of *Psammechinus* as described by Kedes and Birnstiel (1971) and Weinberg *et al.* (1972). *Micrococcus lysodeikticus* (M.L.) served as a desnity marker (left panel). Denatured *Drosophila* DNA or *Psammechinus* DNA was bound to Millipore filters and challenged with an excess of ^{3}H-9S RNA obtained from *Psammechinus* embryos. The media contained 6XSSC, the incubation was overnight at 65°C. The filters were washed but not treated with RNase and the T_m of the hybrids determined (Kedes and Birnstiel, 1971) (right panel). Filled circles, homologous hybrids; open circles, heterologous hybrids.

about 13% mismatching for the cross-hybridizing 9S RNA segments (Fig. 12). Unfortunately, the homology between 9S sequences of sea urchins and the DNA of *Drosophila* involves such a small portion, probably less than 10%, of the RNA that the scatter encountered in a DNA excess reaction obliterates the RNA trace curve and consequently we have not been able to determine the gene reiteration of the 9S DNA complements in this species.

RATE OF DNA EVOLUTION

Paracentrotus and *Psammechinus* are closely related sea urchin species that are thought to have diverged some 25±10 million years ago (D. Nichols, personal communication). This means that nucleotide substitution has occurred at a rate of 3 to 6% over a combined evolutionary time for the two lines of divergence of 5×10^7 years, or $1.8 - 3.6 \times 10^{-9}$ substitutions per codon per generation for the cross-hybridizing RNA segments.

The rate of sequence evolution in structural genes has been estimated from the rate of amino acid substitutions in proteins (Kimura, 1969) or from the incidence of the base substitutions in unique DNA (King and Jukes, 1969; Kohne, 1970). It has been pointed out that the rate of base substitution in nucleic acids is 10 times that of amino acid substitutions in most proteins (Walker, 1969; King and Jukes, 1969; Kohne, 1970), with a few notable exceptions such as the constant half of immunoglobulin light chain and fibrinopeptide A (King and Jukes, 1969). The first method contains the unlikely assumption that all amino acid substitutions are slectively neutral, or nearly so. The second approach is also unsatisfactory since nothing is known about the function of the bulk of the unique DNA.

Here we show that the sequences of the structural genes for 9S mRNA change rapidly in evolution and this supports the general hypthesis that DNA evolves through fixation of "selectively neutral" mutations to synonymous codons (Walker, 1969; King and Jukes, 1969; Kohne, 1970). The rate of sequence evolution in unique DNA is estimated to be 6×10^{-9} substitutions per codon per generation, a value based on the cross-reacting sequences between heterologous DNA's. The rate of sequence evolution in 9S mRNA is approximately that of the unique DNA; in fact, it appears to evolve somewhat more slowly (Table 2). This is interesting because this also corresponds to

Table 2. Evolution of protein and nucleic acid sequences

SUBSTITUTIONS PER CODON

in <u>amino acid</u> sequence: (per year X 10^{11})

histone IV	1	
cytochrome C	42	King & Jukes (1969)
average, 7 proteins	160	
fibrinopeptide A	429	

in <u>nucleotide</u> sequence: (per generation X 10^{11})

unique DNA	500*	Walker (1969)
unique DNA	400-750[†]	Kohne (1970)
9S coding DNA	180-360	this paper

---

*assuming 8 generation per year
[†]data recalculated for 1°C = 0.66% mispaired bases

the theoretical expectation. In genes coding for a protein of immutable amino acid sequence such as histones, only 23% of all base substitutions lead to synonymous codons (Kimura, 1968b), and these would be fixed in evolution, while the remaining 77% would alter the primary structure of the proteins and would be discriminated against by natural selection. In the case of unique DNA, however, it is now thought that much of this DNA may not code for proteins (Crick, 1971). If true, there might then be no restriction on mutational drift and the unique DNA could evolve more rapidly than histone coding sequences.

The rate of amino acid substitution in proteins not conserved in evolution should approximate 3/4 that of the nucleotide substitutions in unique DNA. This is only observed for a select few proteins (Table 2; King and Jukes, 1969; McCarthy and Farquhar, 1971). For all others the rate of amino acid substitution is much lower. This could mean one of three things: 1.) The incidence of nucleotide substitution in histone DNA (and in unique DNA) is not representative for other structural genes; 2.) many amino acid substitutions have a selective disadvantage at the level of the proteins; 3.) amino acid substitutions may or may not have a selective disadvantage at the level of the proteins, but the rate of amino acid substitutions is low, because there are selection pressures at the level of the nucleotide sequence of the mRNA (e.g. by a requirement for specific secondary structure for biological function or a limitation imposed by the concentration of particular isoaccepting tRNA's) and such pressures would cause the DNA to evolve more slowly than unique and histone DNA.

Despite rapid degeneration of the histone coding RNA and DNA sequences, heterologous reactions, such as we observed in sea urchin 9S RNA on *Drosophila*, are quite specific. Our statistical analyses further suggest that even if histone coding sequences were fully randomized there would still be a likelihood of observing some sequence-specific hybridization. The reason for this is that the probability of obtaining matched hybrids with more than the minimal stable length of 15 nucleotide pairs is finite, as shown by our computer studies (Fig. 4). This cross-hybridization would amount to only a few percent of the homologous reaction. Consistent with this it has been found that 9S RNA from sea urchins anneals in a specific way to all eukaryotic DNA studied (Kedes and Birnstiel, 1971; McCarthy and Farquhar, 1971), with the notable exceptions of the DNA's of slime-mold and *Tetrahymena* (Weinberg, Birnstiel, Ashworth and Gorovsky, unpublished results).

NOTE ADDED IN PROOF

A more recent version of Lefevre's map lists band 39E as 39D and 40A as 39E. These changes were made in the text and legends but not in the figures.

REFERENCES

Adesnik, M. and J. E. Darnell. 1972. J. Mol. Biol. 67: 397.

Birnstiel, M. L., B. H. Sells and I. F. Purdom. 1972. J. Mol. Biol. 63: 21.

Borun, T. W., M. D. Sharff and E. Robbins. 1967. Proc. Nat. Acad. Sci. 58: 1977.

Breindl, M. and D. Gallwitz. 1973. Eur. J. Bioch. 32: 381.

Britten, R. J. and D. E. Kohne. 1968. Science 161: 529.

Craig, N., D. E. Kelly and R. P. Perry. 1971. Biochim. Biophys. Acta 246: 493.

Crick, F. 1971. Nature New Biol. 234: 25.

Darnbrough, C., S. Legon, T. Hunt and R. J. Jackson. 1973. J. Mol. Biol. 76: 379.

Delange, R. J., D. M. Frambrough, E. L. Smith and J. Bonner. 1969. J. Biol. Chem. 244: 319.

Delange, R. J. and E. L. Smith. 1971. Ann. Rev. Biochem. 40: 279.

Gallwitz, D. and G. C. Mueller. 1969a. Science 163: 1351.

Gallwitz, D. and G. C. Mueller. 1969b. J. Biol. Chem. 244: 5947.

Gallwitz, D. and G. C. Mueller. 1970. FEBS Lett. 6: 83.

Gallwitz, D. and M. Breindl. 1972. Biochem. Biophys. Res. Comm. 47: 1106.

Greenaway, P. J. and K. Murray. 1971. Nature New Biol. 229: 233.

Gross, K., J. Ruderman, M. Jacobs-Lorena, C. Baglioni and P. R. Gross. 1973. Nature New Biol. 241: 272.

Jacobs-Lorena, M., C. Baglioni and T. W. Borun. 1972. Proc. Nat. Acad. Sci. 69: 2095.

Kedes, L. and P. R. Gross. 1969a. Nature 223: 1335.

Kedes, L. and P. R. Gross. 1969b. J. Mol. Biol. 42: 559.

Kedes, L., P. R. Gross, G. Cognetti and A. L. Hunter. 1969. J. Mol. Biol. 45: 337.

Kedes, L. and M. L. Birnstiel. 1971. Nature New Biol. 230: 165.

Kimura, M. 1968a. Genet. Res. 11: 247.

Kimura, M. 1968b. Nature 217: 624.

Kimura, M. 1969. Proc. Nat. Acad. Sci. 63: 1181.

King, J. L. and T. H. Jukes. 1969. Science 64: 788.

Kinkade, J. M. 1969. J. Biol. Chem. 244: 3375.

Kohne, D. E. 1970. Quart. Rev. Biophys. 33: 327.

McCarthy, B. J. and M. N. Farquhar. 1972. Brookhaven Symposium 23: 1.

Melli, M. L., C. Whitfield, K. Rao, M. Richardson and J. O. Bishop. 1971. Nature New Biol. 231: 8.

Moav, B. and M. Nemer. 1971. Biochem. 10: 881.

Nemer, M. and A. A. Infante. 1965. Science 150: 217.

Panyim, S., R. Chalkley, S. Spiker and D. Oliver. 1970. Biochem. Biophys. Acta 214: 216.

Robbins, E. and T. W. Borun. 1967. Proc. Nat. Acad. Sci. 57: 409.

Schochetman, G. and R. P. Perry. 1972. J. Mol. Biol. 63: 577.

Southern, E. 1971. Nature New Biol. 232: 82.

Ullman, J. S. and B. J. McCarthy. 1973a. Biochim. Biophys. Acta 294: 396.

Ullman, J. S. and B. J. McCarthy. 1973b. Biochim. Biophys. Acta 294: 405.

Ullman, J. S. and B. J. McCarthy. 1973c. Biochim. Biophys. Acta 294: 416.

Walker, P. M. B. 1968. Nature 219: 228.

Walker, P. M. B. 1969. Prog. Nucl. Acid. Res. Mol. Biol. 9: 301.

Weinberg, E. S., M. L. Birnstiel, I. F. Purdom and R. Williamson. 1972. Nature 240: 225.

7. A NEW APPROACH TO THE STUDY OF NUCLEOTIDE SEQUENCES IN DNA'S

Giorgio Bernardi, Stanislav D. Ehrlich and Jean-Paul
Thiery

*Laboratoire de Génétique Moléculaire, Institut de
Biologie Moléculaire, Paris 5°, France*

We wish to outline here a new procedure for studying nucleotide sequences in DNA's. The procedure is based on our recent
demonstration that at least the four deoxyribonucleases (DNases) we
have investigated so far (hog spleen acid DNase, snail hepatopancreas
acid DNase, bovine pancreas DNase and *E. coli* endonuclease I) hy-
drolyze specific sets of short nucleotide sequences.

Using methods described elsewhere (Bernardi *et al.*, 1973) for
the isolation and analysis of the termini, *i.e.* the nucleotides near
the breaks introduced by the enzymes, X↓YZ (the sequence being writ-
ten in the usual 5'→3' direction and the vertical arrow indicating
the position of the break), it is possible to show (Table I) that
the base composition of termini a) differs from the values expected
for random degradation, in which case the composition of each terminus considered should be equal to the average base composition of
the DNA; the 5' penultimate nucleotide is, however, not recognized
by the snail enzyme, as shown by the fact that its composition is
equal to that expected for the nearest neighbors of the 5' terminal
nucleotide; b) differs according to the enzyme used indicating that
different sets of sequences are split by different enzymes; c) does
not vary, as a rule, according to the level of DNA degradation. The
minimum length of the sequences recognized by the nucleases is 4
nucleotides for the spleen enzyme (in which case the 3' penultimate
nucleotides were also analyzed), 3 nucleotides for the pancreatic
DNase and *E. coli* endonuclease I, and 2 nucleotides for the snail
enzyme.

Since these nucleases split specific sets of sequences, the
analysis of termini provides information on the frequency of these
sequences in a given DNA. In fact, the composition of termini is

Table I.   Termini liberated from calf thymus DNA by four DNases

Enzyme		3' term.	5' term.	5' pen.
Spleen DNase*	T	20	11	14
	G	43	43	26
	A	29	18	52
	C	8	28	8
Snail DNase	T	16	14	38
	G	6	45	24
	A	78	10	21
	C	1	31	14
Pan- creatic DNase	T	36	38	13
	G	15	22	36
	A	31	15	30
	C	18	25	21
E. coli endonu- clease I	T	41	24	28
	G	8	35	29
	A	35	17	29
	C	16	23	14

* In this case, the average chain length of oligonucleotides was equal to 15, and 3'-penultimate nucleotides were also analyzed; they were T 22%, G 16%, A 46%, C 16%.

related a) to the average composition of the sequences that can be split by the enzymes; b) to the k_M and V_{max} values associated with each sequence; and c) to their relative amounts in the DNA under consideration.

The latter point is shown by the fact that the composition of termini as obtained from DNA's having different (G+C) contents are different (Fig. 1). If the compositions of termini released from bacterial DNA's are plotted against their (G+C) contents, linear relationships are obtained (Fig. 1). The choice of bacterial DNA's in order to establish such relationships is justified a) by the fact that bacterial DNA's do not contain repetitive sequences and b) by the fact that the doublet frequencies of bacterial DNA's, as determined by the nearest neighbor analysis, show essentially linear relationships with the frequencies predicted for random association, indicating a common type of doublet distribution in these DNA's.

As expected, the composition of termini released from DNA's containing "repetitive" nucleotide sequences deviates, in either direction, from the linear relationship obtained with non-repetitive (bacterial) DNA's. The deviation patterns thus obtained represent

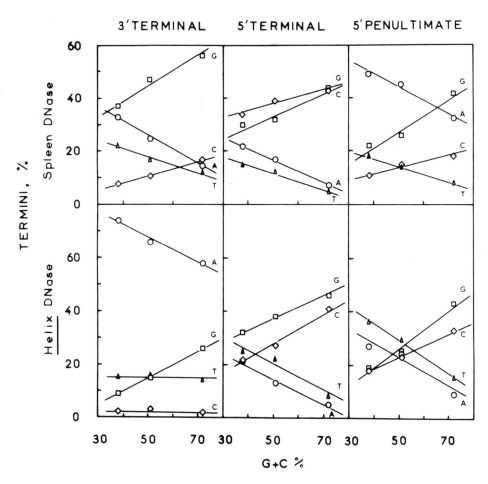

Figure 1. The percentage of A (open circles), G (open squares),
C (open diamonds) and T (open triangles) in the 3'-terminal, 5'-
terminal and 5'-penultimate nucleotides formed by spleen and the
snail DNase from bacterial DNA's, is plotted against the (G+C)
contents of DNA's.

a novel way of characterizing "repetitive" DNA's or, more generally,
DNA's having sequence distributions different from those of the
bacterial DNA's examined here. Fig. 2 shows the deviation patterns
of three DNA's containing short repeated sequences: the satellite
DNA's from mouse and guinea pig and the mitochondrial DNA from yeast
Expectedly, deviation patterns obtained with different enzymes on
the same DNA's are different from each other, as are deviation patterns obtained with the same enzyme on different DNA's.

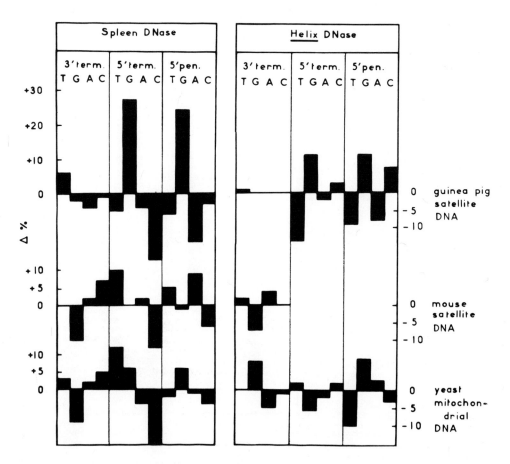

Figure 2. Deviation patterns of three repetitive DNA's. The histograms show the differences between the composition of termini formed
from guinea pig satellite, mouse satellite and yeast mitochondrial
DNA's by spleen and snail DNases and the compositions expected for
bacterial DNA's having the same (G+C) contents. The delta values
represent differences in the percentages of each terminus.

       As another example, Fig. 3 shows deviation patterns obtained
with calf, mouse and guinea pig DNA's and with yeast nuclear DNA.
It is evident that in this case, too, a number of sequences are
present at greater or lower frequencies in the eukaryotic DNA's compared to bacterial DNA's of identical (G+C) composition. Interest-
ingly, the mammalian DNA's have similar deviation patterns whereas
the yeast nuclear DNA pattern is quite different; mammalian DNA's
appear to share the sequence features that are responsible for the
similarity of their deviation patterns and that do not exist in

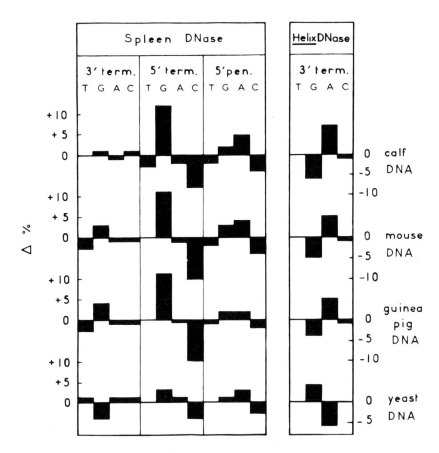

Figure 3. Deviation patterns of four eukaryotic DNA's. The histograms show the differences between the composition of termini formed from eukaryotic DNA's by spleen and snail DNases and the compositions expected for bacterial DNA's having the same (G+C) contents. Delta values represent differences in the percentages of each terminus.

yeast nuclear DNA. The possibility that the deviations observed in the mammalian DNA's arise from their satellite DNA's is ruled out by the completely different deviation patterns exhibited by the latter (Fig. 2).

REFERENCE

Bernardi, G., S. D. Ehrlich and J. P. Thiery. 1973. A new approach to the study of nucleotide sequences in DNA: the analysis of termini formed by DNases. Methods in Enzymol. in press.

8. ON THE STRUCTURE OF PRE-mRNA AND THE TRANSCRIPTIONAL UNIT IN EUKARYOTES

G. P. Georgiev

Institute of Molecular Biology, Academy of Sciences of the USSR, Moscow

THE GENERAL STRUCTURE OF THE TRANSCRIPTIONAL UNIT IN EUKARYOTES

Several years ago I proposed a model (Fig. 1) for the structural organization of the transcriptional unit in eukaryotic cells (Georgiev, 1969) based on studies of the structure of nuclear DNA-like RNA (dRNA), the precursor of mRNA (pre-mRNA) (reviewed in Georgiev, 1972). According to this model, the structural gene(s) is(are) localized at the end of the transcriptional unit, or transcripton. The main part of the transcripton, between the promoter and structural gene(s), does not carry structural information but contains acceptor sites that interact with structural and regulatory proteins of chromatin. Some of the acceptor sites are reiterated and may be present in different transcriptons, allowing one regulatory factor to simultaneously switch on or off many transcriptons. Newly formed giant pre-mRNA is a transcript from the whole transcripton. It consists of an informative part at the 3'-end and a noninformative part. The latter is degraded while the former, corresponding to a true mRNA, is transferred to the cytoplasm.

This model has been tested by several types of experiments. One of the main approaches is analysis of hybridization properties of 3'- and 5'-end sequences in pre-mRNA (Georgiev *et al.*, 1972). The marker at the 5'-end is the existence of a triphosphorylated nucleotide; after alkaline hydrolysis, the labeled nucleoside tetraphosphate (pppNp) could be isolated. The 3'-end is labeled chemically by the periodate oxidation-[3H]borohydride reduction technique (Leppla *et al.*, 1968); after alkaline hydrolysis, it gives a [3H]-labeled nucleoside derivative, which was then purified from non-nucleoside labeled material.

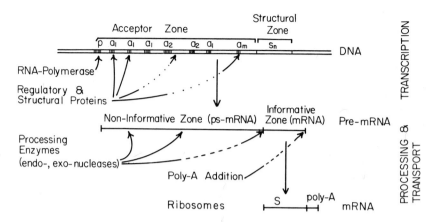

Figure 1. A modified model of the transcriptional unit in eukaryotes (Georgiev, 1969). p=promoter; a_1.....a_m=acceptor sites; S_n=structural gene(s) (usually n=1).

The following results were obtained. 1) Hybridization of the 3'-end sequences of giant pre-mRNA with DNA is very efficiently inhibited by the addition of polysomal RNA. Although the overall competition of the latter with giant pre-mRNA is insignificant, competition with the 3'-end sequences reached 70% in our experiments. 2) 5'-end sequences of giant pre-mRNA, containing pppNp groups, are hybridized very efficiently with DNA, but in this case, polysomal RNA does not compete with the hybridization reaction. Thus, the 5'-end sequences of giant pre-mRNA are represented by reiterated base sequences that do not reach polysomes, but are degraded in the nucleus (Georgiev *et al.*, 1972).

Further information about the localization of mRNA in pre-mRNA was obtained from studies of its poly(A) sequences (Edmonds *et al.*, 1971; Darnell *et al.*, 1971; Lee *et al.*, 1971). It has been shown that long poly(A) stretches are added enzymatically to the 3'-end of newly formed pre-mRNA and then they move, together with the mRNA, to the cytoplasm (Mendecki *et al.*, 1972; Molloy *et al.*, 1972). This confirms the 3'-end localization of mRNA in the precursor molecule. Experiments on hybridization of anti-mDNA (transcribed from hemoglobin mRNA by reverse transcriptase) and pre-mRNA showed that approximately one mRNA molecule is present in one pre-mRNA chain (Imaisumi *et al.*, 1973). This is in good agreement with the data indicating that many structural genes, including those coding for hemoglobin, are represented in the genome by unique sequences (Bishop *et al.*, 1972; Suzuki *et al.*, 1973). Judd *et al.* (1972) have shown, by genetic analysis of the X chromosome of *Drosophila*,

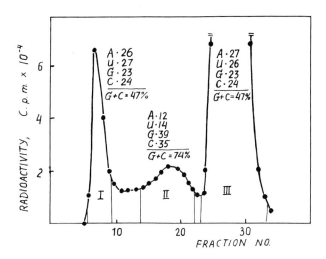

Figure 2. The isolation of long and short hairpins from heavy nuclear pre-mRNA of Ehrlich ascites carcinoma cells (Ryskov *et al.*,
1973a). Nuclear pre-mRNA (>45S) was digested in 2XSSC with pancreatic + T₁ ribonucleases and chromatographed on Sephadex-G75. Peaks
I, II and III were collected, hydrolyzed by alkali and their base
compositions determined. Before hydrolysis, peak I was purified of
poly(A) (∿10% contamination).

that one band contains only one unit of complementation, *i.e.* only
one gene is present in a giant piece of DNA corresponding to a band.
Thus it seems very probably that the transcripton really does contain only one structural gene at one end, and that the remainder
of the molecule does not carry structural information, as predicted
in the model (Fig. 1).

What is the functional role of the non-informative part of the
transcripton? To study this question one needs specific markers of
this region of pre-mRNA. Such markers have been discovered only
recently: 1) reiterated 5'-end sequences containing the pppNp group
(Georgiev *et al.*, 1972); 2) double-stranded hairpin-like structures
(Ryskov *et al.*, 1972, 1973a,b; Jelinek and Darnell, 1972); and
3) uridylate-rich sequences (Burdon and Shenkin, 1972). These
sequences are typical of pre-mRNA and are degraded in the course of
its processing since they are absent from mature mRNA. Investigation of these sequences may give information about the functional
topography of pre-mRNA, in particular about its non-informative
portion. The experiments described below characterize double-
stranded (ds) sequences in pre-mRNA.

HAIRPIN-LIKE STRUCTURE IN PRE-mRNA AND DENATURED DNA

Upon treatment of nuclear RNA with pancreatic plus T_1 ribonucleases, some material is undegraded, and, according to some of its properties, seems to represent double-stranded RNA (dsRNA) (Harel and Montagnier, 1971). Ryskov *et al.* (1972) isolated dsRNA from giant pre-mRNA and showed that this is a part of the latter that is destroyed in the course of processing. Similar results have been published by Jelinek and Darnell (1972).

dsRNA was isolated according to Ryskov *et al.* (1972; 1973a,b). Nuclear pre-mRNA obtained from Ehrlich ascites carcinoma cells, labeled *in vivo* with ^{32}P, can be separated into fractions of different sized molecules. Each fraction was digested with the RNase mixture at an ionic strength of ~ 0.4 and chromatographed on Sephadex G-75 (Fig. 2). Three peaks are obtained: I elutes before tRNA (corresponding mainly to the excluded volume); II elutes as an intermediate wide peak and III is the main peak, containing mono- and oligo-nucleotides (digested material). Peak I isolated from light pre-mRNA (10-20S) consists of poly(A) exclusively. In heavy pre-mRNA, poly(A) comprises only a minor part of peak I. Poly(A) was removed by filtration through a nitrocellulose filter according to Lee *et al.* (1971). The material in peaks I and II was then deproteinized, precipitated with non-labeled carrier and analyzed.

The material of peak I, which comprises about 1% of giant pre-mRNA (>45S), is characterized by a base composition of the (A+U)-type [(A+U)=50-55%]. The material in peak II comprises 2-3% of all pre-mRNA's, regardless of size, and is very (G+C)-rich [(G+C)=75%]. In both cases the base composition is symmetrical, *i.e.* typical of dsRNA. The behavior of peaks I and II on hydroxyapatite columns is also typical of double-stranded material. It is retained on the column under conditions where single-stranded RNA is eluted and the thermal elution curves are sharp and typical of double-stranded material. The melting temperature is higher in the case of peak I, in spite of the lower (G+C) content. Thus, both peaks I and II contain dsRNA.

The length of the dsRNA sequences was measured by means of thin-layer chromatography on Sephadex G-200 and G-75 after melting in the presence of formaldehyde (to prevent formation of secondary structure), using tRNA as a marker. Peak I gives a wide distribution in the region of chains 100-150 nucleotides long; peak II is distributed in the region of shorter chains (15-20 nucleotides long). Thus, peak I contains long dsRNA sequences and peak II contains short dsRNA. If pre-mRNA is melted before RNase treatment, the dsRNA sequences are rapidly reconstituted and 2/3 of them could be recovered after cooling. This suggests that dsRNA sequences in pre-mRNA have hairpin-like structures and that the loop does not

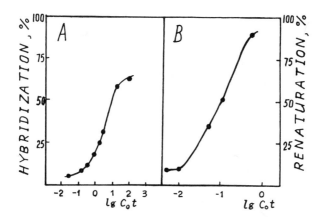

Figure 3. Hybridization and renaturation curves of dsRNA prepared from pre-mRNA of Ehrlich ascites carcinoma. A. Hybridization to an excess of immobilized mouse DNA; C_ot values were corrected by a factor of 10 as the rate of reaction with immobilized DNA is ∿10 times slower than in solution (Ryskov *et al.*, 1973a). B. Renaturation of dsRNA (Ryskov *et al.*, 1973b); dsRNA was melted by heating and annealing was in 2XSSC at 65°C.

survive RNase treatment. For this reason we use the terms "long hairpins" and "short hairpins" for the long and short dsRNA sequences.

After melting, dsRNA sequences are very efficiently hybridized to immobilized DNA (Jelinek and Darnell, 1972). The data in Fig. 3 show that the $C_ot_{1/2}$ is equal to 5-10 moles/liter/sec (Ryskov *et al.*, 1973a,b). If one assumes that 1% of the genome codes for long RNA hairpins, one can calculate that each genome contains about 500 different kinds of such sequences, each repeated about 500 times, on the average.

A more accurate measure of the complexity of hairpins can be obtained from reassociation kinetics of melted dsRNA (Fig. 3). A $C_ot_{1/2}$ of 0.05-0.1 was determined for dsRNA from Ehrlich ascites carcinoma cells. Thus about 250-500 different kinds of hairpins are present in pre-mRNA of these cells, and if one cell contains ∿10^4 hairpins each type of hairpin is represented by ∿40 copies per cell. RNA hairpins, therefore, are transcripts from reiterated DNA base sequences. These sequences are restricted to the nucleus, *i.e.*, they are absent from polysomal mRNA. Long hairpins are also absent from light nuclear pre-mRNA. Finally, neither rRNA nor pre-rRNA contain sequences of this kind.

In order to analyze further the nature of RNA hairpins, we attempted to isolate corresponding DNA sequences (Church and Georgiev,

1973). Highly-labeled denatured DNA was renatured under conditions
where any strand association, even for highly repetitive satellite
DNA, is excluded ($C_0t \leq 10^{-7}$); only linked complementary strands
should be able to reconstitute double-stranded structures in this
case. All single-stranded DNA was digested with DNase Sl; self-
renatured material resistant to this enzyme was collected and purified by chromatography on hydroxyapatite. About 2% of the DNA is
DNase-resistant at infinitely low C_0t value. This material is retained on a hydroxyapatite column and elutes like double-stranded
material. Thermal elution curves are rather sharp, indicating that
the DNase-insensitive material is double-stranded. Melting of dsDNA
does not lead to dissociation of two strands; after cooling the
material retains DNase-stability. The connection between the two
complementary strands is not destroyed by DNase Sl (in contrast to
RNase action on RNA hairpin-like structures).

To prevent self-renaturation the following procedure was developed. The material is melted in the presence of 1-2% formaldehyde,
the latter is removed by rapid gel filtration in the cold, and
DNase Sl is added immediately. About 90% of the DNase-resistant
material is now digested. After a brief incubation (during the time
required to remove HCHO from the DNA), a complete reconstitution
of dsDNA resistant to DNase takes place. Recently, Church (unpublished data) demonstrated that single-strand specific DNase from
Neurospora crassa digests the loop and, after melting, the material
reassociates with kinetics similar to that described above for dsRNA
sequences. It seems probable that the double-stranded material isolated from denatured DNA originates from inverted repetitions present in DNA and that RNA hairpin-like structures are transcripts
from DNA inverted repetitions. To check this idea, hybridization
experiments were done (Ryskov *et al.*, 1973b). DNA hairpins were
melted in the presence of HCHO and fixed on nitrocellulose filters
also in the presence of HCHO. The HCHO was removed by washing and
melted dsRNA was added. After annealing, washing and RNase treatment, the amounts of hybridized RNA and renatured RNA were determined (Table 1). It can be seen that the rate of RNA hybridization and
RNA renaturation are of the same order, *i.e.*, at similar DNA-driven
C_0t and RNA-driven C_0t values the amounts of hybridized and renatured RNA's are similar. These experiments prove that the transcription of dsRNA occurs from inverted repetitions present in the DNA,
and also confirms the hairpin-like structure present in pre-mRNA.

The functions of inverted repetitions in DNA and of hairpins
in pre-mRNA remains obscure. The concentration of long hairpins
in pre-mRNA is about 1% and the length is about 100-150 base pairs.
This corresponds to one hairpin per 20,000-30,000 nucleotides
($7-10 \times 10^6$ daltons), or roughly one hairpin per molecule of giant
pre-mRNA. The same result may be obtained from calculations based
on the amount of inverted repetitions in DNA.

Table 1. Hybridization of pre-mRNA hairpins with DNA hairpins

Exp. No.	Hybridization conditions				Radioactivity			RNA hybridized to DNA, %	RNA re-natured, %
	DNA* hairpins (μg)	RNA* hairpins (μg)	Volume in 6XSSC ml	Time (hr)	Hybridized	Non-hybridized Total	RNase-stable		
1.	0.70	0.30	0.050	2	390	1000	570	28	41
2.	0.30	0.025	0.020	2	350	740	460	32	42
3.	no DNA	0.03	0.050	2	5	1500	—	0.3	—
4.	total DNA (70.0)	0.13	2.0	0.8	400	6300	—	6	—

*Specific activity of RNA was about 50,000 cpm/μg (^{32}P) and that of DNA about 10,000 cpm/μg (^{3}H). RNA driven C_0t value was about 0.05. DNA driven C_0t value was about 0.1.

Several potential functions for these structures can be imagined. Possibly inverted repetitions in DNA correspond to acceptor
sites, reacting with regulatory or structural proteins. Alternatively, the hairpin structure in pre-mRNA may function as a boundary between the functional mRNA and the nucleus-restricted sequences; the
cleavage presumably takes place just in the loop of the hairpin.
Other possibilities are not excluded.

THE ARRANGEMENT OF HISTONES ALONG A DNA STRAND AND ITS POSSIBLE
RELATION TO FUNCTIONAL ORGANIZATION OF THE CHROMOSOME

One very important question in the field of chromosome organization is the relationship between certain sequences in DNA and
structural elements of the chromosome. The only firm fact in this
field is the localization of satellite DNA's in heterochromatic
regions of chromosomes. Some ideas concerning the position of
structural genes in the chromosome have been proposed by Crick
(1971), but experimental data are absent partly because of the
lack of techniques for the separation of different structural parts
of chromosomes and partly because the general principles of chromosome organization are unclear.

Some progress has been made by Varshavsky and Georgiev (1973a,
b). It was found previously that, under certain conditions, it is
possible to transfer, quantitatively, certain histone fractions
from chromatin to tRNA (or DNA). For example, in the presence of
magnesium, only lysine-rich histone F1 and most of the non-histone
proteins are transferred to tRNA; the histones moderately rich in
lysine, F2a2 and F2b, and arginine-rich F2a1 and F3 remain bound
to DNA (Ilyin et $al.$, 1971). The DNP fibril is unfolded under these
conditions and one can study the arrangement of residual histones
along the DNA strand using the CsCl ultracentrifugation technique
(Ilyin and Georgiev, 1969). This technique fractionates DNP according to the protein-to-DNA ratio, as the buoyant densities of protein
and DNA are very different (1.25-1.3 and 1.7 g/cm^3, respectively).

It was found that non-depleted DNP, fixed with formaldehyde,
bands as a single more-or-less homogeneous peak, whereas DNP lacking
histone F1 and some non-histone proteins gives a much more heterogeneous distribution in CsCl. However, extraction with 0.6M NaCl
also leads to a strong redistribution of other histones between DNP
chains (Varshavsky and Ilyin, in preparation). For this reason,
recent experiments utilize another method of histone F1 removal:
transfer to tRNA was performed at low ionic strength under conditions
where the redistribution of remaining histones was minimized.

Chromatin was highly labeled with [^{3}H]thymidine (DNA) and [^{14}C]-
lysine (protein). The chromatin gel was extracted with a ten-fold
excess of tRNA in low ionic strength Mg^{2+}-containing buffer, solu-

bilized carefully and separated from tRNA and tRNA-protein complexes
by gel-filtration. DNP was then fixed, sheared to different chain
lengths and ultracentrifuged to equilibrium in CsCl (Fig. 4). In
these sheared preparations two separate peaks are seen: a peak of
free DNA with a buoyant density of 1.7 and a homogeneous peak of
DNA covered with protein (ρ = 1.46-1.47). The protein to DNA ratio
in the latter peak is not changed from fraction to fraction, confirm-
ing its complete homogeneity. Depending upon the degree of shearing,
a variable amount of material is present between the two peaks.
If the DNA is 500 base pairs long, almost no intermediate material
is present, but if the DNA is ~10,000 base pairs long, all the free
DNA is associated with protein-covered chains and, instead of two
peaks, one finds a main peak with a prominent shoulder toward higher
densities (up to the 1.7 gm/cm^3 zone).

Calculations showed that free DNA constitutes about 20% of the
total DNA in chromatin lacking Fl histone, and that the average
size of free DNA comprises not less than 4000 base pairs (about
3×10^6 daltons). Thus a unit, consisting of one stretch of free
DNA and one stretch of covered DNA, is approximately 20,000 base
pairs long (~15×10^6 daltons), that is, comparable to the size of
an eukaryotic transcription unit.

Control experiments excluded the influence of possible sliding
of histones at the moment of removal of histone Fl. If chromatin
is sheared before extraction and then treated with tRNA, one ob-
serves a very similar picture, *i.e.* the formation of free DNA (Fig.
5a). When the redistribution of proteins before tRNA extraction is
induced by a brief treatment of chromatin with urea, subsequent
removal of histone Fl and non-histone proteins by tRNA treatment
results in no free DNA, even after the most intense shearing (Fig.
5b). These two controls support the idea that the arrangement of
histones found reflects the *in vivo* situation.

It was observed also that during the unfolding, some histones
may be transferred to free DNA under certain conditions. As a
result, stretches of free DNA become shorter, although the amount
of DNA may remain unchanged or increases (Varshavsky and Georgiev,
1973b). It has been suggested that in chromatin the DNP strand is
folded in hairpin-like structures, one branch of which represents
DNA covered with four histones and another that is histone-free
DNA. The first branch is packed in some regular way while the
second branch is more extended (this relates to the 4:1 ratio between covered and free DNA in Fl-depleted chromatin). Histone Fl
either binds to the second branch or joins two branches together
and its presence is important in supporting this packing of the
chromatin strand. In the course of chromatin activation, the interaction of non-histone proteins with chromatin, or histone Fl modification, may lead to separation of the branches and unfolding of
the DNP chain. The main question that arises is the relationship

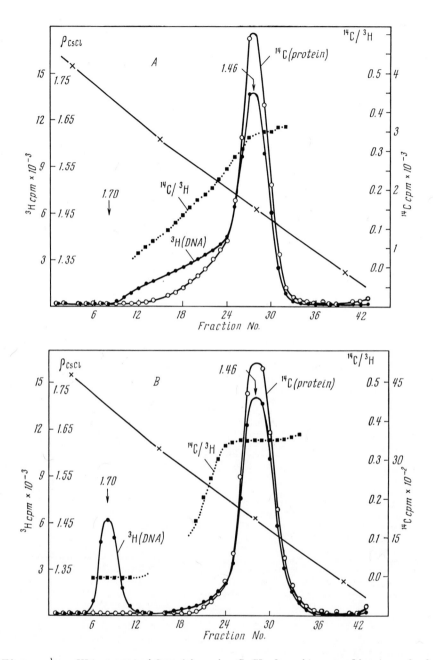

Figure 4. Ultracentrifugation in CsCl density gradients of chromosomal DNP from which histone Fl and most nonhistone proteins were
removed by transfer to tRNA in the presence of 1.0mM Mg^{2+} (Varshavsky and Georgiev, 1973a). A. Fixed, unsheared DNP (average length

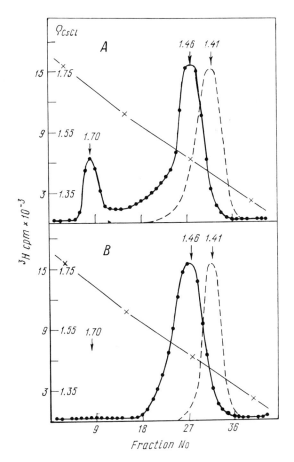

Figure 5. Ultracentrifugation in CsCl density gradients of chromosomal DNP preparations. A. Chromatin was sheared in 1mM TrisCl,
then treated with tRNA in 1.0mM $MgCl_2$ to remove histone F1, fixed
and ultracentrifuged. B. Chromatin was sheared, treated with 4M
urea, dialyzed, treated with tRNA in 1.0mM $MgCl_2$, fixed and ultracentrifuged (Varshavsky and Georgiev, 1973a). Solid circles,
[^{3}H]DNA; X-X-X, density of CsCl; ...., the positions in CsCl
density gradients of original sheared DNP untreated (A) or treated
with urea (B).

of DNA $\sim$10,000 base pairs). B. Fixed and then sheared DNP (average
lengths of DNA $\sim$500 base pairs). Solid circles, [^{3}H]DNA; open
circles, [^{14}C]protein; solid squares, [^{14}C]/[^{3}H]; X-X-X, density.

between the functional genetic elements discussed in the first
section and structural chromosomal elements described here. This
question presently is being studied in our laboratory.

REFERENCES

Bishop, J. O., R. Pemberton and C. Baglioni. 1972. Reiteration
frequency of hemoglobin genes in the duck. Nature New Biol. 235:
531.

Burdon, R. H. and A. Shenkin. 1972. Uridylate rich sequences in
rapidly labeled RNA of mammalian cells. FEBS Lett. 24: 11.

Church, R. B. and G. P. Georgiev. 1973. Double-stranded regions
in denatured DNA from mouse cells. Mol. Biol. submitted.

Crick, F. 1971. General model for the chromosomes of higher
organisms. Nature 234: 25.

Darnell, J. E., R. Wall and R. J. Tushinsky. 1971. An adenylic
acid-rich sequence in messenger RNA of HeLa and its possible relationship to reiterated sites in DNA. Proc. Nat. Acad. Sci. 68:
1321.

Edmonds, M., M. N. Vaughan and H. Nakazoto. 1971. Polyadenylic
acid sequences in the heterogeneous nuclear RNA and rapidly-labeled
polyribosomal RNA of HeLa cells: possible evidence for a precursor
relationship. Proc. Nat. Acad. Sci. 68: 1336.

Georgiev, G. P. 1969. On the structural organization of operon
and the regulation of RNA synthesis in animal cells. J. Theoret.
Biol. 25: 473.

Georgiev, G. P. 1972. The structure of transcriptional unit in
eukaryotic cells. Current Topics Devel. Biol. 6: 1.

Georgiev, G. P., A. P. Ryskov, Ch. Coutelle, V. L. Mantieva and
E. R. Avakyan. 1972. On the structure of transcriptional unit in
mammalian cells. Biochim. Biophys. Acta 259: 259.

Harel, L. and L. Montagnier. 1971. Homology of double stranded RNA
from rat liver cells with the cellular genome. Nature New Biol.
229: 106.

Ilyin, Yu. V. and G. P. Georgiev. 1969. Heterogeneity of deoxyribonucleoprotein particles as evidenced by ultracentrifugation in
cesium chloride density gradient. J. Mol. Biol. 41: 299.

Ilyin, Yu. V., A. Ja. Varshavsky, U. N. Mickelsaar and G. P. Georgiev. 1971. Studies on deoxyribonucleoprotein structure. Redistribution of proteins in mixtures of deoxyribonucleoproteins, DNA and RNA. Europ. J. Biochem. 22: 235.

Imaizumi, T., H. Diggelman and K. Scherrer. 1973. Demonstration of globin messenger sequences in giant nuclear precursors to mRNA of avian erythroblasts. Proc. Nat. Acad. Sci. 70: 1122.

Jelinek, W. and J. E. Darnell. 1972. The occurrence of double-stranded regions in HeLa cell heterogeneous nuclear RNA. Proc. Nat. Acad. Sci. 69: 2537.

Judd, B. H., M. W. Shen and T. C. Kaufman. 1972. The anatomy and function of a segment of the x-chromosome of *Drosophila melanogaster*. Genetics 71: 139.

Lee, S. Y., J. Mendecki and G. Brawerman. 1971. A polynucleotide segment rich in adenylic acid in the rapidly-labeled polyribosomal RNA component of mouse sarcoma 180 ascites cells. Proc. Nat. Acad. Sci. 68: 1331.

Leppla, S. H., B. Bjoraker and R. M. Bock. 1968. Borohydride reduction of periodate-oxidized chain ends. Methods in Enzymol. 12: 236.

Mendecki, J., S. Y. Lee and G. Brawerman. 1972. Characteristics of the polyadenylic acid segment associated with messenger ribonucleic acid in mouse sarcoma 180 ascitic cells. Biochemistry 11: 792.

Molloy, G. R., M. B. Sporn, D. E. Kelley and R. P. Perry. 1972a. Localization of polyadenylic acid sequences in messenger ribonucleic acid of mammalian cells. Biochemistry 11: 3256.

Molloy, G. R., W. L. Thomas and J. E. Darnell. 1972b. Occurrence of uridylate-rich oligonucleotide regions in heterogeneous nuclear RNA of HeLa cells. Proc. Nat. Acad. Sci. 69: 3684.

Ryskov, A. P., V. R. Farashyan and G. P. Georgiev. 1972. Ribonuclease-stable base sequences specific exclusively for giant dRNA. Biochim. Biophys. Acta 262: 568.

Ryskov, A. P., G. F. Saunders, V. R. Farashyan and G. P. Georgiev. 1973a. Double-helical regions in nuclear precursor of mRNA (pre-mRNA). Biochim. Biophys. Acta in press.

Ryskov, A. P., R. B. Church, G. Bajszar and G. P. Georgiev. 1973b. Inverted repetitions in mammalian DNA transcribed into nuclear restricted hairpin-like structures of pre-mRNA. Biochim. Biophys. Acta in press.

Suzuki, Y., L. P. Gage and D. D. Brown. 1972. The genes for silk fibroin in *Bombyx mori*. J. Mol. Biol. 70: 637.

Varshavsky, A. Ja. and G. P. Georgiev. 1973a. Structure of chromatin: very long stretches of free DNA in chromatin lacking histone Fl. Nature in press.

Varshavsky, A. Ja. and G. P. Georgiev. 1973b. Unfolding of chromosomal deoxyribonucleoproteins. Nature in press.

9. PURIFICATION OF INDIVIDUAL HISTONE mRNA'S AND EVOLUTION OF
THEIR SEQUENCES AND SIZES

Michael Grunstein*, Paul Schedl[†] and Larry Kedes*

*Departments of *Medicine and †Biochemistry, Stanford University School of Medicine, and *Veterans Administration Hospital, Palo Alto, California*

The isolation and purification of the histone messenger RNA's (mRNA's) is an important step in the analysis of eukaryotic gene organization and structure. First, histone messengers can be isolated easily and labelled to high specific activity using both tritiated uridine (Kedes and Gross, 1969) and ^{32}P (Grunstein, unpublished). Second, the DNA complementary to the messengers is moderately repetitive (Kedes and Birnstiel, 1971; Weinberg *et al.*, 1972) with 400-1200 copies per haploid DNA content. Third, sheared DNA complementary to the histone messengers has a unique buoyant density as measured by CsCl equilibrium centrifugation (Kedes and Birnstiel, 1971). Thus, the reiterated DNA exists as one or a few clusters that can be separated from bulk DNA and further analyzed structurally. Last, the knowledge that several of the histone proteins themselves exhibit nearly absolute evolutionary sequence stability (DeLange *et al.*, 1969) will allow investigation into the extent of sequence divergence of the histone messenger RNA's both "longitudinally", between species, and "horizontally", amongst the several-hundred-fold reiterated DNA complements of a single species.

The evidence that the heterogeneous 9S class of RNA's isolated from light polysomes of sea urchin embryos are indeed histone messengers has been presented elsewhere (Kedes and Gross, 1969). Recently, it has been shown that total polysomal 9S RNA of the sea urchin can direct the synthesis of the full range of histone proteins *in vitro* (Gross *et al.*, 1973). Furthermore, recent work in this laboratory has shown that individual histone mRNA's can direct the synthesis of individual histone proteins in the *in vitro* ascites cell-free system (Levy and Kedes, in preparation).

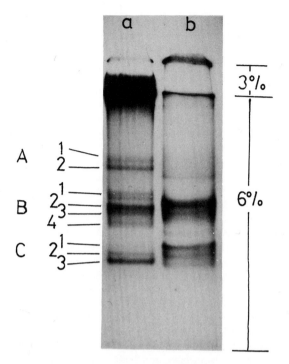

Plate I.   Autoradiograph of dried acrylamide slab gel (discontinuous 3%/6%) showing the banding patterns of (a) *L. pictus* and (b) *A. punctulata* ^{32}P-labelled 9S RNA.   Embryos were labelled with carrier-free [32]P (50 µCi/ml, artificial sea water) until the 64-128 cell stage.   Polysomal 9S RNA was extracted, dissolved in 1mM EDTA, 40% glycerol and layered onto the slab gel.   Electrophoresis took place in the 0.039M phosphate buffer of Loening (1969) for 15 hr at 20mA/slab.   Details of RNA extraction, electrophoresis and autoradiography will be published elsewhere.

We report here the separation of heterogeneous 9S RNA into homogeneous histone mRNA's.   In addition, we present data demonstrating the evolutionary divergence of the histone mRNA sequences.

SEPARATION OF HETEROGENEOUS 9S RNA INTO DISCRETE SUBGROUPS

When ^{32}P-labelled polysomal RNA of the sea urchin *Lytechinus pictus* is resolved by electrophoresis on a discontinuous polyacrylamide 3%/6% slab gel, the autoradiographic banding pattern shown in Plate I is obtained.   9S RNA is separated into 3 main groups (A, B and C where A is the slowest migrating group).   Each of these groups is resolved into several subgroups.   Note that the B group bands are arbitrarily designated as B1, B2, etc.   It is possible however, that

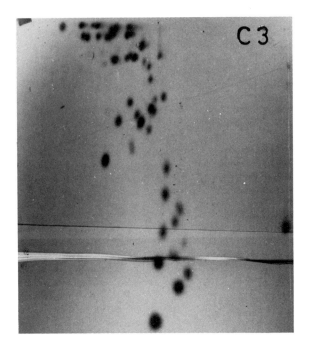

Plate II. Fingerprinting of ribonuclease T$_1$ digest of *L. pictus* ^{32}P-labelled 9S RNA C3. Ribonuclease digestion and ionophoresis conditions are those of Sanger *et al.* (1965) with a ribonuclease to RNA ratio of 1:20 (37°C, 30 min).

there are more than 4 bands within this group. When each band is eluted and rerun on 6% polyacrylamide slab gels (not shown), it is evident that slower bands of each cluster are contaminated with faster migrating RNA's of the same cluster. Band C3 is the purest species isolated to date, lacking notable contamination.

FINGERPRINT ANALYSIS OF INDIVIDUAL RNA'S

Plate II is an autoradiograph of a two-dimensional "fingerprint" of the fastest migrating RNA, *L. pictus* C3, after digestion with T$_1$ ribonuclease. This is a relatively simple fingerprint whose complexity corresponds to that of a molecule approximately 370 nucleotides long. Considering the probable presence of untranslated sequences serving at least for ribosome attachment and translation start and stop signals, this is a size one might expect for the RNA template of the smallest histone protein, histone IV (f2a$_1$) which contains 102 amino acids (DeLange *et al.*, 1969). All other histones would require templates longer than 370 nucleotides. It should be

Table 1. Base composition analysis of L. *pictus* 9S RNA. Each value represents the average of three separate determinations. Each 9S RNA band was extracted from the gel by the method of DeWachter and Fiers (1971) and digested in 0.2M KOH at 37°C for 18 hr. The hydrolyzed nucleotides were separaed on Whatman 3 MM paper by high voltage electrophoresis in pyridine-acetic acid buffer, pH 3.5 (Smith, 1968).

Band Number	Percent				Percent
	C	A	G	U	C + G
A1	26.2	30.0	25.4	18.3	51.6
A2	26.7	28.2	26.8	18.3	53.5
B1	30.2	27.3	23.1	19.4	53.3
B2	29.5	28.6	22.6	19.3	52.1
B3	31.3	25.4	22.9	20.3	54.2
B4	28.7	25.8	24.7	20.6	53.4
C1	27.8	25.1	29.3	17.8	57.1
C2	27.6	25.9	28.9	17.6	56.5
C3	26.5	24.6	31.6	17.2	58.1

noted that there is a small but reproducible degree of nucleotide heterogeneity in the C3 fingerprint. Some nucleotides are consistently found in less than molar yield. This suggests that there are sequences present in some C3 molecules but not in other molecules within this band. This may arise from gene heterogeneity within the gene family coding for C3 RNA. Alternatively, since these RNA's have been prepared from 10^7 embryos collected from 5-10 female sea urchins, genetic polymorphism within the L. *pictus* population could account for this result.

"Fingerprint" analysis of each of the other gel bands (not shown) reveals that each is a distinct sequence, and that the complexity of the fingerprint increases, in general, with greater sequence length.

BASE COMPOSITION OF FRACTIONATED RNA'S

Table 1 lists the nucleotide base compositin of each of the ^{32}P-labelled RNA fractions obtained from L. *pictus* 9S RNA. The base compositions correspond in general to those predicted for

histone messengers (Grunstein and Kedes, unpublished data). Also,
the high (G+C)-content agrees satisfactorily with that calculated
from the buoyant density of the DNA complementary to 9S RNA (Kedes
and Birnstiel, 1971) and to the thermal stability (T_m) of the 9S
RNA·DNA hybrids (Grunstein, unpublished data).

HYBRIDIZATION PROPERTIES OF 9S RNA

When minute amounts of highly labelled RNA are hybridized with
a vast excess of DNA and then treated with ribonuclease, the labelled RNA in hybrid form traces the reaction of the complementary DNA
renaturation (Melli *et al.*, 1971). This technique can be used for
both homologous and heterologous hybridization using the DNA of one
organism and the RNA of another (Grunstein, 1971; Weinberg *et al.*,
1972). In both cases one would expect that well matched hybrids
will be resistant to ribonuclease activity. Poorly matched hybrids
will either not form at all due to the instability in nucleation
sites (Walker, 1969; Southern, 1971) or if they do form, they may
be attacked by ribonuclease.

The kinetics of homologous hybridization of *L. pictus* 9S RNA
in conditions of DNA excess is presented in Fig. 1 and plotted according to the convention of Britten and Kohne (1968). The reactions
of RNA's from both groups B and C with *L. pictus* DNA show virtually
ideal second-order kinetics with indistinguishable reaction profiles. The reaction rate observed ($C_0t_{1/2}$ = 5-7) represents some
400-550 sequence repeats for each RNA sequence. This result further
suggests that the majority of 9S RNA sequences must be represented
by a very similar level of DNA sequence reiteration. This degree
of reiteration could allow widespread divergence within each family
of sequences. However, the T_m of these hybrids is 85-87°C in 0.12M
phosphate (data not shown). This is close to the stability expected of very well-matched hybrids containing homogeneous paired
sequences of approximately 50-58% (G+C) content (Mandel and Marmur,
1968). It is quite possible, however, that a low degree of divergence exists that would not be detected in an RNA·DNA hybridization
reaction. An an example, the microheterogeneity of RNA C3 (Plate
II) is undetected by such hybridization in DNA excess experiments.

THE DIVERGENCE OF 9S SEQUENCES: HYBRIDIZATION

The evolution of 9S sequences was examined by cross-hybridization using the 9S RNA of *L. pictus* and the DNA of two other sea
urchins, *Strongylocentrotus purpuratus,* which shared a common ancestor with *L. pictus* some 60 million years ago, and *Arbacia punctulata,* which diverged 200 million years ago (Durham and Melville,
1957). The results of experiments published by Weinberg *et al.*

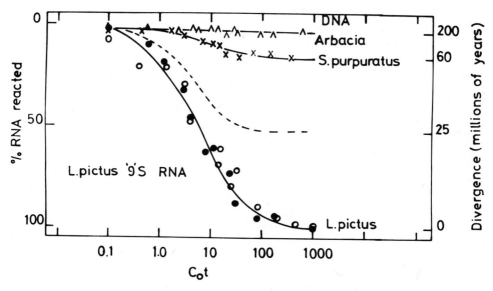

Figure 1.   Hybridization of ^{3}H-labelled *L. pictus* 9S RNA with a
variety of sea urchin DNA's (sonicated to a single-stranded molecular weight of approximately 200,000) in conditions of DNA excess
(Melli *et al.*, 1971). Open circles, *L. pictus* peak B RNA reacted
with *L. pictus* DNA; filled circles, *L. pictus* peak C RNA reacted
with *L. pictus* DNA; X-X-X, *L. pictus* peak B RNA reacted with *S.
purpuratus* DNA; ⋏-⋏-⋏, *L. pictus* peak B RNA reacted with *A. punctulata* DNA. In all cases the incubation medium consisted of 2 ml
0.12M phosphate (equimolar volumes of NaH_2PO_4 and Na_2HPO_4) at 67°C.
The DNA concentration was 3 mg/ml. The dotted line represents a
similar 9S cross-hybridization between *Paracentrotus lividus* and
Psammechinus milarus for comparison, from Weinberg *et al.* (1972).

(1972), who examined *Paracentrotus lividis* and *Psammechinus milaris*,
are included for comparison. The results are shown in Fig. 1.

     It is evident that there is a hierarchical degree of homology.
Organisms closer in evolution show a greater degree of cross-hybridization of their histone mRNA's. What is most striking, however,
is the low degree of cross-hybridization. While ribosomal RNA show
70% cross-reaction (as a percentage of the homologous reaction) between *L. pictus* and *S. purpuratus* (Grunstein, unpublished), only
16% of the 9S RNA (B group) cross-hybridizes. Cross-hybridization
of B group *L. pictus* RNA to *Arbacia* DNA shows less than 4% reaction
(Fig. 1). If indeed the histone proteins are as conserved among
sea urchin species as pea and calf histones, an explanation for the
lack of cross-hybridization of these histone templates must lie in
the degeneracy of the genetic triplet code. This is supported by

the observation that band C3 of L. *pictus* and A. *punctulata* show
very different fingerprint patterns (not shown) suggesting that extensive base changes have occurred along the molecule.

Theoretically, a single base mismatch within the minimal stable
length (MSL) necessary for hybridization to occur may preclude the
possibility of reaction at that site (Southern, 1971). Under our
conditions of hybridization (0.12M phosphate, 67°C) the MSL is approximately 10 nucleotides long (Sutton and McCallum, 1971). Hence
10% random base changes could cause a near total lack of cross-hybridization. However, since 10% random mutation, especially if restricted to third position changes, is likely to give rise to a few
oligonucleotides equal to or longer than the MSL, some hybridization
will be expected. Thus the failure of the hybridization test to
demonstrate homology between templates that may code for almost
identical proteins can be explained by the lack of sensitivity of
the hybridization method. Nevertheless, the method does demonstrate
a marked difference between the homologous and the heterologous reactions shown in Fig. 1. The homologous reaction behaves as would
be expected for a single or small number of sequences. With some
400 DNA repeats coding for an mRNA class, one might expect a large
degree of horizontal divergence in the homologus sequences as well.
Why there is so little heterogeneity within the gene family cannot
yet be explained.

The main problem in interpreting with greater precision reassociation data of this kind lies in the fact that we do not know
the exact effect of ribonuclease on partially matched hybrids, nor
the exact effect of sequence divergence on either the rate or extent
of reassociation. Without this information one can make only very
general assumptions as to the nature and degree of evolutionary
changes.

THE DIVERGENCE OF 9S SEQUENCES: MOLECULAR SIZE

L. *pictus* and A. *punctulata* shared a common ancestor over 200
million years ago. The evidence presented above demonstates that
the nucleotide sequence of the 9S RNA's of these sea urchins has
diverged. Comparison of the electrophoretic mobility of the fractionated 9S RNA's from these two species allows us to examine the
evolution of the RNA in another manner. Plate I is an autoradiograph of the ^{32}P-labelled 9S RNA's from these two species of urchins
after separation on a 3%/6% discontinuous polyacrylamide slab gel.
The two RNA preparations share the A, B and C clustering pattern
but the *Arbacia* messengers migrate somewhat more rapidly than those
of *Lytechinus*. If we assume a direct correspondence between the
RNA fractions of the two species, the mobility differences may reflect absolute molecular weight differences among the templates for
a specific histone. Since the amino-acid sequence of some histones

is rigidly conserved in evolution, we propose that these species-dependent molecular-weight differences may represent sequence-length differences in untranslated portions of the mRNA molecule. Proof of this proposal must await further sequence analysis of the mRNA's.

ACKNOWLEDGMENT

     This work was supported in part by grants from the Veterans Administration, and the USPHS GM HD17995. M.G. is a Fellow and L.K. a scholar of the Leukemia Society of America. P.S. is the recipient of a Biochemistry Training Grant USPHS GM 00196.

REFERENCES

Britten, R. J. and D. E. Kohne. 1968. Repeated sequences in DNA. Science 161: 529.

DeLange, R. J., D. M. Fambrough, E. L. Smith and J. Bonner. 1969. Calf and pea histone IV. J. Biol. Chem. 244: 319.

DeWachter, R. and W. Fiers. 1971. Fractionation of RNA by electro-phoresis on polyacrylamide gel slabs. In (L. Grossman and K. Moldave, eds.) Methods in Enzymology, Vol. XXI, Part D. p. 167. Academic Press, New York and London.

Durham, J. W. and R. V. Melville. 1957. A classification of echinoids. J. of Paleontology 31: 242.

Gross, K., J. Ruderman, M. Jacobs-Lorena, C. Baglioni and P. R. Gross. 1973. Cell-free synthesis of histones directed by messenger RNA from sea urchin embryos. Nature New Biol. 241: 272.

Grunstein, M. 1971. Structure and evolution of the ribosomal RNA genes. Ph.D. Thesis, University of Edinburgh.

Kedes, L. H. and M. L. Birnstiel. 1971. Reiteration and clustering of DNA sequences complementary to histone messenger RNA. Nature New Biol. 230: 165.

Loening, U. E. 1969. The determination of the molecular weight of ribonucleic acid by polyacrylamide gel electrophoresis. Biochem. J. 113: 131.

Mandel, M. and J. Marmur. 1968. Use of ultraviolet absorbance-temperature profile for determining the guanine plus cytosine con-tent of DNA. In (L. Grossman and K. Moldave, eds.) Methods in Enzymology, Vol. XII, Part B. p. 195. Academic Press, New York and London.

Melli, M., C. Whitfield, K. V. Rao, M. Richardson and J. D. Bishop. 1971. DNA-RNA hybridization in vast DNA excess. Nature New Biol. 231: 8.

Sanger, F., G. G. Brownlee and B. G. Barrell. 1965. A two-dimensional fractionation procedure for radioactive nucleotides. J. Mol. Biol. 13: 373.

Smith, J. D. 1967. Paper electrophoresis of nucleic acid components. In (L. Grossman and K. Moldave, eds.) Methods in Enzymology, Vol. XII, Part A. p. 350. Academic Press, New York and London.

Southern, E. M. 1971. Effects of sequence divergence on the reassociation properties of repetitive DNA's. Nature New Biol. 232: 82.

Sutton, W. D. and M. McCallum. 1971. Mismatching and the reassociation rate of mouse satellite DNA. Nature New Biol. 232: 83.

Walker, P. M. B. 1969. The specificity of molecular hybridization in relation to studies on higher organisms. Prog. in Nucl. Acid Res. and Mol. Biol. 9: 301.

Weinberg, E. S., M. L. Birnstiel, I. F. Purdom and R. Williamson. 1972. Genes coding for polysomal 9S RNA of sea urchins: Conservation and divergence. Nature New Biol. 240: 225.

10. REITERATION OF DNA CODING FOR COLLAGEN MESSENGER RNA

R. Brentani, N. Marques, J. Balsamo, L. Wang, M. Myiashita
and A. M. S. Stolf

*Laboratório de Oncologia Experimental, Faculdade de
Medicina, Universidade de São Paulo, São Paulo, Brasil*

Early morphological evidence (Schultz, 1965) led to the conclusion that, during cell differentiation, either loss or selective
replication of genetic material can occur.

When eukaryotic DNA was shown to possess repeated sequences,
besides unique species (Britten and Kohne, 1968), it seemed that the
molecular correspondent of selective gene replication had been found.
So far, however, reiterative DNA classes are present in centromeric
DNA (Pardue and Gall, 1970) or code for such ubiquitous materials
as rRNA (Birnstiel *et al.*, 1971) or histone mRNA (Kedes and Birnstiel, 1971). On the other hand, work with highly differentiated
cells has demonstrated that hemoglobin mRNA (Bishop *et al.*, 1972)
and fibroin mRNA (Suzuki *et al.*, 1972) are transcribed from unique
sequences.

We have attempted here to understand the redundancy discrepancy
of genes coding for different mRNA species and to show that genes
coding for specific proteins may be selectively amplified in those
cells that express these genes. Collagen mRNA was chosen as a model
because it has already been characterized (Brentani *et al.*, 1973)
by the ability of chick embryo RNA to affect proline incorporation
by rat liver ribosomes.

Collagen synthesizing ribosomes were separated from the bulk
of the ribosomal population, from guinea pig granulomas, by low-
speed centrifugation, taking advantage of the fact that the collagen-
synthesizing aggregation is supposed to contain 100 ribosomes (Gould,
1968).

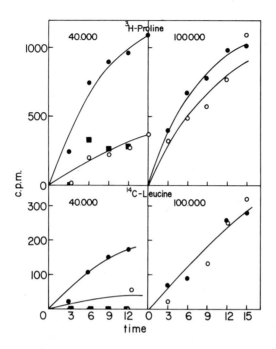

Figure 1. Amino acid incorporation by granuloma cytoplasmic fractions. Granulomas were induced in guinea pigs by subcutaneous injections of carrageenan (Robertson and Schwartz, 1953). After ho-
mogenization, the tissue was detergent-treated as if to prepare
polysomes (Borun *et al.*, 1967). Nuclei and cell debris were spun
out at 1,000g and the suspension was centrifuged at 40,000g for one
hour. After saving the 40,000g pellet, the supernatant was re-
centrifuged at 100,000g for two hours to yield the 100,000g pellet.
Conditions of incubation and radioactivity determination have been
previously described (Brentani *et al.*, 1973).

The product of amino acid incorporation (Fig. 1) by the 40,000g
pellet was tentatively identified as collagen because of the effect
of collagenase on the incorporation, and because of its solubility
in hot trichloroacetic acid. The product of incorporation by the
100,000g pellet is richer in leucine content and also insoluble in
hot trichloroacetic acid.

Labeled RNA, obtained from the 40,000g pellet was next hybridized to DNA fractions separated by centrifuging purified chromatin
DNA in CsCl gradients. Fig. 2 shows that most of the hybridization
takes place with DNA of very high (G+C) content [estimated (G+C) =
83%] providing further evidence that this cytoplasmic fraction is
involved in collagen synthesis. Indeed, collagen mRNA would be ex-

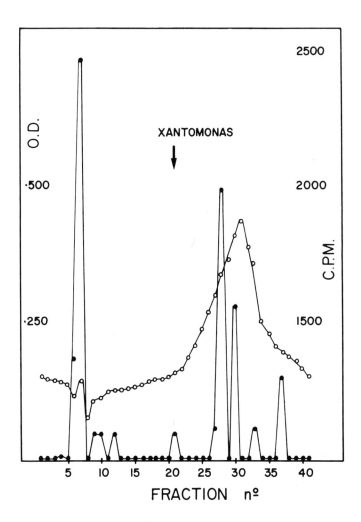

Figure 2. Hybridization of 40,000g pellet RNA to chromatin DNA.
RNA was extracted (Perry *et al.*, 1972) from 40,000g pellets obtained
after incubating granuloma slices with $^{32}P_i$ for one hour. DNA was
purified from chromatin prepared by salt extraction of granuloma
nuclei (Steele *et al.*, 1965). Centrifugation on CsCl gradients, denaturation and immobilization of gradient fractions on filters and
hybridization conditions have been described (Brentani *et al.*, 1973).

pected to contain more than 80% (G+C), from the protein's amino acid
composition (Eastoe, 1968). It is also clear that rRNA does not
participate in the hybridization reaction (Fig. 2).

Table I.   Detection of Poly(A) Sequences in 40,000g Pellet RNA

	Millipore	Poly(U)
Input radioactivity	100	100
Filter-retained radioactivity	48.3	48.1
Enzyme-resistant radioactivity	9.1	9.5
Alkali-resistant radioactivity	0.72	1.17

Estimation of poly(A) content was performed utilizing both retention by Millipore filters (Lee et al., 1971) and by glass fiber-poly(U) filters (Sheldon et al., 1972). Enzyme digestion with 10μg RNase and 50 units RNase T_1, was carried out for 30 minutes at 37°C. RNA was hydrolyzed with KOH (final concentration = 0.3M) for 18 hours at 37°C.

Examination of 40,000g pellet RNA for its poly(A) content reveals (Table I) that about 50% of the fraction's radioactivity is retained by filters under conditions in which poly(A) containing messengers are bound. The poly(A) chain comprises about 20% of the polymer's total length and is of a ribonucleotide nature, since it is alkali-labile.

Hybridization of labeled 40,000g pellet RNA with chromatin DNA, under conditions of vast DNA excess, shows that when granuloma DNA is employed, most of the RNA is rendered RNase-resistant at C_ot values between 10 and 1,000 [average $C_ot_{1/2}$ (50% resistance) = 100-150], whereas when liver DNA is substituted for granuloma DNA, only 20% of the RNA anneals at C_ot values smaller than 100 (Fig. 3). The $C_ot_{1/2}$ value for liver chromatin DNA is around 8,000. Since the amount of radioactivity rendered RNase resistant (Fig. 3) is roughly equivalent to that bound by filters (Table I) these results can be interpreted as indicating that genes coding for collagen mRNA are 100 to 150 times repeated in granuloma DNA and less than 5-fold repeated in liver DNA, considering the structural complexity of guinea pig DNA (Sparrow et al., 1972).

From actinomycin D inhibition experiments (Bekhor et al., 1965) collagen mRNA appears to be markedly unstable and therefore our results suggest that selective gene amplification may take place in cells synthesizing specific proteins translated from unstable messengers.

ACKNOWLEDGMENTS

This work was supported by grants from the Projeto Bioq/FAPESP and CNPQ. We also acknowledge the able technical assistance of Mr. A. M. Olmo. Permanent address of RB and JB: Departamento de Bioquímica, Instituto de Química, USP.

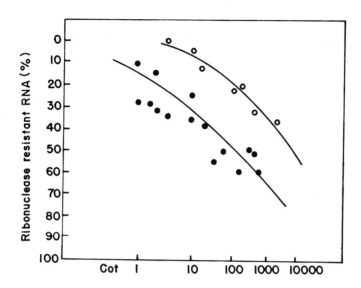

Figure 3. Time course of reassociation of granuloma DNA and liver
DNA in the presence of cytoplasmic RNA fractions. Sonicated DNA at
a concentration of 5 mg/ml (usually 2.0 ml) was heat denatured and
10 µg of radioactive 40,000g pellet RNA was added after cooling.
The mixture was incubated at 65°C and at intervals 0.1 ml aliquots
were withdrawn and delivered into 2 ml ice-cold 1XSSC and quickly
frozen. Upon termination of the experiment, one half of each sample
was treated with 10 µg pancreatic RNase and 50 units RNase T$_1$ for
30 minutes at 37°C. Both treated and untreated samples were precipitated with trichloroacetic acid in the presence of 100 µg carrier RNA and collected on Millipore filters.

REFERENCES

Bekhor, I. J., Z. Mohseni, N. E. Nimni and L. A. Bavetta. 1965.
The biosynthesis of microsomal-bound collagen precursor in rabbit
embryo skin *in vitro*. Proc. Nat. Acad. Sci. 54: 615.

Birnstiel, M. L., M. Chipchase and J. Speirs. 1971. The ribosomal
RNA cistrons. Prog. Nucleic Acid Res. Mol. Biol. 11: 351.

Bishop, J. O., R. Pemberton and C. Baglioni. 1972. Reiteration
frequency of haemoglobin genes in the duck. Nature New Biol. 235:
231.

Borun, T. W., M. D. Scharff and E. Robbins. 1967. Preparation of
mammalian polyribosomes with detergent Nonidet P40. Biochim. Biophys. Acta 149: 302.

Brentani, R., C. S. Peres, L. Wang and C. H. Oda. 1973. Messenger RNA processing in vertebrate cells. In (F. T. Kenney, B. Hamkalo, G. Favelukes and J. T. August, eds.) Gene Expression and Its Regulation. p. 169. Plenum Press, New York.

Britten, R. J. and D. E. Kohne. 1968. Repeated sequences in DNA. Science 161: 529.

Eastoe, J. E. 1968. Composition of collagen and allied proteins. In (G. N. Ramachandran, ed.) Treatise on Collagen vol II part A p. 19. Academic Press, New York.

Gould, B. S. 1968. Collagen biosynthesis. In (G. N. Ramachandran, ed.) Treatise on Collagen vol II part A p. 39. Academic Press, New York.

Kedes, L. H. and M. L. Birnstiel. 1971. Reiteration and clustering of DNA sequences complementary to histone messenger RNA. Nature New Biol. 230: 165.

Lee, S. Y., J. Mendecki and G. Brawerman. 1971. A polynucleotide segment rich in adenylic acid in the rapidly labeled polyribosomal RNA component of mouse sarcoma 180 ascites cells. Proc. Nat. Acad. Sci. 68: 1371.

Pardue, M. L. and J. G. Gall. 1970. Chromosomal localization of mouse satelite DNA. Science 168: 1356.

Perry, R. P., J. LaTorre, D. E. Kelley and J. R. Greenberg. 1972. On the lability of poly(A)sequences during extraction of messenger RNA from polyribosomes. Biochim. Biophys. Acta 262: 220.

Robertson, W. van B. and B. Schwartz. 1953. Ascorbic acid and the formation of collagen. J. Biol. Chem. 201: 689.

Schultz, J. 1965. Genes, differentiation and animal development. Brookhaven Symp. Biol. 18: 116.

Sheldon, R., C. Jurale and J. Kates. 1972. Detection of polyadenylic acid sequences in viral and eucaryotic RNA. Proc. Nat. Acad. Sci. 69: 417.

Sparrow, A. H., H. J. Price and A. G. Underbrink. 1972. A survey of DNA content per cell and per chromosome of procaryotic and eucaryotic organisms: some evolutionary considerations. Brookhaven Symp. Biol. 23: 451.

Steele, W. J., Jr., M. Okamura and H. Busch. 1965. Effects of thioacetamide on the composition and biosynthesis of nucleolar and nuclear RNA in rat liver. J. Biol. Chem. 240: 1742.

Suzuki, Y., L. P. Page and D. D. Brown. 1972. The genes for silk fibroin in *Bombyx mori*. J. Mol. Biol. <u>70</u>: 637.

11. ON THE ROLE OF POLY A SEQUENCES IN mRNA METABOLISM

R. P. Perry

The Institute for Cancer Research, Fox Chase Center for Cancer and Medical Sciences, Philadelphia, Pennsylvania

In this brief report I shall discuss some experiments designed to examine critically two hypotheses concerning the role of poly-adenylic acid (poly A) sequences in messenger RNA (mRNA) metabolism. One hypothesis specifies a nuclear function for poly A in the processing of heterogeneous nuclear RNA (HnRNA) into mRNA; the other postulates a cytoplasmic role for poly A in stabilizing mRNA after it becomes incorporated into polyribosomes.

Experiments performed in several laboratories (Mendecki *et al.*, 1972; Molloy *et al.*, 1972; Sheldon *et al.*, 1972; Nakazato *et al.*, 1973; Adesnik and Darnell, 1972; Greenberg and Perry, 1972a; Adesnik *et al.*, 1972; Perry *et al.*, 1973) have indicated (i) that poly A sequences are located at the 3'-OH termini of some HnRNA molecules and of essentially all species of mRNA except those coding for histones; and (ii) that both polyadenylation of HnRNA and entry into polyribosomes of newly synthesized mRNA are inhibited by the drug 3'-deoxyadenosine (cordycepin). These observations suggested that polyadenylation might be required for the proper processing of most kinds of mRNA, and led us to consider the hypothesis that polyadenylation of an HnRNA molecule ensures that it will be eventually processed and transported to the cytoplasm. Poly-adenylation would thus be associated with transcript selection. This hypothesis, at least in its simplest form, predicts that poly A segments should be conserved during the HnRNA→mRNA transition, a situation which is in marked contrast to the large intranuclear turnover of the total HnRNA (Darnell, 1968). In some respects, the conservation of poly A would be analogous to the conservation of methylated nucleotides that characterize the processing of ribosomal RNA (Perry, 1969).

It has also been observed that the length of the poly A segment in mRNA decreases as the mRNA ages in the cytoplasm (Mendecki
et al., 1972; Greenberg and Perry, 1972b; Sheiness and Darnell,
1973). This fact, plus indications from earlier experiments with
actinomycin-treated cells that the histone message, which lacks
poly A, is less stable than other mRNA (Borun *et al.*, 1967; Gallwitz and Mueller, 1969; Craig *et al.*, 1971), gave rise to the idea
that poly A may in some way be implicated in the regulation of mRNA
turnover. If this hypothesis were true, one might expect that the
histone messages would have considerably higher rates of turnover
compared to other mRNA's, and furthermore that the turnover rate of
the poly A-containing mRNA [poly A(+)mRNA] would increase with age
of the message.

The predictions stated above were tested in a series of experiments in which we measured the kinetics of incorporation of radioactive precursors into mRNA, HnRNA and poly A segments in both
nuclear and cytoplasmic fractions of growing L cells. The results
of such experiments, summarized below and described in detail elsewhere (Greenberg, 1972; Perry and Kelley, submitted; Perry, Kelley
and LaTorre, submitted) indicate that there is no quantitative
transfer of poly A from nucleus to cytoplasm, and hence that the
"transcript selection" hypothesis is essentially untenable. Moreover, the results of mRNA turnover measurements tend to argue against
a simple relationship between the stability of a particular mRNA
molecule and the relative length of its poly A segment.

REQUISITE CONDITIONS FOR MEANINGFUL KINETIC STUDIES

In order for kinetic data to be correctly interpreted in terms
of reaction rates and steady state concentrations of intermediates
and products, several restrictive conditions must be met (McCarthy
and Britten, 1962). In experiments in which growing cells are
allowed to incorporate radioactive precursor continuously into metabolically stable and unstable products, it is essential that the
labeling procedure not cause any significant perturbations in the
physiological state of the cells, and that there be no change in
the specific radioactivity of the precursor pools over the course
of the experiment. The former condition can be verified in an
exponentially growing population of cells by demonstrating that the
culture remains in steady exponential growth at its characteristic
doubling time. The latter condition can be achieved by using precursors of low specific activity so that the amount of exogenous
precursor is always large relative to the amount utilized. In our
experiments, for example, we have found it necessary to use at least
9 femtamoles of adenosine per cell for experiments of 90 minutes
duration, and more than 375 femtamoles per cell for experiments
lasting 24 hours. I am emphasizing this point because it may help

explain the difference between some of the kinetic data presented
here and that from similar experiments on HeLa cells mentioned
earlier by Darnell (Jelenik *et al.*, 1973).

KINETICS OF ADENOSINE INCORPORATION INTO THE POLY A SEGMENT
AND NON-POLY A PORTION OF mRNA

In the experiments shown in Fig. 1, we isolated polyribosomal
RNA from cells labeled for various periods of time with [³H]adeno-
sine and measured the incorporation into the poly A(+)mRNA and into
the poly A segment, excised from the poly A(+)mRNA by appropriate
ribonuclease treatment. It is seen that there is a much more rapid
entry of label into the poly A segment than into the non-poly A
portion of the molecule. This fact, also observed in earlier experiments by Brawerman and coworkers (Mendecki *et al.*, 1972), confirms the post-transcriptional nature of the poly A addition (Darnell *et al.*, 1971). A constant rate of labeling of the poly A segment is reached within less than 10 minutes, whereas more than 25
minutes are required to attain a constant rate of labeling of the
non-poly A region. This indicates that the polyadenylation of mRNA
is a relatively late event, *i.e.*, that it occurs during the latter
portion of the interval between transcription of mRNA precursor and
appearance of the mRNA in the cytoplasmic polyribosomes.

COMPARATIVE KINETICS OF LABELING OF NUCLEAR AND CYTOPLASMIC POLY A

The very rapid achievement of a constant rate of labeling of
the poly A in mRNA would lead one to predict that the precursor of
this poly A, presumably the poly A in HnRNA, should approach its
maximum specific activity within a very short time.[1] However, contrary to this expectation, when the kinetics of labeling of the
poly A in HnRNA were measured (Fig. 2), the specific activity continued to increase for at least one hour. The failure to obtain
kinetic data consistent with a simple precursor-product relationship was confirmed and extended in another experiment (Fig. 3) in
which we followed the time course of labeling of total nuclear
and cytoplasmic poly A over a period equivalent to several cell
generations. A quantitative analysis of these data indicates that

---

[1] This expectation follows from the rate equations governing
radioactive labeling (Perry, Kelley and LaTorre, submitted). The
rate of labeling of a product at early times, when product turnover
can be ignored, is proportional to the specific activity of its
immediate precursor.

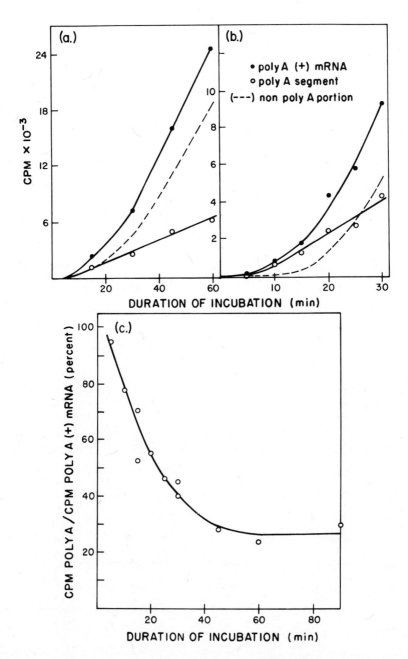

Figure 1. Kinetics of incorporation of [³H]adenosine into poly A
segments and into total poly A(+)mRNA in polyribosomes. Panels (a)
and (b) illustrate two similar experiments. Exponentially growing
cells were concentrated to 2.8 X 10⁶ cells/ml and incubated with
20 µCi/ml [³H]adenosine (21.3 µM total adenosine concentration). At

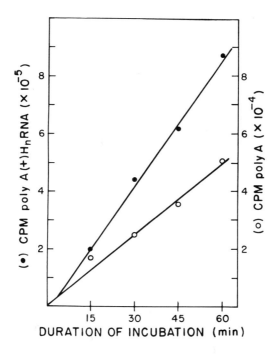

Figure 2. Kinetics of incorporation into poly A segments of HnRNA
and total poly A (+)HnRNA. RNA was extracted from the nuclei of
the experiment shown in Fig. 1a and assayed for poly A and poly
A(+)mRNA as described in Fig. 1. The ordinate effectively represents
specific activity since each sample contained approximately the
same number of cells.

selected time intervals, samples containing approximately 2.2×10^7
cells (a), or 3.7×10^7 cells (b) were harvested, the cells lysed
by treatment with 0.05% Triton X-100 and polyribosomes isolated from
the cytoplasmic fraction by sucrose gradient centrifugation. RNA
was extracted from the polyribosomes with sodium dodecyl sulfate-
chloroform-phenol and either assayed directly on poly U-impregnated
glass fiber filters for poly A(+)mRNA, or treated with a mixture of
ribonucleases A and T_1 and then assayed on poly U-filters for poly
A. The activity in the non-poly A portion of the mRNA was obtained
by difference: poly A(+)mRNA minus poly A. In panel (c) the data
from several experiments are expressed as a ratio of the radioactivity in the poly A segment to the radioactivity in the total poly
A(+)mRNA and plotted as a function of incubation time.

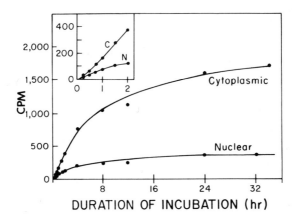

Figure 3.   Kinetics of incorporation into poly A in nuclear and
cytoplasmic compartments.   A 1300 ml culture of exponentially growing L cells at an initial concentration of 1.25 X 10^5 cells/ml was
labeled with 2 µCi/ml [^{3}H]adenosine (60µM total adenosine concentration).   To maintain a constant supply of exogeneous precursor
and a roughly comparable cell density over the entire course of the
experiment, the culture was diluted at 12 and 25 hr with 0.7 volume
of fresh medium containing 26 µCi/ml [^{3}H]adenosine and 79 µM total
adenosine.   The slightly higher concentrations were used to replen-
ish the precursor consumed by the cells.   At selected time intervals,
100 to 200 ml of culture was harvested and the cells fractionated
into nuclei, cytoplasm and a nuclear wash fraction.   A constant
amount of commercial [^{14}C]-labeled poly A was added to each sample
and RNA extracted with sodium dodecyl sulfate-chloroform-phenol.
Each RNA sample was treated with appropriate nucleases and poly A
assayed on poly U-glass fiber filters.   The [^{3}H]data were corrected
for yield by normalizing to a constant amount of [^{14}C].   The kinetics
of the cytoplasm and nuclear fractions were indistinguishable and
therefore the data for these were combined and plotted as a single
fraction designated "cytoplasmic".

only a relatively small fraction of the poly A found in the nucleus
could actually serve as precursor to the poly A in mRNA; the remainder would presumably turn over with the nucleus.   This lack of
conservation of poly A would seem to disfavor the "transcript selection" hypothesis.   Moreover, the observed initial rate of labeling of nuclear poly A appears to be insufficient to account for the
observed rate of labeling of total cytoplasmic poly A, suggesting
that there may be some polyadenylation which occurs concurrently
with, or even subsequent to, emergence of RNA into the cytoplasm.

TURNOVER OF POLY A-CONTAINING MESSENGER RNA

Measurements of steady state labeling kinetics can also be used to obtain information about the metabolic lifetime and mode of decay of mRNA (Greenberg, 1972; Perry and Kelley, submitted). In the case of metabolically stable RNA components, such as ribosomal RNA (rRNA) or transfer RNA (tRNA), the normalized incorporation rate is determined solely by the growth rate of the cells, so that after a small initial lag the RNA attains 50% of its maximum specific activity after one doubling time, 75% after two doubling times, 87.5% after three, etc. For metabolically unstable components which decay by a first order (stochastic) process the incorporation curves have a similar shape except that a given percent of maximum specific activity is attained in a shorter time. The time required to reach 50% maximum specific activity is equal to $T_D \times T_{1/2}/(T_D + T_{1/2})$ where T_D is the doubling time of the cell population, and $T_{1/2}$ is the halflife of the unstable RNA component. From an analysis of such data (Fig. 4) we have estimated the mean lifetime ($T_m = T_{1/2}/\ln 2$) of the poly A(+)mRNA in L cells to be approximately 15 hr. In cells growing more slowly (at lower temperatures) the mean lifetime of poly A(+)mRNA was observed to be proportionally longer.

The fact that the data for rRNA follows the theoretically predicted curve for a stable RNA component verifies that the intracellular precursor pool used for synthesis remained at a constant specific activity over the course of the experiment. The fact that the data for the poly A(+)mRNA in this and several other similar experiments follow curves derived for a first-order decay process suggests that the turnover of poly A(+)mRNA may be a stochastic phenomenon. However, this method of analysis is relatively insensitive for distinguishing between the situation in which all components decay with a single mean lifetime *versus* there being several classes of components, each of which decays with a distinctive mean lifetime. In fact, the results of recent experiments in which the decay of differentially labeled pulse-and steady-state-labeled poly A(+)mRNA was followed during a chase in unlabeled medium (Singer and Penman, 1973; E. Bard, unpublished observations) do indeed suggest that there is a class of short-lived mRNA components in addition to the longer-lived components described above.

The important observation insofar as the hypothetical role of poly A is concerned is that the life expectancy of old mRNA molecules, which have relatively short poly A segments, does not appear to be *less* than that of new mRNA molecules which have maximum-sized poly A segments. If such were the case, one would expect the incorporation curves for poly A(+)mRNA to have a sigmoid shape such as the dotted curve shown in Fig. 6, and in chase experiments one would expect the data to show increasingly negative deviations from exponential decay as time proceeds. Since this does not seem to be the case, we can conclude that the length of the poly A segment, *per se,* is not a determinant of mRNA stability.

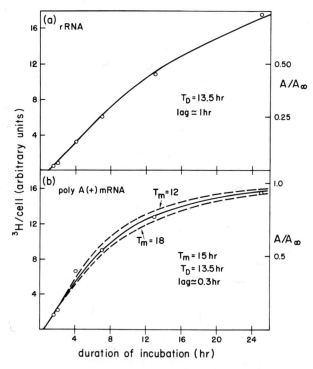

Figure 4.   Kinetics of uridine incorporation into ribosomal RNA and poly A(+)mRNA. A culture of exponentially growing L cells (doubling time T_D=13.5 hr) was incubated with 2 μCi/ml [^{3}H]uridine (11.5 μM total uridine concentration). Cell density was maintained between 1.2 and 2.4 X 10^5 cells/ml by a 1:1 dilution with fresh labeled medium at 13 hr. At various periods of time, samples of from 2 to 4 X 10^7 cells were harvested, mixed with a constant amount (1.8 X 10^7 of cells labeled for 21 hr with 1 μCi/ml [^{32}P]orthophosphate and used for the isolation of polyribosomal RNA as described in Fig. 1. The RNA was assayed with respect to (a) total trichloro-acetic acid-insoluble radioactivity, which, for incubations greater than a few hours, consists almost entirely of rRNA and (b) poly A(+)mRNA as measured by the poly U-filter method. The [^{3}H]data were corrected for yield by normalizing to a constant amount of ^{32}P. Solid curves are theoretical curves obeying the equation $A/A_\infty = 1-e^{-(k_D+k_T)t}$ where A and A_∞ represent the radioactivity per cell in the particular RNA species under consideration at time t and t→∞, respectively. The time $t=t_i-t_{lag}$ is the time necessary to reach maximal incorporation rate; k_D is the growth constant of the cell culture (k_D=ln2/T_D); and k_T is the turnover rate constant (k_T+1/T_m= ln2/$T_{1/2}$ where T_m and $T_{1/2}$ are the mean lifetime and halflife, re-spectively). For rRNA (a) the parameters used were k_D=0.0513 hr^{-1}, k_T=0 and t_{lag}=1 hr; for poly A(+)mRNA (b) the parameters are k_D= 0.0513 hr^{-1}, k_T=0.0666 hr^{-1} (T_m=15 hr) and t_{lag}=0.3 hr. In (b) two

TURNOVER CHARACTERISTICS OF HISTONE mRNA

We have also determined the lifetime and mode of decay of histone mRNA. Since we could not resort to methods based on poly A
selectivity for the isolation of this mRNA species we had to devise
a reliable way of identifying the histone message in the presence
of large quantities of other RNA components which are labeled after
relatively long incubation times. We made use of the selective
disappearance of histone mRNA from the polyribosomes soon after the
synthesis of DNA is inhibited with a drug such as cytosine arabinoside (araC) (Borun *et al.*, 1967). By analyzing the mRNA with acryl-
amide-gel electrophoresis and measuring the difference between the
radioactivity in a designated set of gel fractions of RNA from control cells and the same fractions of RNA from cells treated with
araC one hour before harvesting, we could effectively measure an
activity which represents histone mRNA (Fig. 5).

The steady state labeling kinetics obtained using this technique did not follow curves based on first-order decay as was observed for the poly A(+)mRNA, but rather seemed to follow curves
representing an age-dependent decay or a zero-ordered process with
a fixed lifetime of about 11 hrs (Fig. 6). A model which gives a
good fit to the data considers that the histone messages persist
for a fixed duration of the cell cycle, *e.g.*, the DNA synthetic
phase, and are then destroyed in a "sensitive period" after this
phase.

The noteworthy observation here is that the histone messages,
which, as far as we know, totally lack poly A sequences, do *not*
have unusually short lifetimes. This would seem to support the con-
tention that the poly A segment *per se* does not stabilize mRNA with
respect to random degradative events. However, at the moment one
could still entertain the possibility that the lack of poly A on the
histone messages might render them uniquely sensitive to destruction
during a restricted period of the cell cycle.

CONCLUSIONS AND PERSPECTIVES

The above experiments were designed to test certain hypotheses
formulated on the basis of current notions about the role of poly
A in mRNA metabolism. Although we have not yet definitively established the physiological significance of poly A, the results obtain-

---

other theoretical curves (dashed lines) are shown for k_D=0.0513 hr^{-1},
t_{lag}=0.3 hr and either k_T=0.0833 hr^{-1} (T_m=12 hr) or k_T=0.0555 hr^{-1}
(T_m=18 hr).

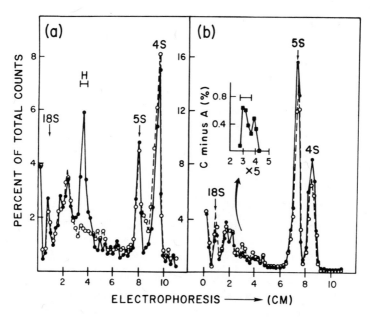

Figure 5. Polyacrylamide gel profiles of low molecular weight polyribosomal RNA from control cells (solid curves) and cells treated
with araC (dashed curves). In the experiment described in Fig. 4,
an equivalent sample of cells at each time point was incubated with
40 µg cytosine arabinoside (araC)/ml for one hour before harvesting.
The polyribosomal RNA from control and araC-treated cells was centrifuged on 15-25% (w/w) sucrose gradients and the low molecular
weight components (∼4-15S) analyzed by polyacrylamide gel electrophoresis. (a) Cells labeled for 2 hr; (b) cells labeled for 25 hr.
In (b) the difference between the percent radioactivities in control and araC cells in the region of the histone mRNA (horizontal
bar designated "H") is plotted on a 5-fold enlarged scale (solid
squares). Electrophoresis for 3.75 hr at 5 mA per gel on 6%, 9 mm
diameter, polyacryalmide gels.

ed to date allow us to place certain restrictions on the possibilities. Thus, we can state, for example, that although polyadenylation of certain types of HnRNA molecules may be necessary for their
proper processing into functionally active mRNA, the polyadenylation
of a particular HnRNA molecule is not sufficient to ensure that it
will be processed. We can also state with reasonable certainty
that the stability of a particular mRNA molecule with respect to
random degradation is not appreciably diminished when the poly A
segment is of decreased length or even totally absent.

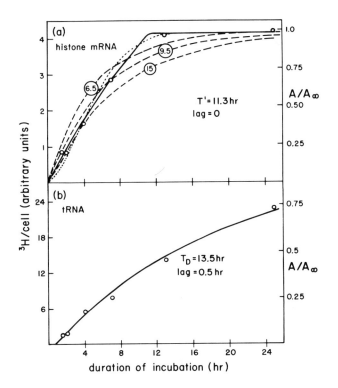

Figure 6. Kinetics of uridine incorporation into histone mRNA (a) and tRNA (b). Data are derived by summing the radioactivity in appropriate gel fractions such as those illustrated in Fig. 5. The [^{3}H]values were corrected for yield by normalizing to a constant amount of ^{32}P. For histone mRNA the ordinate represents the difference in corrected [^{3}H]radioactivity between control and araC-treated cells; for tRNA the ordinate represents the average of control and araC-treated cells. In (a) the solid curve is drawn according to the equation $A/A_\infty=(1-e^{-k_Dt})/(1-e^{-k_DT'})$, $0<t<T'$, $A/A_\infty=1$, $t>T'$, which describes an ordered decay of a molecule with a fixed lifetime, T', in a population of cells growing exponentially with a growth constant, k_D. The curve is drawn for the values: $T'=11.3$ hr and $k_D=0.0513$ hr^{-1}. The dotted, sigmoidal curve is drawn according to the equation $A/A_\infty=1-e^{-(k_D+k_Tt)t}$ which describes a linearly aging function with $k_D=0.0513$ hr^{-1} and $k_T=0.0201$ hr^{-1} ($T_m=6.25$ hr). The dashed curves are drawn according to the equation in Fig. 4 with $k_D=0.0513$ hr^{-1} and either $k_T=0.154$ hr^{-1} ($T_m=6.5$ hr), $k_T=0.105$ hr^{-1} ($T_m=9.5$ hr) or $k_T=0.666$ hr^{-1} ($T_m=15$ hr). The theoretical curve in (b) is drawn according to the equation of Fig. 4 with $k_D=0.0513$ hr^{-1}, $k_T=0$ and a lag of 0.5 hr.

ACKNOWLEDGMENT

Experiments from this laboratory were carried out in collaboration with Dr. J. LaTorre and Ms. D. E. Kelley. The research was supported by grant No. GB30721X1 from the National Science Foundation, grant Nos. CA06927 and RR05539 from the National Institutes of Health, and an appropriation from the Commonwealth of Pennsylvania.

REFERENCES

Adesnik, M. and J. E. Darnell. 1972. Biogenesis and characterization of histone messenger RNA in HeLa cells. J. Mol. Biol. 67: 397.

Adesnik, M., M. Salditt, W. Thomas and J. E. Darnell. 1972. Evidence that all messenger RNA molecules (except histone messenger RNA) contain poly A sequences and that the poly A has a nuclear function. J. Mol. Biol. 71: 21.

Borun, T. W., M. D. Scharff and E. Robbins. 1967. Rapidly labeled, polyribosome-associated RNA having the properties of histone messenger. Proc. Nat. Acad. Sci. 58: 1977.

Craig, N. C., D. E. Kelley and R. P. Perry. 1971. Lifetime of the messenger RNA's which code for ribosomal proteins in L cells. Biochim. Biophys. Acta 246: 493.

Darnell, J. E. 1968. Ribonucleic acids from animal cells. Bact. Rev. 32: 262.

Darnell, J. E., L. Philipson, R. Wall and M. Adesnik. 1971. Polyadenylic acid sequences: Role in conversion of nuclear RNA into messenger RNA. Science 174: 507.

Gallwitz, D. and G. Mueller. 1969. Histone synthesis *in vitro* on HeLa cell microsomes. J. Biol. Chem. 244: 5947.

Greenberg, J. R. 1972. High stability of messenger RNA in growing cultured cells. Nature 240: 102.

Greenberg, J. R. and R. P. Perry. 1972a. Relative occurrence of polyadenylic acid sequences in messenger and heterogeneous nuclear RNA of L cells as determined by poly (U)-hydroxylapatite chromatography. J. Mol. Biol. 72: 91.

Greenberg, J. R. and Perry, R. P. 1972b. The isolation and characterization of steady state labeled messenger RNA from L cells. Biochim. Biophys. Acta 287: 361.

Jelenik, W., M. Adesnik, M. Salditt, D. Sheiness, R. Wall, G. Molloy, L. Philipson and J. G. Darnell. 1973. Further evidence on the nuclear origin and transfer to the cytoplasm of polyadenylic acid sequences in mammalian cell RNA. J. Mol. Biol. 75: 515.

McCarthy, B. J. and R. J. Britten. 1962. The synthesis of ribosomes in *E. coli*. I. The incorporation of ^{14}C-Uracil into the metabolic pool and RNA. Biophys. J. 2: 35.

Mendecki, J., S. Y. Lee and G. Brawerman. 1972. Characteristics of the polyadenylic acid segment associated with messenger ribonucleic acid in mouse sarcoma 180 ascites cells. Biochemistry 11: 792.

Molloy, G. R., M. B. Sporn, D. E. Kelley and R. P. Perry. 1972. Localization of polyadenylic acid sequences in messenger RNA of mammalian cells. Biochemistry 11: 3256.

Nakazato, H., D. W. Kopp and M. Edmonds. 1973. Localization of the polyadenylate sequences in messenger ribonucleic acid and in the heterogeneous nuclear ribonucleic acid of HeLa cells. J. Biol. Chem. 248: 1472.

Perry, R. P. 1969. Nucleoli: The cellular sites of ribosome production. In (A. Lima-de-Faria, ed.) Handbook of Molecular Cytology. p. 620. North-Holland, Amsterdam.

Perry, R. P., J. R. Greenberg, D. E. Kelley, J. LaTorre and G. Schochetman. 1973. Messenger RNA: Its origin and fate in mammalian cells. In (F. T. Kenney, B. A. Hamkalo, G. Favelukas and J. T. August, eds.) Gene Expression and Its Regulation. p. 149. Plenum Press, New York.

Perry, R. P. and D. E. Kelley. mRNA turnover in L cells. Submitted to J. Mol. Biol.

Perry, R. P., D. E. Kelley and J. LaTorre. On the synthesis and turnover of nuclear and cytoplasmic polyadenylic acid in L cells. Submitted to J. Mol. Biol.

Sheiness, D. and J. E. Darnell. 1973. Polyadenylic acid segment in mRNA becomes shorter with age. Nature New Biol. 241: 265.

Sheldon, R., J. Kates, D. E. Kelley and R. P. Perry. 1972. Polyadenylic acid sequences on 3' termini of vaccinia messenger RNA and mammalian nuclear and messenger RNA. Biochemistry 11: 3829.

Singer, R. H. and S. Penman. Messenger RNA in HeLa cells: Kinetics of formation and decay. J. Mol. Biol. in press.

12. NONHISTONE PROTEINS OF THE NEWT GERMINAL VESICLE

Ronald J. Hill*, K. G. Maundrell and H. G. Callan

Department of Zoology, Bute Buildings, The University, St. Andrews, Fife, Scotland

The problem of assignment of intranuclear location and function to the nonhistone proteins is very much in a state of flux at present. Nonhistone proteins of the newt germinal vesicle offer a potentially interesting focus of inquiry. This giant oocyte nucleus may be isolated by microdissection in an operation monitored directly under the microscope and performed much more rapidly than classical bulk biochemical separations. Furthermore, there is a vast body of cytological information available; within the isolated nuclei peripheral nucleoli and a central mass of lampbrush chromosomes are demonstrable by phase microscopy (Gall, 1954; Callan and Lloyd, 1960).

Removal of the nuclear envelope releases the lampbrush chromosomes, nucleoplasmic granules and a variable proportion of the nucleoli. A typical portion of such a preparation from *Triturus cristatus carnifex* after centrifugation is illustrated in Fig. 1a. In an attempt to achieve molecular dispersion of these structures for analysis as performed by Hill *et al.* (1971), aqueous guanidine hydrochloride, buffered at pH 8.0, was added to a final concentration of 4 M. The optical contrast of the preparation decreased considerably (Fig. 1b) but all cytological structures of the original preparation are still apparent.

A far more dramatic effect is observed when this experiment is repeated with the modification of incorporation 0.1 M mercaptoethanol in the final solvent (Figs. 1c and d). Dissolution has gone to

---

* Present address: CSIRO, Division of Animal Genetics, P.O. Box 90, Epping, N.S.W., Australia, 2121.

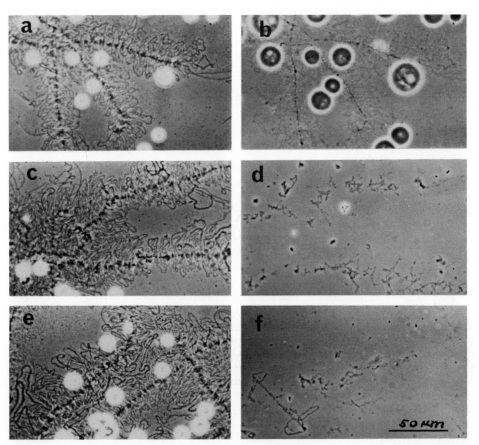

Figure 1. Effects of guanidine hydrochloride and disulfide reducing agents on lampbrush chromosomes and nucleoli from *Triturus cristatus carnifex*. a) Before treatment with 4M guanidine hydrochloride; b) after exposure; c) before exposure to guanidine hydrochloride in 0.1M mercaptoethanol; d) after exposure; e) before treatment with guanidine hydrochloride in 0.1M dithiothreitol; f) after exposure.

near completion and the original cytological structures have collapsed. Traces of cores are all that remain of the nucleoli. The chromosome axes can be traced as barely recognizable strings, no doubt held together by the DNA backbone. Replacing mercaptoethanol with dithiothreitol or with thioglycollate leads to more complete dissolution of the structures (Figs. 1e and f).

All three of the reagents utilized (mercaptoethanol, dithiothreitol and thioglycollate) are well established as specific reagents for the reductive cleavage of disulfide bonds. These observations thus provide circumstantial evidence that disulfide-bond cross-

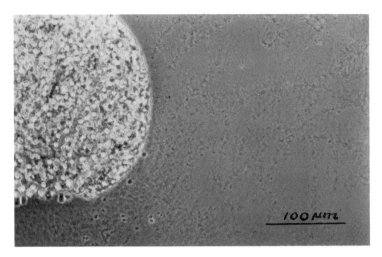

Figure 2. Oocyte "chromatin" prepared from a manually isolated germinal vesicle which was allowed to rupture in 0.075M KCl-0.025M NaCl and subsequently fractionated by centrifugation. Lampbrush chromosomes have partially emerged from the herniated nucleus. The bright objects associated with the nuclear membrane are nucleoli.

links contribute to the morphological stability of isolated nucleoli and lampbrush chromosomes.

It has been known for some time that the germinal vesicle is rich in protein sulfhydryl groups (Brachet, 1938). Since sulfhydryl groups, including those of proteins, are subject to aerial oxidation, it is quite possible that the disulfide crosslinks manifesting themselves in the above effect are progressively formed during isolation and subseqeunt manipulations of the germinal vesicle. Indeed, such a reaction would explain our observations that lampbrush chromosomes become more refractory to dissolution as time passes, and a similar phenomenon exhibited by amphibian oocyte nucleoli (O. Miller, personal communication, 1971; Miller and Beatty, 1969).

In order to obtain proteins for electrophoretic examination, hand-isolated germinal vesicles were massed and fractionated into nucleoplasm and chromatin. Their membranes were allowed to rupture spontaneously on standing in a solution of 0.075 M KCl and 0.025 M NaCl. After gently mixing, centrifugation at 1000g for 10 minutes gave a nucleoplasm supernatant over a pellet of chromatin. Fig. 2 shows the microscopic appearance of the centrifugable product when these operations were performed in a bored slide. The resulting chromatin consists of lampbrush chromosomes spilling out through a ruptured nuclear envelope to which nucleoli remain attached.

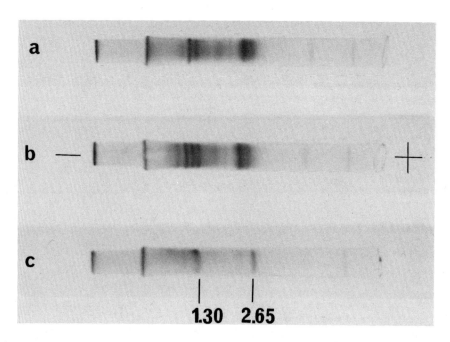

Figure 3. Gel electropherograms given by solubilized, reduced and
S-carboxymethylated proteins: a) nucleoplasmic proteins; b) total
nuclear proteins; c) chromatin proteins. The numbers associated
with bands indicate relative mobilities. Electrophoresis according
to the system of Davis (1964) with the inclusion of 7M urea.

Nuclear proteins were prepared from total nuclei, nucleoplasm
and washed chromatin by treatment with 2 µg/ml pancreatic ribonuclease in 2 M urea (introduced as a precaution to degrade RNA and min-
imize any possible RNA-protein interactions during electrophoresis),
followed by dissolution of all structures in 4 M guanidine hydro-
chloride/0.1 M mercaptoethanol. Finally the proteins were S-carboxymethylated essentially by the procedure of Crestfield *et al.* (1963).
Gel electropherograms at pH 9 in 7 M urea are depicted in Fig. 3.
Total nuclear protein is resolved into some twelve bands. Of these,
one (1.30) is very much depleted in the nucleoplasmic fraction. A
second (2.65) appears to be present in slightly decreased proportions in the nucleoplasm. Both of these components are very much
enriched in the chromatin fraction. The mobility of these two
species towards the anode at pH 9 eliminates them from the histone
class.

Further fractionations of the nuclear components by microdissection are currently in progress. To date they have shown, as pre-

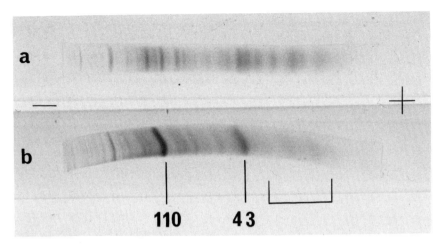

Figure 4.   Gel electropherograms in 0.1M sodium dodecyl sulfate
(Shapiro *et al.*, 1967) of S-carboxymethylated proteins: a) total
germinal vesicle proteins;   b) chromatin proteins. The bracket de-
lineates the region where histones would be expected to run.   The
molecular weights, in kilodaltons, of the two major nonhistones are
indicated.

dicted by calculation, that the nuclear membranes are not contribut-
ing to the major nonhistone proteins. On the other hand, nucleoli
give a pattern similar to that displayed by whole chromatin and thus
contain both major polypeptides. Semi-bulk preparations of isolated
lampbrush chromosomes have, as yet, not provided sufficient material
to give a distinctive electropherogram.

Both basic and acidic proteins adopt a high net negative charge
on exposure to sodium dodecyl sulfate. A total display of nuclear
proteins is thus obtained on electrophoresis in the presence of this
detergent (Fig. 4). Again the chromatin protein pattern differs
markedly from the whole nuclear pattern and once more demonstrates
the presence of the two distinct major components. The molecular
weights of these major components, calculated from sodium dodecyl
sulfate electrophoresis, are 110,000 and 43,000. The region where
histones would be expected to run is indicated by the bracket. This
class of proteins thus, at most, makes only a minor contribution to
the overall protein population. The two major nonhistones therefore
predominate over all other proteins.

This level of simplicity in the oocyte chromatin protein population is outstanding. We may have a clue as to the role of at
least one of the major nonhistones. An unusual feature of oocyte
chromatin (both nucleoli and lampbrush chromosomes) is the high

content of RNA relative to DNA (Macgregor, 1972; Edstron and Gall, 1963). In fact, the enrichment of the RNA to DNA ratio compared with somatic chromatin (see, *e.g.* Hill *et al.*, 1971) is of the order of ten to one hundredfold. Thus much of the protein of germinal vesicle chromatin is likely to be associated with nascent RNA. In other words, nascent chromosomal RNA-associated proteins are likely to be amplified relative to the other nonhistones of somatic chromatin. At this point it may be germane to recall the very simple pattern given by fully dissociated "informatin" protein in the hands of Krichevskaya and Georgiev (1969). This protein, which is believed to associate with nuclear RNA and be involved in its processing, gives a single band on gel electrophoresis. Its molecular weight has been quoted as 40,000-45,000. It may be of interest that informatin polymerizes via disulfide bond formation.

Somatic chromatin complexes, in which the RNA is a minor component relative to DNA, generally give a complex pattern of nonhistones (see *e.g.* MacGillivray *et al.*, 1971; Hill *et al.*, 1971). However, when RNA synthesis in rat liver cells is stimulated by cortisol there is a concomitant response in a single chromatin acidic protein. This species has a molecular weight of 41,000 (Shelton and Allfrey, 1970). On ecdysone-induced puffing of *Drosophila* polytene chromosomes there occurs an accumulation of a specific nonhistone of molecular weight 42,000 (Helmsing and Berendes, 1971). There is an interesting possibility that the nonhistone species from newt germinal vesicles, rat liver and *Drosophila* polytene nuclei, all with molecular weights measured to be in the range 41,000-43,000 and all associated with stimulated transcription, may represent informatin functioning at the chromosomal level.

REFERENCES

Brachet, J. 1938. Bull. Acad. Roy. Belg. Classe des Sciences, 499.

Callan, H. G. and L. Lloyd. 1960. Phil. Trans. Royl. Soc. London B 243: 135.

Crestfield, A. M., S. Moore and W. H. Stein. 1963. J. Biol. Chem. 238: 622.

Davis, B. J. 1964. Annals New York Acad. Sci. 121: 404.

Edström, J. E. and J. G. Gall. 1963. J. Cell Biol. 19: 279.

Helmsing, P. J. and H. D. Berendes. 1971. J. Cell Biol. 50: 893.

Hill, R. J., D. L. Poccia and P. Doty. 1971. J. Mol. Biol. 61: 445.

Krichevskaya, A. A. and G. P. Georgiev. 1969. Biochim. Biophys. Acta 194: 619.

MacGillivray, A. J., D. Carroll and J. Paul. 1971. FEBS Lett. 13: 204.

Macgregor, H. C. 1972. Biol. Rev. 47: 177.

Miller, O. L., Jr. and B. R. Beatty. 1969. Science 164: 955.

Shapiro, A. L., E. Vinuela and J. V. Maizel, Jr. 1967. Biochem. Biophys. Res. Comm. 28: 815.

Shelton, K. R. and V. G. Allfrey. 1970. Nature 228: 132.

13. THE GIANT RNA TRANSCRIPT IN A BALBIANI RING OF *CHIRONOMUS*

TENTANS

B. Daneholt

Department of Histology, Karolinska Institutet, S 104 01 Stockholm 60, Sweden

Several years ago Beermann (1952), Breuer and Pavan (1953) and Mechelke (1953) described transient changes in the structure of giant chromosomes in insects. The modifications, designated puffs, were dependent on the cell type and developmental stage studied. These early investigations indicated that the puffs might be mor- phological manifestations of gene activity. Although it is likely that the puffs do represent differentially activated genes, the concept is primarily based on correlative data between chromosome structure and different cellular functions in cytoplasm. With the advent of molecular biology and the knowledge of the basic features of gene expression, it seems possible to test the puffing concept in a more straightforward way. The most likely hypothesis is that RNA is synthesized in the puffs, transported to cytoplasm and there specifies protein synthesis. Such studies have been initiated and will be discussed below.

BALBIANI RING 2 OF *CHIRONOMUS TENTANS*

Since the giant chromosomes consist of many thousand of iden- tical chromatids, side by side, their dimensions make them suitable for microdissection. The giant puffs attain such a large size that they can be isolated and analyzed separately (Daneholt *et al.*, 1970). Most experiments have been carried out on one particular giant puff (called Balbiani ring 2) on chromosome IV in the larval salivary glands of *Chironomus tentans*. This puff is specific to this tissue and probably linked to the production of salivary pro- teins (Beermann, 1961; Grossbach, 1969), the main product of these cells. Like other puffs, a Balbiani ring usually originates from one single chromosome band. The closely packed deoxyribonucleo-

protein fibrils in the band uncoil, RNA as well as protein accumulate, and the chromosome region becomes expanded (puffed).

TRANSCRIPTION IN BALBIANI RING 2

When salivary glands of *Chironomus tentans* are exposed to
radioactive precursors to RNA, the RNA in Balbiani ring 2 (BR 2)
is heavily labelled. This is true also after short pulses, indicating a local synthesis of this RNA (Pelling, 1964). That the
rapidly labelled RNA species is indeed transcribed within the
ring has been adequately demonstrated by *in situ* hybridization
(Lambert *et al.*, 1972). Labelled RNA from BR 2 hybridized to the
BR 2 region but not to the remainder of the chromosome set (Fig. 1).
High molecular weight RNA from chromosomes I-III and nucleolar RNA
did not show this preferential binding to BR 2.

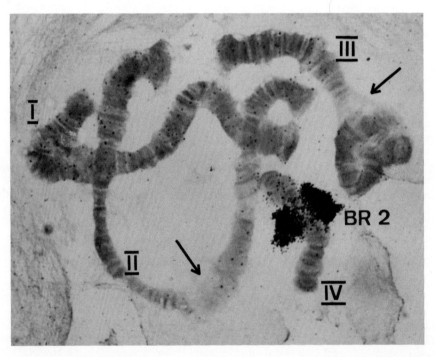

Figure 1. *In situ* hybridization of BR 2 RNA. The autoradiograph
shows a chromosome set of *Chironomus tentans* after hybridization of
BR 2 RNA, obtained from salivary glands labelled *in vitro* for 90
min. Roman numerals designate the four polytene chromosomes. Arrows indicate the nucleolar organizers. (Courtesy of Dr. B.
Lambert.)

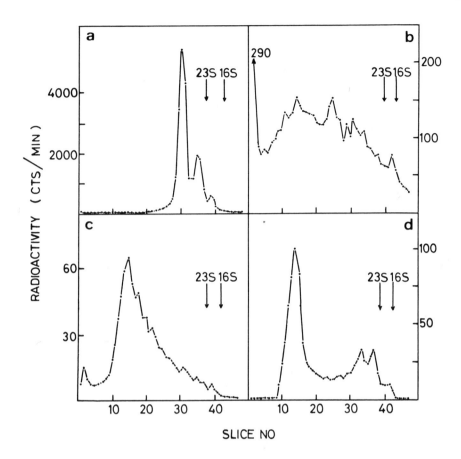

Figure 2. Electrophoretic analyses of labelled RNA from nucleoli (a), chromosomes I-III (b), Balbiani ring 2 (c) and nuclear sap (d). Salivary glands were labelled *in vitro* for 90 min at 18°C and afterwards fixed and prepared for microdissection. Nuclear components from 30 cells were isolated. The labelled RNA from each sample was released in a sodium dodecyl sulfate-Pronase solution and directly analyzed by electrophoresis in 1% agarose gels.

Labelled RNA from Balbiani ring 2 has been analysed by electrophoresis in agarose gels and by sucrose gradient sedimentation (Daneholt, 1972). Contrary to the broad distribution of activity in chromosomes I-III, and the pattern of defined multiple fractions in the nucleoli, there is only one main RNA peak in Balbiani ring 2 (Fig. 2). This RNA species has a sedimentation value of 75S. Although there is only one main peak in BR 2, the distribution of molecules is not symmetric around this peak. The slope on the high molecular weight side is always steep, while that on the low molecular weight side is not. There seems to be a continuous spectrum

of molecules of all sizes up to 75S with no reproducible enrichment
of molecules of a particular size class other than 75S RNA. As the
BR RNA is transcribed in the ring itself, one might propose that
the wide spectrum of molecular sizes represent RNA molecules *in
statu nascendi*. The finished product should then be 75S RNA. A
conspicuous RNA species of that size is also recorded in nuclear
sap (Fig. 2). BR 2 RNA sequences are readily detected in nuclear
sap by *in situ* hybridization (Lambert *et al.*, 1972). Furthermore,
base composition data (Daneholt and Svedhem, 1971) indicate that
RNA delivered from Balbiani ring 2 constitutes the main part of the
high molecular weight, rapidly labelled RNA in the nuclear sap.
Therefore it is supported that the completed transcript in Balbiani
ring 2 is 75S RNA and that this is released into nuclear sap without a major cahnge in size. If, in Balbiani ring 2, the RNA molecules smaller than 75S do represent growing molecules, they should
not be recorded in nuclear sap. It is then interesting to note
that the nuclear sap 75S RNA fraction is more symmetric than the
BR 2 75S RNA profile, and evidently lacks most of the molecules on
the low molecular weight side present in BR 2. This difference between BR 2 and nuclear sap RNA makes other possible explanations to
the asymmetric BR 2 profile less attractive, such as degradation
(*in vivo* or preparative) or variable initiation/termination of
transcription of 75S RNA.

If the interpretation of the BR 2 profile as a nascent RNA
profile is correct, it is to be expected that the BR 2 contains
transcription complexes of a type related to those demonstrated
for lampbrush chromosome loops in *Triturus viridescens* (Miller *et
al.*, 1970). These loops consist of a central deoxyribonucleoprotein
(DNP) axis with ribonucleoprotein (RNP) fibrils of gradually increasing length attached to the DNP axis. The technique of Miller
and coworkers has not been adopted to Balbiani rings. There is,
however, some information available from electron microscope studies
on sectioned BR's (Beermann and Bahr, 1954; Stevens and Swift,
1966; Vazquez-Nin and Bernhard, 1971). The Balbiani rings are
characterized by a great number of loop structures, which appear
to consist of a thin DNP axis and many large RNP granules, each
attached to the axis by a ribonucleoprotein fibril. Unfortunately
only short sections (maximally 5-10 μm long) of the loop can be
visualized in thin section. However, it seems plausible that the
granules with the connecting fibril represent growing ribonucleoprotein complexes in analogy with the fine structure of the loops
in *Triturus*. Spherical granules of the large size specific to the
Balbiani rings can be frequently recorded in nuclear sap. They
lack the projecting fibril characteristic for granules in the ring,
and thus probably constitute completed and released Balbiani ring
RNP particles. It is therefore evident that the present information
on RNP particles as well as on RNA support the idea of transcription
complexes as a dominating structure in Balbiani ring 2.

The 75S transcript is a very large molecule; its mass has
been estimated as 35 X 10^6 daltons from electrophoretic mobility
and as 15 X 10^6 daltons from sedimentation velocity (Daneholt,
1972). Although these two determinations do not agree, they both
indicate that the transcript in BR 2 is of giant size. It is of
interest to compare the size of this transcript with the amount of
DNA in the corresponding chromomere (a chromomere is the equivalent
on the chromatid level to the band on the chromosome level). The
DNA content of the BR 2 chromomere has not been estimated directly,
but the amount of DNA in an average chromomere has been determined
to be 60 X 10^6 dlatons (Daneholt and Edström, 1967). As the BR 2
chromomere is of intermediate size (Beermann, 1952), it is likely
that the average chromomere value is a reasonable estimate of the
DNA content in the BR 2 chromomere. Thus, a transcript of the
whole BR 2 chromomere would then be on the order of that recorded
in BR 2. At least a substantial part of the BR 2 chromomere is
therefore transcribed into one single transcript. In fact it cannot be excluded that the whole chromomere is transcribed into one
single RNA molecule. Comparative morphological studies have earlier
suggested that a chromomere is a unit of transcription (Beermann,
1964). Available data then indicate that such a concept might be
adopted also in a more precise molecular sense. On the basis of
present knowledge, it cannot be decided whether or not transcription
starts and/or terminates in interchromomere regions. Most of the
75S RNA molecule is, however, likely to be transcribed on chromomere DNA. This is obvious from the fact that less than 5% of the
chromosomal DNA is in interchromomere regions (Beermann, 1972);
it is unlikely that the BR 2 region is exceptional in this respect.

TRANSPORT OF RNA FROM BALBIANI RING 2 VIA NUCLEAR SAP TO CYTOPLASM

By *in situ* hybridization technique it has been possible to
demonstrate that BR 2 RNA sequences are present in nuclear sap as
well as in cytoplasm (Lambert, 1973), implying that BR 2 delivers
RNA to nuclear sap and further to cytoplasm. Some features of this
transport have been revealed in an electrophoretic study of RNA
from different nuclear components as well as cytoplasm after different labelling times (Daneholt and Hosick, 1973). When nuclear sap
was studied after 90 min labelling (Fig. 2), a prominent fraction
migrating as 75S was found. Such a distinct peak could not be detected in the cytoplasm at that time (Fig. 3a), but could be observed after 90 min additional incubation (Fig. 3b). During *in vivo*
labelling for one week this fraction accumulated in the cytoplasm.
It was even feasible to record it with optical density measurements
(Fig. 4), which showed that it comprises as much as 1.5% of the
total RNA. Thus, a 75S RNA fraction appears in nuclear sap and
after some delay time also in cytoplasm, where it remains stable
for a considerable time. Over a 180 min labeling period, BR 2 RNA

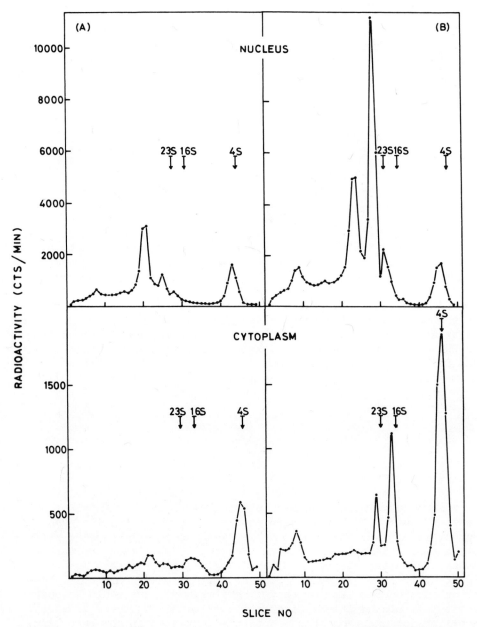

Figure 3. Electrophoresis in 1% agarose gels of labelled RNA from
nucleus and cytoplasm after 90 min (A) and 180 min (B) incubation
of explanted salivary glands at 18°C. Nucleus and cytoplasm were
dissected from 15 cells. Each sample was dissolved in a sodium
dodecyl sulfate-Pronase solution, precipitated in ethanol overnight,
redissolved and analyzed by electrophoresis.

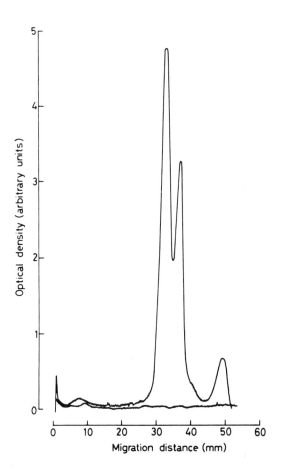

Figure 4. Electrophoresis in 1% agarose gels of total salivary
gland RNA extracted from about 60 glands. Fixed glands were dissolved in a sodium dodecyl sulfate-Pronase solution, precipitated
in ethanol, redissolved and run in the gels. The electrophoretic
separation was scanned at 254 nm (upper tracing). The gel was
then incubated overnight in an RNase solution and afterwards
scanned (lower tracing).

is preserved to a large extent (perhaps completely), while the major
part of RNA from chromosomes I-III, is turning over (Daneholt *et
al.*, 1970; Daneholt and Svedhem, 1971). This fact together with
the successful demonstration of BR 2 sequences in cytoplasmic RNA
labelled for seven days (Lambert, 1973), suggest that most of the
75S RNA is delivered from BR 2. The transfer of 75S RNA from BR 2
via nuclear sap to cytoplasm is likely to occur without a substantial size change.

The most interesting feature of the RNA molecule in the cytoplasm is its giant size. This is an unusual situation, as in most
cases in eukaryotic cells the giant RNA molecule is probably cleaved
prior to the delivery of the messenger RNA to the cytoplasm (e.g.
Darnell et al., 1970). However, non-ribosomal RNA of very high
molecular weight in cytoplasm of *Chironomus tentans,* does not seem
to be a unique finding. In *Bombyx mori,* for example, Suzuki and
Brown (1972) have recently established that there is a rapidly
sedimenting RNA (45-65S) that has been proven to be the fibroin
messenger. So, although not frequently recorded, the presence of
giant RNA in cytoplasm of *Chironomus tentans* might not be a highly
exclusive phenomenon.

In considering the transport of BR 2 RNA, it is interesting
to follow the fate of the Balbiani ring granules. As mentioned
above, the BR specific granules are frequently recorded in the
nuclear sap, but they are also found in the nuclear pores. Occasionally in *Chironomus thummi* (Stevens and Swift, 1966), but rather
frequently in *Chironomus tentans* (Hyde, personal communication),
BR granules can be detected in a cytoplasmic zone close to the
nuclear envelope. Thus, the electron microscope data indicate that
there is a transport from nucleus to cytoplasm of the whole RNP
complex without any obvious dimensional changes. However, when
biochemical and morphological data are put together, it seems likely
that most 75S RNA-protein complexes change conformation when they
are transferred further out into the cytoplasm. One obvious possibility is that 75S RNA (with or without proteins) is incorporated
into polyribosome structures, which then sooner or later become
associated with the endoplasmic reticulum, as do most polyribosomes in these secretory cells (Kloetzel and Laufer, 1969).

STRUCTURE AND INFORMATION CONTENT OF 75S RNA

Although cytogenetic data (Beermann, 1961; Grossbach, 1969)
strongly indicate that the tissue specific BR's of salivary glands
generate messenger for salivary proteins, there are no results
available that prove that BR RNA contains such messenger sequences.
However, it is interesting to note that the cytoplasmic 75S RNA
species, presumably of BR origin, display certain predicted properties for a salivary polypeptide messenger. First, because salivary
protein synthesis makes up more than 80% of the total protein synthesis (Doyle and Laufer, 1969a), the corresponding messenger must
be a main, non-ribosomal and non-transfer RNA species in cytoplasm.
75S RNA comprises as much as 1.5% of the total RNA, and this figure
can be compared, for example, with that for the fibroin messenger,
about 1% (Suzuki and Brown, 1972). Furthermore, the messenger for
salivary polypeptides must be stable. This can be inferred from
actinomycin D experiments, in which it has been possible to maintain

protein synthesis for more than 24 hours without a main reduction in protein synthesis (Clever *et al.*, 1969; Clever, 1969; Doyle and Laufer, 1969b). The half life time for 75S RNA is likely to exceed 35 hours (Daneholt and Hosick, 1973).

Since both cytogenetic and biochemical data suggest that BR 2 RNA contains genetic information for salivary polypeptides, it might be worthwhile to discuss the size and structure of the BR 2 transcript in relation to that assumption.

The mass of 75S RNA has been estimated to be 15-35 X 10^6 daltons (Daneholt, 1972). Because the molecular weight of the largest salivary polypeptide probably does not substantially exceed 500,000 (Grossbach, 1971), the giant RNA molecules could contain genetic information for more than one polypeptide. Thus, the RNA transcript might be mono- as well as polycistronic. It is of course quite conceivable that a part of the transcript does not encode proteins.

Although incomplete, there is some information on the structure of the transcript. It is known that rapidly labelled BR 2 RNA has a very peculiar base composition (Daneholt, 1970). RNA in the main peak was compared in this respect with other fractions of the BR 2 spectrum that contain shorter RNA molecules. The conclusions from this study was that molecules of different sizes in BR 2 have a similar, BR 2 specific, structure. Tentatively, this result could then be applied to the most likely explanation for the BR 2 profile, that it represents RNA molecules *in statu nascendi*. The inference would then be that the transcript contains a similar, BR 2 specific, base composition, more or less along its whole extension.

Recently, *in situ* and biochemical hybridization (Lambert, 1972; Lambert *et al.*, 1972; Sachs and Clever, 1972) have been applied in studies of BR RNA. Both types of experiments indicate that BR 2 RNA contains repeated sequences. The number of binding sites has been estimated in hybridization rate experiments, in which nucleolar RNA has served as a standard (Lambert, 1972). It was found that BR 2 RNA has twice as many binding sites as nucleolar RNA, *i.e.* about 200 (nucleolar RNA has about 100 according to Lambert *et al.*, 1973). It was concluded from these experiments that the 75S RNA transcript contains sequences repeated within the molecule.

The nature of the repeated sequences is unknown. A repeated structure might, for example, be due to a serial arrangement of several similar or identical cistrons. It is interesting, however, to note also that there can be a substantial internal sequence redundancy within a cistron, which has been nicely demonstrated for the fibroin messenger (Suzuki and Brown, 1972). This might be

important to recall in the case of *Chironomus tentans*, as the main
products of the salivary gland cells of *Chironomus tentans* and
Bombyx mori are similar in function; the construction of a tube
surrounding the larvae, and the formation of a cocoon respectively.
Certainly, it has not been settled whether or not the repeated
sequences in the BR 2 transcript represent repeated genetic information (in the conventional sense). They do comprise, however, a
large proportion of the molecule, well above 15% and probably the
major part (Lambert, 1972).

Since the 75S RNA molecule is the transcript of a very considerable part of the BR 2 chromomere, the futher revelation of
its structure will also provide important information on the
structure of this particular chromomere. Whether the BR 2 chromomere shares essential features with chromomeres in general, can
hardly be predicted at the present time.

ACKNOWLEDGMENTS

The author's work discussed in this review was supported from
the Swedish Cancer Society, Magnus Bergvalls Stiftelse and Karolinska Institutet (Reservationsanslaget).

REFERENCES

Beermann, W. 1952. Chromosoma 5: 139.

Beermann, W. 1961. Chromosoma 12: 1.

Beermann, W. 1964. In Genetics Today, p. 375. Pergamon Press,
Oxford.

Beermann, W. 1972. In Results and Problems of Cellular Differentiation, Vol. 4 (W. Beermann, ed.), p. 1. Springer-Verlag, Berlin.

Beermann, W. and G. F. Bahr. 1954. Exptl. Cell Res. 6: 195.

Breuer, M. and C. Pavan. 1953. Caryologia Suppl. 6: 778.

Clever, U. 1969. Exptl. Cell Res. 55: 317.

Clever, U., I. Storbeck and C. G. Romball. 1969. Exptl. Cell
Res. 55: 306.

Daneholt, B. 1970. J. Mol. Biol. 49: 381.

Daneholt, B. 1972. Nature New Biol. 240: 229.

Daneholt, B., J.-E. Edström, E. Egyházi, B. Lambert and U. Ringborg.
1970. Cold Spring Harbor Symp. Quant. Biol. 35: 513.

Daneholt, B. and H. Hosick. 1973. Proc. Nat. Acad. Sci. 70: 442.

Daneholt, B. and L. Svedhem. 1971. Exptl. Cell Res. 67: 263.

Darnell, J. E., G. N. Pagoulatos, U. Lindberg and R. Balint. 1970.
Cold Spring Harbor Symp. Quant. Biol. 35: 555.

Doyle, D. and H. Laufer. 1969a. J. Cell Biol. 40: 61.

Doyle, D. and H. Laufer. 1969b. Exptl. Cell Res. 57: 205.

Grossbach, U. 1969. Chromosoma 28: 136.

Grossbach, U. 1971. Habilitationsschrift (Universität Stuttgart-
Hohenheim).

Kloetzel, J. A. and H. Laufer. 1969. J. Ultrastruct. Res. 29: 15.

Lambert, B. 1972. J. Mol. Biol. 72: 65.

Lambert, B. 1973. Nature 242: 51.

Lambert, B., E. Egyházi, B. Daneholt and U. Ringborg. 1973. Exptl.
Cell Res. 76: 369.

Lambert, B., L. Wieslander, B. Daneholt, E. Egyházi and U. Ringborg.
1972. J. Cell Biol. 53: 407.

Mechelke, F. 1953. Chromosoma 5: 511.

Miller, O. L., Jr., B. R. Beatty, B. A. Hamkalo and C. A. Thomas,
Jr. 1970. Cold Spring Harbor Symp. Quant. Biol. 35: 505.

Pelling, C. 1964. Chromosoma 15: 71.

Sachs, R. I. and U. Clever. 1972. Exptl. Cell Res. 74: 587.

Stevens, B. J. and H. Swift. 1966. J. Cell Biol. 31: 55.

Suzuki, Y. and D. D. Brown. 1972. J. Mol. Biol. 63: 409.

Vazquez-Nin, G. and W. Bernhard. 1971. J. ULtrastruct. Res. 36:
842.

14. STUDIES ON THE TEMPLATE SPECIFICITIES OF EUKARYOTIC DNA-

DEPENDENT RNA POLYMERASES *IN VITRO*

Sarah Jane Flint, David I. de Pomerai, C. James Chesterton
and Peter H. W. Butterworth

*The Departments of Biochemistry of University College
London and King's College London, U.K.*

Investigations of bacteriophage infection of *Escherichia coli*
have established a role for the DNA-dependent RNA polymerase in the
regulation of gene expression. It is now generally accepted that
host *E. coli* RNA polymerase transcribes at least a part of the
phage genome (the 'early' regions) whereas a modified host RNA
polymerase (in the case of T4) or even a new phage-specified polymerase (as in the case of T7) transcribes the 'late' regions
(Travers, 1971; Bautz, 1972). These observations suggest that
the host *E. coli* RNA polymerase, the modified T4 polymerase and the
new phage-specified polymerase recognize different nucleotide sequences and thus bind to and transcribe from different initial
binding sites (promoter sites) on the phage DNA. Thus at least
one "positive" control mechanism resides in the ability of different polymerase species to recognize different promoter sites.

During the last three years, our knowledge concerning the
machinery of RNA synthesis in eukaryotes has increased greatly.
The major stimulus to research in this area was the publication by
Roeder and Rutter (1969) of a system for the solubilization of the
rate liver DNA-dependent RNA polymerase activity and its resolution
into two species (termed forms A and B or I and II). Forms A and
B are conveniently distinguished by the inhibition of form B by
α-amanitin (Kedinger *et al.*, 1970). Since this initial discovery
of multiple eukaryotic RNA polymerases, the numbers of polymerase
forms has continued to increase. It now appears that there are at
least three form A polymerases: forms AI and AII, which are restricted to the nucleolus (Roeder and Rutter, 1970; Chesterton
and Butterworth, 1971a,b), and form AIII, which is thought to be

167

nucleoplasmic (Roeder and Rutter, 1970). Form B polymerase is exclusively nucleoplasmic and at least two forms (BI and BII) have
been recognized (Kedinger *et al.*, 1971).

The presence of multiple DNA-dependent RNA polymerases in the
cells of higher organisms may suggest that there is a role for the
polymerases in the control of gene expression analogous to that
described for prokaryotes above; that is, the different polymerase
species may have different initial binding site ("promoter" site?)
specificities, thus transcribing different classes of genes.

The different eukaryotic RNA polymerases can be characterized
by their different elution properties from ion exchange celluloses;
the different conditions of ionic strength and divalent metal ion
concentration required to give optimal activity *in vitro;* their
ability to transcribe native and/or denatured DNA; their sensitivity to the toadstool toxin α-amanitin; their intracellular localization and, to a certain extent, their subunit structure. But much
of the evidence concerning differential template specificity of
these enzymes is vague, negative or indirect. As the form A polymerases (excluding AIII) are restricted to the nucleolus (Roeder
and Rutter, 1969; Chesterton and Butterworth, 1971a) which is the
locus of the ribosomal cistrons, this polymerase is thought to be
responsible for the synthesis of ribosomal RNA: the best evidence
for this comes from an analysis of stage IV oocytes of *Xenopus
laevis* where 95% of RNA synthesis is of ribosomal RNA. Since RNA
synthesis in these cells is not inhibited by α-amanitin the involvement of form A polymerase is implied (Tocchini-Valentini and Crippa,
1970). On the other hand, form B RNA polymerases are nucleoplasmic
and are therefore thought to be responsible for the synthesis of
most forms of RNA excluding ribosomal RNA.

The major problem facing those interested in the template
specificity of each of the multiple RNA polymerases of eukaryotic
cells is the choice and preparation of a suitable template for these
studies. Much of our knowledge concerning the specificities of prokaryotic RNA polymerase has been derived from studies using simple
bacteriophage DNA's, elegant genetic analysis and meaningful RNA·
DNA hybridization studies on the *in vitro* synthesized products.
However, any approach to the study of differential template specificities of the eukaryotic RNA polymerases is hampered by the
gross complexity of the eukaryotic genome and the hopes that animal
viral templates might prove as useful as bacteriophage DNA's have
yet to be realized. Two possibilities therefore are open to us:
either the nucleoprotein complex "chromatin" can be used as a template for these studies or attempts may be made to deproteinize the
chromatin to yield 'native' DNA.

TEMPLATES

Chromatin

Studies using rat liver chromatin and purified rat liver DNA-
dependent RNA polymerases in our laboratory (Butterworth *et al.*,
1971) have yielded several important findings. Chromatin preparations were found to contain endogenous form B RNA polymerase. This
activity was not inhibited by rifampicin AF/0-13 and is thus thought
to be involved in the elongation of RNA chains only. The lack of
any α-amanitin-resistant activity is taken to mean that nucleolar
chromatin, which is known to contain form A polymerase (Roeder and
Rutter, 1969; Chesterton and Butterworth, 1971a; Grummt, 1972),
is absent from these preparations. Chromatin was found to be transcribed by added purified form B polymerase (BI and BII) whereas
form AI polymerase does not transcribe this template. This result
suggests that there are discrete differences in the template specificities of these two groups of polymerases. By competition
studies it was clearly demonstrated that form B rat liver RNA polymerases and a bacterial polymerase (derived from *Micrococcus lysodeikticus*) bind to and transcribe from different sites of the
chromatin DNA.

There is little doubt that chromatin might be an 'ideal' template for studies on the specificities of the different forms B
polymerase, which have yet to be resolved preparatively from rat
liver nuclei. However, further extension of this work may be
severely restricted by our lack of understanding concerning the
structure of "chromatin". It is also clear that nucleolar chromatin
might be the template of choice for the form A polymerases and we
are currently investigating this possibility.

Native DNA

It seems to be inevitable that, for the present anyway, studies
on the template specificities of the mammalian RNA polymerases will
have to resort to the use of protein-free ('native') DNA. The DNA
isolated from eukaryotic nuclei is of high but heterogeneous molecular weight and the isolation procedures unavoidably result in a
certain amount of shearing of the DNA and the insertion of a number
of single-stranded breaks ('nicks'). It is known that certain types
of 'nicks' act as pseudo-promoters for some RNA polymerases (Vogt,
1969; Dausse *et al.*, 1972). Therefore, before one can study the
template specificity of the different eukaryotic RNA polymerases,
it is necessary to ascertain first the effect of changes in the
integrity of the DNA on the activity of the various classes of these
enzymes. The study of the effect of artificially-induced changes
in the integrity of the DNA template on the activity of the mam-

malian polymerases is difficult because at least two opposing effects are evident: activation by the insertion of single-stranded
breaks ('nicks') and an inhibition that is probably due to the binding of polymerase to 'ends'. The data discussed below attempt to
resolve these two effects.

METHODOLOGY

RNA Polymerase Preparation and Assay

Form AI rat liver RNA polymerase was prepared by the procedure
of Butterworth *et al*. (1971); form B (a mixture of forms BI and
BII) rat liver RNA polymerase was purified according to Chesterton
and Butterworth (1971c). Assays were carried out and processed as
described previously (Chesterton and Butterworth, 1971b).

DNA Preparation

Preparation of DNA from rat liver nuclei was carried out
either by the procedure of Paul and Gilmour (1968), or by a modification of this procedure used to prepare higher molecular weight
DNA - all alcohol precipitation steps were eliminated; Pronase
digestion was carried out in 0.5% sodium dodecyl sulfate; depro-
teinization was carried out using 1 volume of a 1:1 mixture of
chloroform/octanol (24:1) and water-saturated phenol; DNA concentration was achieved by sedimentation through 4M CsCl. This procedure will be published in detail elsewhere.

DNA Molecular Weight Determinations and Assays for 'Nicks'

Molecular weight determinations were carried out either by
Studier analysis by analytical ultracentrifugation on an MSE
Centriscan 75 (Studier, 1965) or by the "end-labelling" technique
using polynucleotide kinase of Weiss *et al*. (1968). This technique
was also used to assay DNA for 'nicks'. Both techniques give good
agreement for the molecular weights of discrete DNA species (fractions from glycerol gradient fractionation of DNA). However,
Studier analysis can only be used to assess the molecular weights
of the principal component of a mixture of DNA species (*e.g.* in
bulk DNA preparations) and the "end-labelling" technique will give
the *average* molecular weight of DNA species in a mixture.

EXPERIMENTAL RESULTS

Treatment of Rat Liver DNA with Pancreatic Deoxyribonuclease (DNase I)

Fig. 1 shows that treatment by low concentrations of DNase I
(generating increasing numbers of 'nicks') activates the template
towards the form A polymerase whereas the activity of the form B

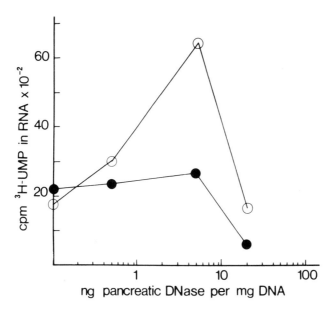

Figure 1. Effect of pancreatic deoxyribonuclease treatment of DNA
on the activity of form AI and form B rat liver RNA polymerases.
Partially purified, nuclease-free, form AI was prepared according
to Butterworth *et al.* (1971); purification of form B and the assays
for RNA synthesis were carried out as previously described (Chesterton and Butterworth, 1971b). Pancreatic DNase (Sigma) treatment
followed the procedure of Aposhian and Kornberg (1962). The number
of 'nicks' in the DNA was assayed for using the end-labelling technique of Weiss *et al.* (1968). The number of 'nicks' per 100 µg DNA
were: untreated DNA, 44; DNA treated with 0.5 ng DNase/mg DNA,
742; DNA treated with 5.0 ng DNase/mg DNA, 1074; DNA treated with
20 ng DNase was not assayed. Form AI activity, open circles; form
B activity, filled circles.

polymerase changes little. Higher concentrations of nuclease
appear to reduce the activity of both forms of the enzyme. [It
should be pointed out that there is an intriguing similarity between these results and those of Dausse *et al.* (1972) and Hinkle
et al. (1972) using E. *coli* 'core' and 'holo' RNA polymerase.]
Although it would be tempting to speculate that the form AI polymerase will form productive complexes at 'nicks' inserted by DNase
I whereas form B polymerases will not, consideration must first be
given to other changes taking place in the structure of the template upon nuclease treatment.

Using the "end-labelling" technique (Weiss *et al.*, 1968) to
assess "average" molecular weight of DNA species, it was found that
a DNA preparation having an average molecular weight of 1.05 X 10^7

was reduced in size to 1.74×10^6 on treatment with 0.5 ng nuclease
(DNase I) per mg DNA. This reduction in average molecular weight
is probably due to the production of large amounts of low molecular
weight DNA species. Therefore, nuclease treatment introduces a
further parameter, one of DNA size $o\hbar$ the number of DNA 'ends'.
These results prompted us to investigate further the effect of DNA
size on template activity for the mammalian RNA polymerases.

Sepharose Fractionation of DNA

        In the simplest case, we fractionated DNA that had not been
nuclease treated on Sepharose 4B. The DNA was heterogeneous and
fractions were bulked over three ranges of molecular weight (Fig.
2). Each bulked fraction was assayed for its template properties.
Fifteen percent of the DNA was not recovered from the column and
is thought to be of low molecular weight. The data are summarized
in Table 1. It can be seen that the activity of the form B polymerase did not change markedly on fractionation of the DNA. However, the activity of the form A polymerase increased on fractionation of the DNA and this is thought to be due to the removal of low
molecular weight DNA by the gel-filtration procedure. The activity

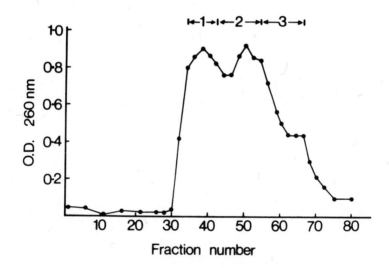

Figure 2.   Fractionation of DNA on Sepharose 4B. DNA was prepared
by a minor modification of the technique of Paul and Gilmour (1968).
DNA at 500 μg/ml was applied to a Sepharose 4B (Pharmacia) column,
equilibrated with 0.01M TrisCl pH 8, 0.1 mM EDTA and 0.1 M KCl.
Fractions were bulked and concentrated using polyethylene glycol
6000.

of the form A polymerase decreased as the molecular weight of the DNA decreased. Unfortunately, a definitive interpretation of this data is difficult because of the variation in the number of 'nicks' in the separate fractions, the lowest molecular weight fraction containing vastly more 'nicks' than the others.

Table 1. Effect of fractionation of bulk DNA on the activity of form AI and form B RNA polymerases.

DNA Fraction	M.W.[a]	'Nicks'/ 100 μg DNA	RNA Polymerase Activity (cpm)	
			AI	B
Bulk DNA before fractionation	(1.05×10^7)	44.0	1786	2239
Sepharose Fraction 1	1.85×10^7	6.5	4059	1720
Sepharose Fraction 2	6.5×10^6	28.2	3455	1854
Sepharose Fraction 3	3.2×10^6	319.0	2718	1954

[a] Molecular weight determinations were carried out by the "end-labelling" technique using polynucleotide kinase (Weiss *et al.*, 1968). The figure for the molecular weight of the "bulk DNA before fractionation" is given in brackets because the bulk fraction is highly heterogeneous and this technique will give a low average figure for M.W.

Effect of DNA "Ends"

For a true study of the effect of DNA molecular weight on template activity, a large number of DNA preparations were fractionated on Sepharose and the template activity of DNA fractions having different molecular weights but about the same low number of 'nicks' (about 20 'nicks' per 100 μg DNA) was studied with forms AI and B RNA polymerases. Fig. 3 shows that for both enzymes there is a sharp decrease in polymerase activity as the DNA molecular weight drops below 5×10^6. This could be due to one of several effects. We favor the notion that the polymerases form abortive complexes at 'ends' and that there is a competition between 'nicks' and 'ends' for the binding of either RNA polymerase type because DNA having molecular weights in the region of 3×10^6 but containing high numbers of 'nicks' (about 300 'nicks' per 100 μg DNA) is a good template for both form AI and form B polymerases.

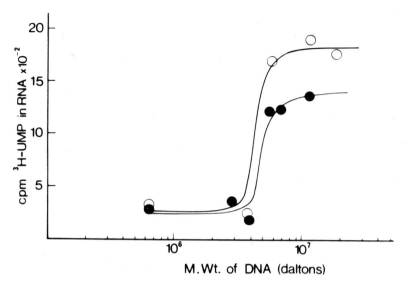

Figure 3. The effect of DNA molecular weight on activities of forms
A and B RNA polymerases. Several preparations of DNA were fractionated on Sepharose 4B columns. Using the end-labelling technique (Weiss *et al.*, 1968) the molecular weight and 'nick' content
were compared. For the data presented in this figure, the major
variable is DNA molecular weight, each DNA having a low 'nick'
content. Assays for template activity were carried out as described in the legend to Fig. 1. Form AI activity, open circles; form
B activity, filled circles.

Reassessment of the Effect of 'Nicks' on Template Activity of DNA

     In the previous experiment, the effect of 'ends' could be
studied in isolation as the numbers of 'nicks' in the different DNA
species was kept approximately constant. A similar approach may
now be adopted to study the effect of 'nicks', where the molecular
weight of the DNA is maintained constant. Table 2 shows that the
effect of 'nicks' on the template activity of the DNA for *both*
enzymes is markedly increased. The fact that the activities of
the enzymes do not increase in proportion to the number of 'nicks'
is due to the use of limiting amounts of enzyme in the assay for
the template activity of the highly 'nicked' DNA.

                    Studies on High Molecular Weight DNA

     A second, more practical method of minimizing the effect of
'ends' on the analysis of template activity is to use high molecu-

Table 2. Effect of 'nicks' on template activity of DNA's of similar molecular weight[a]

DNA Sample	M.W.	'Nicks'/100 μg DNA	RNA Polymerase Activity (cpm)	
			AI	B
1	6.5×10^6	28.2	3455	1854
2	6.4×10^6	228.0	7415	4134

[a] Two samples of a bulk rat liver DNA preparation were taken; one sample was treated with DNase I [20 ng/mg DNA according to the procedure of Aposhian and Kornberg (1962)] and both samples were fractionated independently on Sepharose 4B (as described in the legend to Fig. 1). Fractions of DNA from the column of similar molecular weight [assayed by "end-labelling" (Weiss *et al.*, 1968)] are compared for template activity.

lar weight DNA. The routine procedures for DNA isolation rarely produce DNA preparations in which a significant proportion of the DNA has a molecular weight in excess of 10^7 and these preparations are highly heterogeneous. Two higher molecular weight DNA preparations are compared in Table 3. Studier analysis (1965) of both preparations showed that neither contained a significant amount of DNA having molecular weights lower than that of the principal component and both preparations (particularly DNA 3) had a considerable quantity of species much larger than that of the principal component. A qualitative assessment of the numbers of single-stranded scissions (by comparison of native and denatured DNA molecular weights: N/D in Table 3) indicates that DNA 4 contains many more 'nicks' than

Table 3. Molecular weights of native and denatured DNA derived from Studier analysis[a]

DNA Sample	Native M.W. (N)	Denatured M.W. (D)	N/D	RNA Polymerase Activity (cpm)	
				AI	B
3	3.2×10^7	8.1×10^6	3.9	1186	1658
4	2.2×10^7	1.4×10^6	16.0	3256	3098

[a] It must be emphasized that the Studier technique (1965) for the assay of DNA molecular weight can only be used to assess the molecular weight of the principal component of a mixture of DNA species.

DNA 3; a mathematical analysis of the Studier data to give an assessment of the actual number of 'nicks' was not attempted owing to
the heterogeneous nature of the species present.

A comparison of the template activities of these two higher
molecular weight DNA preparations for the form AI and forms B RNA
polymerases again shows that 'nicks' increase the activity of *both*
forms of the enzyme. Also it is interesting to note that although
the rate of RNA synthesis is higher on the more 'nicked' DNA (DNA
4), the RNA product (Fig. 4) is of much higher molecular weight on
the less 'nicked' DNA, DNA 3 (800-8000 nucleotides). For DNA 4,
the product size was in the range between 100 and 800 nucleotides.
Although this result would have been anticipated, its significance
in terms of the design of experiments to ascertain template specificity cannot be underestimated.

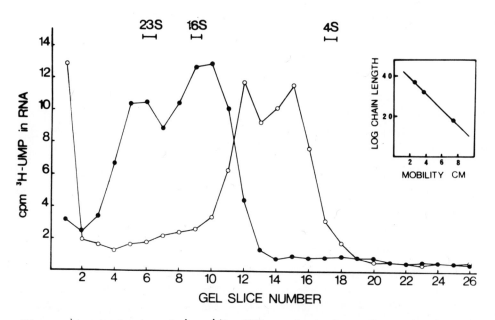

Figure 4. Analysis of *in vitro* RNA products by polyacrylamide gel
electrophoresis. Large scale *in vitro* incubations were carried out
using either DNA 3 or DNA 4 as template (see Table 3) and purified
rat liver form B RNA polymerase. Labelled RNA was extracted by the
technique of Hecht and Birnstiel (1972) and was subjected to electrophoresis on 2.5% polyacrylamide gels according to Loening (1967).
Gels were sliced as described by Mondal *et al.* (1972) and assayed
for radioactivity. *E. coli* rRNA and tRNA were used as molecular
weight markers. A plot of log chain length (nucleotides) against
mobility in the gels of the markers allows calculation of the chain

CONCLUSIONS

It is probably reasonable to predict that there are hierarchies of binding sites for polymerases on DNA: true initial binding sites ("promoters") and single-stranded scissions (at least of the type inserted by DNase I), both which produce productive complexes; and 'ends' (probably double-stranded), which produce abortive complexes. It would be expected that the polymerase has the highest affinity for "promoters". As DNA preparations from eukaryotic cell nuclei are heterogeneous with respect to molecular weight (and therefore contain a highly variable number of 'ends') and inevitably contain some single-stranded scissions, it was deemed necessary to investigate the effect of artificially induced changes in template integrity on the activity of the different RNA polymerase species. As a working hypothesis, we speculated that the form AI polymerase has few "promoters" in bulk DNA (assuming that its function is the expression of the ribosomal cistrons): therefore its activity might be expected to change as the degree of modification of the DNA template increases; on the other hand, if the form B polymerases are responsible for the transcription of all non-nucleolar DNA, it would be anticipated that there would be relatively large numbers of "promoters" for this enzyme for which the enzyme would be expected to have a high affinity. Therefore, the activity of this polymerase would be affected to a lesser extent by changes in template integrity. Until very recently, we thought that there were sufficient data to allow for the tentative acceptance of this broad concept (Butterworth *et al.*, 1973a,b), and it was suggested that "so long as assays are carried out at limiting enzyme concentration, the effect of factors such as 'nicks' in the DNA on the activity of the form B polymerases may be minimal". However, it is felt that a reappraisal of these conclusions is necessary as there is no doubt that the inhibitory effect of 'ends' (generated by the reduction of DNA size by DNase I, for example) has been underestimated. In the later experiments described in this paper where the effect of 'ends' was eliminated (Table 2) or minimized (Table 3), increasing numbers of 'nicks' showed a pronounced activation on the activity of the form B RNA polymerases. Similar data on the effect of sonication of DNA (not described in this paper) also show that 'nicks' inserted into the DNA by this treatment result in an increased template activity for both forms of the enzyme *so long as* care is taken to normalize the effect of increasing numbers of 'ends' due to the reduction in size of the DNA on sonication.

---

length range of the *in vitro* synthesized products (see insert). Product using DNA 3 as template, filled circles; product using DNA 4 as template, open circles.

It is felt that the general picture of the effects of changes in DNA template integrity on the activities of the different polymerase species is still a developing one and it would be dangerous to attempt to be definitive at this time. It is evident that a major problem exists in the differentiation between initiation at 'nicks' and at putative "promoter" sites. While intensive efforts are being made to design experiments to make this distinction, the obvious conclusion from the data presented here would dictate that high molecular weight DNA having few, if any, single-stranded scissions must be the obligatory template for critical experiments designed to define the absolute template specificities of the multiple eukaryotic DNA-dependent RNA polymerases.

ACKNOWLEDGMENTS

We are grateful for the excellent technical assistance of Miss Karen Pollock and Mr. Brian Jenkins. This work was supported by grants from the Science Research Council (B/SR7803 and B/SR/7804) and the Wellcome Foundation.

REFERENCES

Aposhian, H. V. and A. Kornberg. 1962. J. Biol. Chem. 237: 519.

Bautz, E. K. F. 1972. Prog. Nucleic Acid Res. and Mol. Biol. 12: 129.

Butterworth, P. H. W., R. F. Cox and C. J. Chesterton. 1971. Eur. J. Biochem. 23: 229.

Butterworth, P. H. W., S. J. Flint and C. J. Chesterton. 1973a. Trans. Biochem. Soc. in press.

Butterworth, P. H. W., S. J. Flint and C. J. Chesterton. 1973b. In (B. B. Biswas, A. Stevens, R. K. Mandal and W. E. Cohn, eds.) Control of Transcription. Plenum Press, New York. In press.

Chesterton, C. J. and P. H. W. Butterworth. 1971a. Eur. J. Biochem. 19: 232.

Chesterton, C. J. and P. H. W. Butterworth. 1971b. FEBS Lett. 12: 301.

Chesterton, C. J. and P. H. W. Butterworth. 1971c. FEBS Lett. 15: 181.

Dausse, J.-P., A. Sentenac and P. Fromageot. 1972. Eur. J. Biochem. 31: 394.

Grummt, I. 1972. Studia Biophysica, Band 31/32.

Hecht, R. M. and M. L. Birnstiel. 1972. Eur. J. Biochem. 29: 489.

Hinkle, D. C., J. Ring and M. J. Chamberlin. 1972. J. Mol. Biol. 70: 197.

Kedinger, C., M. Gniadowski, J. L. Mandel, Jr., F. Gissinger and P. Chambon. 1970. Biochem. Biophys. Res. Comm. 38: 165.

Kedinger, C., P. Nuret and P. Chambon. 1971. FEBS Lett. 15: 169.

Loening, U. E. 1967. Biochem. J. 102: 251.

Mondal, H., A. Ganguly, A. Das, R. K. Mandal, and B. B. Biswas. 1972. Eur. J. Biochem. 28: 143.

Paul, J. and R. E. Gilmour. 1968. J. Mol. Biol. 34: 305.

Roeder, R. G. and W. J. Rutter. 1969. Nature 224: 234.

Roeder, R. G. and W. J. Rutter. 1970. Proc. Nat. Acad. Sci. 65: 675.

Studier, F. W. 1965. J. Mol. Biol. 11: 373.

Travers, A. 1971. Nature New Biol. 229: 69.

Tocchini-Valentini, G. P. and M. Crippa. 1970. Nature 228: 993.

Vogt, V. 1969. Nature 223: 854.

Weiss, B., T. R. Live and C. C. Richardson. 1968. J. Biol. Chem. 243: 4530.

Henry R. Mahler

Department of Chemistry, Indiana University, Bloomington, Indiana

As a result of studies during the past ten years, the presence in the mitochondria of all "ordinary" eukaryotic cells - from protists to the most complex metazoa, including man - of a system for the storage, transmission and expression of genetic information can now be considered to rest on a firm experimental foundation (Ashwell and Work, 1970; Rabinowitz and Swift, 1970; Schatz, 1970; Preer, 1971; Boardman *et al.*, 1971; Borst, 1972; Linnane *et al.*, 1972; Sager, 1972; Mahler, 1973a). These investigations have also established that, although this second system is distinct and separate from the primary (nuclear-cell sap) system in the same cell - by virtue not only of its sequestration within the organelle but also by the properties of its components and of the reactions that they catalyze - it is by no means independent of it. Since these conclusions and the experiments on which they rest have been repeatedly and recently reviewed (see above), this presentation is restricted to a consideration of the nature, extent and limits of the biogenetic autonomy of the mitochondria of just one organism, *Saccharomyces cerevisiae*, baker's yeast. It will make use of our own data, both published and some yet unpublished, as well as on studies by several groups here and abroad who are making use of the same experimental system. It will be convenient to broach the question in such a way as to work backwards from the gene products to the genes and to start with the translational products unique to mitochondria.

AUTONOMY OF TRANSLATION

Mitochondria contain their own system for protein synthesis, consisting of a distinct population of polysomes attached to the

inner mitochondrial membrane, tRNA's, aminoacyl-tRNA ligases and
initiation, elongation and - presumably - termination factors (reviewed in the above references plus Borst and Grivell, 1971; Kroon
et al., 1972; Dawidowicz and Mahler, 1973). What are the products
formed by this system? This question has been answered by a combination of techniques, among them the following:

a) The use of site specific inhibitors, such as cycloheximide
for protein synthesis in the cell sap, and chloramphenicol or
erythromycin for this event in mitochondria to measure the extent,
and identify the nature and function, of the entities formed by the
two systems (*e.g.* Mahler *et al.*, 1971b; Mason *et al.*, 1972; Sager,
1972). This paradigm necessarily relies on the disjunction of what
are probably two tightly coupled systems in a fully functional cell.
It cannot be used to probe any regulatory interplay between them
and may lead to faulty inferences even in its absence.

b) The unambiguous identification of such entitites synthesized *outside* the mitochondria by the use of a class of mutants
(cytoplasmic *petites* or ρ^-) that lack the protein synthesizing
system and sometimes are deficient either in meaningful or in *any*
mitochondrial DNA (mtDNA) (Mahler *et al.*, 1971b; Linnane and Haslam, 1970; Linnane *et al.*, 1972; Sager, 1972). The utility of
this approach is not restricted to mitochondrial enzymes or other
such entities of known structure and function but can be extended
to related molecules by suitable immunological techniques, etc.
(Kraml and Mahler, 1967; Shakespeare and Mahler, 1972; Mason *et
al.*, 1972).

c) The use of labeled formate as a specific factor for polypeptide chain initiation by, as well as for nascent chains on,
mitochondrial polysomes. This technique, developed by K. Dawidowicz (1972), is based on the fact that the occurrence of fMet-
tRNA^{fMet} and chain initiation by this molecule is restricted to
mitochondria (Smith and Marcker, 1970; Galper and Darnell, 1971;
Mahler *et al.*, 1972; Dawidowicz and Mahler, 1973; Mahler and
Dawidowicz, 1973). An example is shown in Fig. 1 in which mitochondrial (Fig. 1A) and cell sap polysomes (Fig. 1B) isolated from
spheroplasts of strain A364A are compared with regard to their
response to a 10 min pulse of labeled leucine and formate *in vivo*.
The results show that while the nascent polypeptides on either set
of polysomes can be labeled with leucine, labeling by formate is
restricted to the mitochondrial one. Such labeled formate can be
discharged by RNase at relatively high concentration, or transferred
to puromycin forming fMet-Puro, and formation of this compound can
be used as a specific and convenient assay for chain initiation.
Formate incorporation is prevented by prior incubation with chlor-
amphenicol or ethidium bromide (EtdBr). This N-terminal formate
on polypeptides is retained by at least some of the completed chains
after their release from the ribosome and their integration into

the mitochondrion proper (Mahler *et al.*, 1972), and Dr. F. Feldman
is currently trying to take advantage of this fact for their identification.

Current estimates using the various techniques are in agreement in assigning an upper limit of about ten percent of the total
protein (or ≤15% of the proteins of the inner membrane) as the
intramitochondrial contribution (Sager, 1972; Mason *et al.*, 1972;
Linnane *et al.*, 1972; Tzagoloff and Akai, 1972; Mahler, 1973a).
The polypeptides in question are probably localized entirely in
the hydrophobic core of these membranes. After their complete dissociation in hot sodium dodecyl sulfate-mercaptoethanol, followed
by electrophoresis on acrylamide gels, they appear restricted to
some half dozen molecular weight classes. As shown in Table 1,
their function is concerned with the biogenesis, integration or
regulation of only three of the multienzyme complexes of mitochondrial electron and energy transfer (above references plus Mahler
and Perlman, 1971a; Tzagoloff *et al.*, 1972; Weiss, 1972; Jagow
and Klingenberg, 1972; Jagow *et al.*, 1973). Although some of the
data concerning the molecular weights of the complexes come from
studies on beef heart by Hatefi and his collaborators (1973),
there is sufficient analogy in both structure and function as to
make a similar assignment for yeast highly probable. Since the
five complexes account for roughly half of the proteins of the
inner membrane we may draw the rather surprising inference that
these polypeptides probably account for the majority of the products of mitochondrial translation. That is not to rule out the
possible existence of other products, particularly certain minority
species present in less than stoichiometric amounts – and therefore
regulated independently of the bulk constituents of the inner membrane. In fact we shall have occasion to refer to a component of
the mitochondrial system of damage repair for DNA as one such possible product. The possibility must be entertained, therefore,
that at least some of the products known to be specified by mitochondrial genes, including ones producing certain antibiotic resistant phenotypes (Bolotin *et al.*, 1971; Saunders *et al.*, 1971)
may also or principally affect the structure of the inner membrane.
Indeed this hypothesis is in accord with similar suggestions made
previously by Linnane and his collaborators (see Linnane *et al.*,
1972). Finally, it now appears certain that mitochondria make
little, and possibly no, direct contributions to proteins involved
in the *biosynthesis* of their own macromolecules, by they DNA, RNA
or proteins.

AUTONOMY OF TRANSCRIPTION

Studies in a number of laboratories are now in agreement that
the base sequences specifying the stable mitochondrial RNA's are

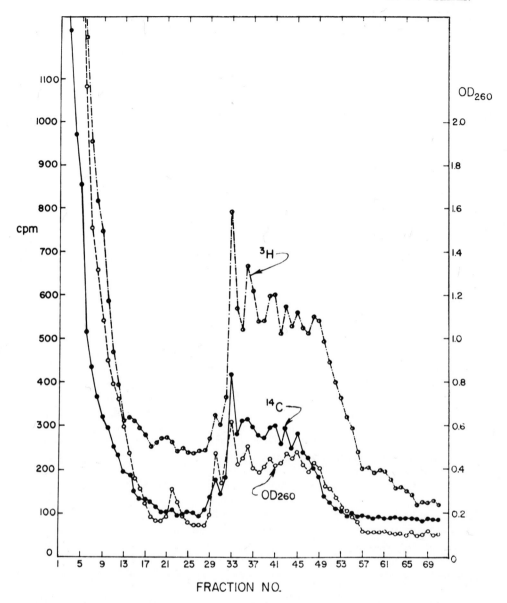

Figure 1. Comparison of mitochondrial (A) and cell sap (B) polysomes from spheroplasts of strain A364A obtained from cells growing
exponentially in YM-1, 3% lactate. Procedures used are described
in Mahler *et al*. (1972) and Mahler and Dawidowicz (1973). Labeling was at 23°C in YM-5 3% lactate by exposure to [^{3}H]leucine
(5 µCi/ml) and [^{14}C]formate (2.5 µCi/ml) for 10 min. The reaction
was stopped by simultaneous addition of cycloheximide (100 µg/ml)
and chloramphenicol (4 mg/ml). Spheroplasts were lysed by blending

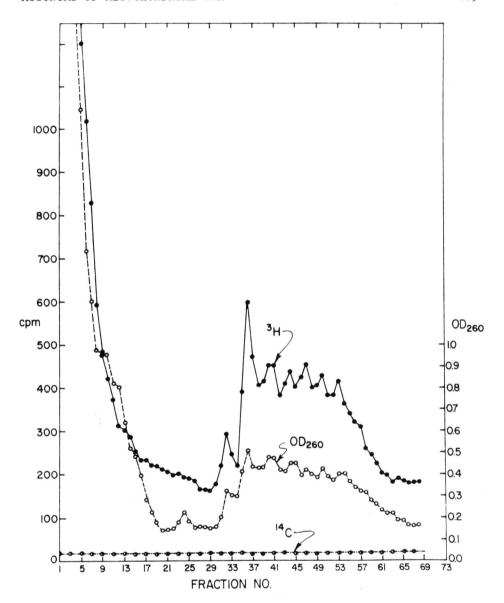

in 0.5M sorbitol-NMT (100mM NH$_4$Cl, 10mM MgCl$_2$ and 10mM TrisCl, pH
7.4), mitochondrial and cell sap fractions were isolated and mitochondria were washed with EDTA and lysed in 2% Triton X-100, NMT.
Lysates were analyzed in linear 0.3M to 1.4M sucrose-NMT gradients
by centrifugation for 4 hrs at 26,000 rpm in the SW27 rotor of a
Beckman L2 centrifuge. Samples were collected from the top and
A$_{260}$ and radioactivity insoluble in hot trichloroacetic acid (TCA)
were determined.

Table 1. Mitochondrial specification of mitochondrial respiratory chain

Complex	Description	M.W.x10^{-6}	% synth in mitos	M.W.x10^{-6}
I	NADH-ubiquinone reductase	0.7	0	
II	Succinate-ubiquinone reductase	0.2	0	
III	Ubiquinone-cytochrome C reductase	0.23	~15 (1)	0.03
IV	Cytochrome C oxidase	3x0.20	~50 (3)	0.30
V	Membrane-bound, oligo-mycin sensitive ATPase complex	0.47	20 (2-3)	0.08
Totals		2.20		0.41

The values shown for the molecular weights of complexes I-IV are those cited by Hatefi *et al.* (1973) for heart muscle; however, currently accepted values for *S. cerevisiae*, where known, do not appear to differ greatly. The estimate for the fraction of the complexes synthesized by mitochondria are based on the references cited in the text, as are the number of polypeptides per complex, shown in parenthesis.

inscribed as single copies exclusively in mtDNA (review in Borst, 1972; Borst and Flavell, 1972; Mahler, 1973a,b); these include the two rRNA's (M.W. = 1.2-1.3 and ~0.65 X 10^6 in *Ascomycetes*) and tRNA's (probably >20 in *Ascomycetes*) but no distinct 5S RNA. However before any conclusion can be drawn concerning the mitochondrial *specification* of the mitochondrial proteins discussed in the previous section, we must set limits on the mitochondrial contribution to the mRNA translated by the particles. A *priori*, this value may vary from 100 to zero percent, and the specter of the latter possibility has been raised explicitly and most cogently by Dawid (1972a,b). Dawidowicz and I therefore set out to subject it to an experimental test (Mahler and Dawidowicz, 1973) by performing the experiment outlined in Table 2 with the results shown in Table 3. The required specific blocks were constituted by a) a temperature sensitive mutant (ts⁻136) of strain 364A, kindly provided by Prof. Leland Hartwell which at the nonpermissive temperature of 36°C shuts off supply of all nuclear transcripts, including mRNA, to the cell sap, leading to a decay of polysomes with a half-life of 21 min (Hutchison *et al.*, 1969; Hartwell *et al.*, 1970), and b) by

Table 2. How to determine the origin of mitochondrial mRNA

	MODEL mRNA	I 〰〰 (mt)	II 〰〰〰 (n)	III 〰〰〰 〰〰〰 both
STAGE A	mt 〰〰〰〰 n 〰X〰	+	↓ to 0	↓
B	mt〰〰X〰 n 〰X〰	↓ to 0	0	↓ to 0
C	mt〰〰X〰 n 〰〰〰	0	↑	↓

+	full	ura*
0	no	f* Met puro
↑	increasing	leu*
↓	decreasing	polysomes

The paradigm involves the response to the application and removal of specific blocks on the supply of mRNA; with the X marking the location of the postulated blocks of nuclear transcripts (Stage A), of both nuclear and mitochondrial transcripts (Stage B), and the release of the nuclear block (Stage C): ura* - uracil incorporation into RNA, f* Met puro (and f*) - incorporation of formate into formylmethionyl puromycin and nascent polypeptide chains, and leu* - incorporation of leucine into the latter.

EtdBr, which as can be seen, shuts off mitochondrial RNA synthesis. Formation and retention of polysomes and their ability to carry out initiation and elongation of polypeptide chains were used as an operational measure of functional mRNA. We found no evidence for the import of any such RNA into mitochondria under conditions where there is restoration of activity in the cell sap. Conversely, the prior shift to 36°C even for prolonged periods, which completely eliminates mRNA function in the cell sap, does not interfere with this function in the mitochondria. This activity *is*, however, inhibited by prior incubation with EtdBr, a treatment that has no effect on cell sap functions, even at that temperature, in the wild type (or at the permissive temperature in the mutant). We have concluded therefore that under these conditions the programming of the mitochondrial polysomes appear restricted to mitochondrial transcripts, and that only polypeptide products translated by the organelle are the ones encoded in its DNA. Other evidence for the mitochondrial provenance of its mRNA has recently also been furnished by the studies of Reijnders *et al.* (1972) and by Perlman, Abelson and Penman (1973).

Table 3. Response of functional mRNA to selective blocks

t (°C)	EtdBr	RNA Synthesis[a] Mt	Cell Sap	Polysomes[b] Mt	Cell Sap	Protein Synthesis[c] Mt	Cell Sap	Initiation (Mt)[c] Formate	fMet–Puro
36°	−	2500	100[d]	+	−	92	3.5	100	75
	+	0[d,e]		−	−	2	f	29	22
36→23°	−	1000	10,000[d]	+	+	100	17	100	100
	+	<20	8,000[d]	−	+	f	f	f	100

Mt = mitochondria

a incorporation of uracil into RNA (cpm X 20 min^{-1} in cell fraction)

b presence of active polysomes (cf Fig. 1 for properties)

c as percent of wild type activity at that temperature; incorporation of [^{3}H]leucine and [^{14}C]formate

d after a lag of 20–30 min

e decay of counts previously incorporated, with a $t_{1/2} \simeq 20$ min

f not done

Application of the paradigm of Table 2 by the use of ts-136. For a complete description and experimental details see Dawidowicz (1972) and Mahler and Dawidowicz (1973).

AUTONOMY OF GENE MAINTENANCE

Gene Dosage and Mitochondrial Number

One of the recurrent problems in all studies on mitochondrial
genetics and autonomy is an almost complete absence of quantitative
information on the actual number of mitochondria and their DNA per
cell (see Williamson, 1970 for earlier results). Since such data
constitute an essential prerequisite for determining the effect
on the mitochondrial and cellular genome of such parameters as
physiological and genetic constitution, my colleagues Drs. G.
Grimes, P. Perlman and I have begun a collaborative effort in
this direction. For this program we are using quantitative evaluation of serial sections in electron micrographs, together with
quantitative determinations of total cellular DNA and the fraction
of it constituted by mtDNA.

The first set of questions we have asked concerns the effect
of nuclear gene dosage on mitochondrial mass and the number of
genomes per cell. For this purpose we have obtained three isogenic
strains: two haploids (2180A and 2180B) that differ only in their
mating type allele (a vs α), and the diploid (HOH) derived from
their mating. All cells were grown to mid-exponential phase (3-4
X 10^6 cells/ml) with lactate as a carbon source to eliminate catabolite repression. The analytical data for their DNA and the various quantitative relationships that can be derived from these
data plus the fraction of the cellular volume constituted by the
mitochondria are shown in Table 4. Using the currently accepted
values for the size of the nuclear (Schweizer and Halvorson, 1969;
Bicknell and Douglas, 1970; Christiansen et $al.$, 1971) and mitochondrial (Borst, 1972; Borst and Flavell, 1972; Blamire et $al.$,
1972) genomes we see that the diploid - which is twice as large,
and also contains twice the dry mass of its haploid parents -
disposes of twice as many mitochondrial genomes in twice the
mitochondrial volume (and hence twice the mitochondrial mass).
Since the largest number of mitochondria per cell, excluding buds,
was 29 in the case of HOH and 17 in the case of the haploid examined, it is evident that the total complement of mt genomes is
sufficient to provide each mitochondrion, on the average with at
least two molecules of mtDNA. The content of mtDNA in all cells,
regardless of ploidy is of the order of 1.7 X 10^{-4} pg/particle.

Evidence for the absolute dependence of the dosage of mtDNA
per cell on some form of nuclear regulation is provided by the
observation that stable cytoplasmic mutant cell lines fall into
only two classes (Goldring et $al.$, 1972): those that do not contain mtDNA in detectable amounts (DNA° or $\rho°$ petites) and those
that do; the proportion of mtDNA in the latter is indistinguishable from that found in the wild type. Interesting from the point

Table 4.   Characteristics of isogenic cells

Cell	Nuclear		Mitochondrial		Volume	
	DNA (pg $\times 10^2$)	Genomes[a]	DNA (pg $\times 10^3$)	Genomes[b] (per N chromosomes)	Cell (μm^3)	Mitos (%)
HOH (Diploid)	3.7	2.4	4.5	55 (23)	26.0	11.9
2180A (Haploid)	1.6	1.1	2.7	33 (30)	14.1	12.2
2180B (Haploid)	1.5	1.0	2.3	28 (28)		

[a] taken as 10×10^9 daltons = 1.5×10^{-2} pg

[b] taken as 50×10^6 daltons = 8.25×10^{-5} pg

Total cellular DNA was isolated and purified from spheroplasts of 400–500 ml cells grown on a semi-synthetic medium with 3% lactate as a carbon source to a cell density (determined accurately by hematocytometer counts) of 1×10^7/ml. DNA concentration of the final preparation was estimated both by A_{260} and the diphenylamine reaction and averaged. The proportion of nuclear and mitochondrial DNA was determined in the Beckman Model E analytical ultracentifuge equipped with UV optics, scanner and multiplexer by integration under the well-separated peaks with the "γ-DNA" included in the nuclear DNA. All values shown are the means of two separate sets of experiments. Mitochondrial and cellular volumes were determined with the electron microscope by serial sections and stereology. Six complete cells were examined for HOH [containing 15, 19, 23, 23, 24 and 29 (17 + 12 in a bud) mitochondria] and five for 2180A (containing 7, 8, 8, 10 and 17 mitochondria). Other details are given in the text.

of evolution are the observations that rodent fibroblasts (L cells) have been reported to contain 7.5 X 10^{-3} pg of mtDNA per cell (Nass, 1970) and that the mitochondrial volume in such cells and in human HeLa cells accounts for 7.1 and 8.9% of the cytoplasmic volume, respectively (King *et al.*, 1972).

The Use of Ethidium Bromide as a Probe for Mitochondrial Genetic Activity

Since all cytoplasmic petite mutants that retain mtDNA, even the ones with no useful genetic information (Mehrotra and Mahler, 1968; Bernardi *et al.*, 1968; Sanders *et al.*, 1973), evidently also contain a system for its replication and control, we have searched for alternatives useful in determining the mitochondrial contribution to their genetic continuity in replication, repair and recombination. One possibility is to introduce a perturbation that can lead to the disruption of this continuity - or its possible restoration. This is a feasible approach for in ethidium bromide (EtdBr) we have available a mutagen that a) can convert a population of cells rapidly and quantitatively into cytoplasmic petites without any lethality or other detectable effects at the chromosomal or cellular level, and can do so even upon exposure of starved cells in buffer in the complete absence of cell growth or division (Slonimski *et al.*, 1968; Mahler *et al.*, 1971b; Goldring *et al.*, 1970; Mahler and Perlman, 1972a); b) it can generate the complete spectrum of mutants exhibiting the petite phenotype (Bolotin *et al.*, 1971; Goldring *et al.*, 1971; Mahler *et al.*, 1971c; Nagley and Linnane, 1972; Hollenberg *et al.*, 1972). These mutants range from ones characterized by a substantial retention of the wild type genome, its base composition and sequences as well as its genetic information [various antibiotic resistance markers, tRNA's and rRNA's (Cohen *et al.*, 1972; Cohen and Rabinowitz, 1973)], through others in which this retention is restricted only to a small portion of the genome - which may or may not be meaningful in terms of identifiable gene products - to ones which no longer retain any part of the genome (for reviews see Borst, 1972; Linnane *et al.*, 1972; Mahler, 1973a). This heterogeneity can be detected not only on the level of a cell population exposed to the mutagen (Perlman and Mahler, 1971a) but also on that of the individual cell (Slonimski, P., private communication; Perlman, P., private communication; Nagley and Linnane, 1972). And finally, c) the eventual expression of these mutagenic alterations is neither absolute nor irreversible. Instead it may be modulated by various cellular, and particularly mitochondrial events and entities (for review see Mahler, 1973a). As we shall see this fact may provide us with an alternative means for effecting genetic exchanges that do not require mating and zygote formation.

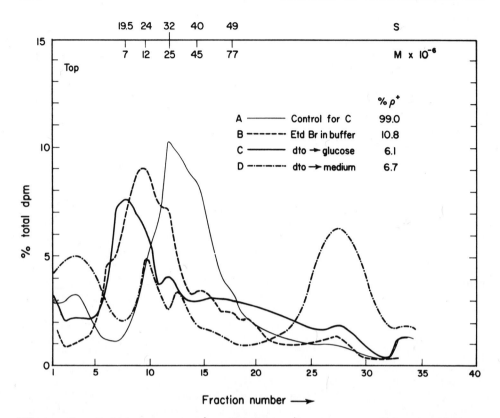

Figure 2. Initial events (registration) after exposure of mtDNA to EtdBr. Cells of IL-8-8C, a *his⁻try⁻* auxotroph were grown on 1% glucose to $A_{600}=0.3$ and labeled with $[^{14}C]$-(4 μCi/ml) or $[^{3}H]$-(196 μCi/ml) adenine for 2 hr in the presence of 100 μg/ml of cycloheximide as described in Mahler and Perlman (1972b). Cells were washed, transferred to 0.1M phosphate buffer and starved by aeration for 60 min at 30°C. EtdBr (25 μM) was then added to cells labeled with $[^{14}C]$ and the incubation continued for 4 hr when mutagenesis had reached the level indicated. Aliquots were removed for analysis, for incubation in buffer (similar to A, not shown), in buffer plus 1% glucose, in complete glucose medium, and in medium plus cycloheximide (100 μg/ml) (similar to C, not shown) and subjected to incubation for an additional 150 min. Samples were mixed with $[^{3}H]$labeled controls treated similarly but with EtdBr omitted. Cells were lysed as described previously (Perlman and Mahler, 1971a) and subjected to analysis by sedimentation in 5-20% neutral sucrose gradients for 18 hr at 18,000 rpm at 5°C in the SW27 rotor. Samples were hydrolyzed in 0.1N NaOH overnight precipitated with 10% TCA, plated on glass fiber discs and counted. All controls gave similar patterns. The zero time control was standardized against $[^{3}H]$labeled DNA from bacteriophage T7 (Freifelder, 1970). The labeled component was identified as mtDNA by equilibrium banding in CsCl and by virtue of its identity with the DNA isolated from highly purified mitochondria.

Steps in Mutagenesis by Ethidium Bromide

Prior exposure of non-growing cells of S. *cerevisiae* to EtdBr
in the mutagenic range of $\geq$2 μM leads to the following consequences
detectable once growth is restored (Perlman and Mahler, 1971a;
Mahler and Perlman, 1972a): a) a rapidly developed (<30 min of
initial exposure) block of specifically mitochondrial DNA replication and transcription, and b) a fragmentation of the genome leading eventually to its complete destruction. Removal of the mutagen
prior to transfer to medium results in resumption of synthesis of
mtDNA with progeny molecules that utilize as templates the population of mtDNA fragments remaining in any cell *at that particular
time*.

We have tried to see whether we can distinguish the prerequi-
sites and the different steps that lead to this characteristic
EtdBr-induced fragmentation of mtDNA. As is shown by the results
of Fig. 2, exposure of starved cells (previously labeled preferentially for mtDNA in the presence of cycloheximide) to a mutagenic
dose in buffer produces a diminution of the size of mtDNA without
a substantive loss ($\leq$20%) of the total counts: Most of the mtDNA
examined by us and others in sucrose gradients (Blamire *et al.*,
1972) exhibits a M.W. $\simeq$ 25 X 10^6 for control cells, and thus corresponds to a population containing mainly linear half-molecules.
This size distribution is shifted toward molecules half that size
(*i.e.* "quarter"-molecules, M.W. $\simeq$ 12 X 10^6) by a 2 hr exposure to
EtdBr. More extensive exposure to the mutagen in buffer, or removal
of this compound followed by further incubation in buffer (up to
24 hrs) has no additional deleterious effect. This result, which
may be regarded as a *registration* of the original mutagenic exposure, can probably be explained in terms of a single cut in both
strands (or "chop"-Koch, 1973) of the circular molecule by an
endonuclease capable of recognizing its distortion by EtdBr. The
further cleavage attendant upon its isolation then leads to the
size distribution observed. To produce additional degradation -
again apparently by a chopping reaction - requires the provision of
an energy source (transfer to buffer plus glucose). Finally the
extensive degradation to small fragments observed here and in
earlier studies (Goldring *et al.*, 1970; Perlman and Mahler, 1971)
- whether again predominantly endonucleolytic is not known - requires
some attributes present only in growing cells. It occurs in complete medium but not when protein synthesis is blocked by cycloheximide. We have also made an attempt to determine whether these
events are peculiar to EtdBr by comparing its action with that of
many other mutagens (Mahler, 1973b). Of the large number examined
only EtdBr and certain closely related phenanthridinium derivatives

---

The accumulation of counts in the heavy (nDNA) region of the gradient
is due to the utilization of ribonucleotides as precursors of mtDNA
synthesis under these conditions.

are capable of mutagenizing starved cells in buffer - none of the
structurally analogous acridinium dyes (*i.e.* euflavine and other
alkyl-proflavines) are capable of doing so. Two compounds, although ineffective under these conditions, do turn out to be highly
efficient mutagens but only in the presence of an energy source:
they are 10-allylproflavine (2,8-diamino-10-allyl acridinium chloride) and Berenil [di-(4-aminodiphenyl)-triazine-(N-1,3)diaceturate]
which as shown by Waring (1971) does not intercalate into DNA
(Mahler and Perlman, 1973; Perlman and Mahler, 1973). Experiments
to determine this influence on the fate of mtDNA show that they
have no effect when cells are exposed in buffer alone, but that
degradation *is* initiated by them in the presence of an energy source,
perhaps by a ATP-requiring endonuclease. Thus, EtdBr (and its
close relatives) is unique in deforming intramitochondrial DNA
sufficiently to render it susceptible to an alteration in primary
structure in the absence of any additional requirements.

                         Modulation by Repair

     The results just presented suggest that mutagenesis may per-
haps be explained in terms of the "unleashing" of various enzymes
usually concerned with damage repair (Shankel and Molholt, 1973),
either of the excision or post-replication variety (or both).
There is corroborative evidence for this suggestion which had already been advanced earlier (Mehrotra and Mahler, 1968; Borst,
1972; Mahler and Perlman, 1972b). For instance, the kinetics of
mutagenesis by EtdBr (Slonimski *et al.*, 1968; Mahler *et al.*,
1971a), exhibit the common pattern - familiar, for example, from
studies of petite induction by ultraviolet light (Allen and Mac-
Quillan, 1969) - of a lag or shoulder followed by a pseudo-first
order reaction. Such behavior can be, and in some of the earlier
studies has been, interpreted in terms of a multiple target-single
hit model. This inference, although potentially attractive in
providing a clue concerning the number of genetically competent
copies of mtDNA, is probably not entirely correct: the complete
kinetics, *including* the lag, can be profoundly affected by a variety
of treatments or agents (review in Mahler, 1973a) among them most
simply - as found by my student R. Bastos and shown in Fig. 3 -
the length of starvation of cells in buffer prior to a mutagenic
exposure to 10 μM EtdBr. It is doubtful whether such a treatment
is really sufficient to alter the number of targets. Instead an
alternative explanation in terms of a modification in the repair-
ability of lesions appears much more attractive.

     More direct evidence comes from a study of three strains, one
wild type (N123), and two mutants (*uvs* p5 and *uvs* p72), originally
isolated and studied by E. Moustacchi (1969, 1971) at Orsay,
France, and kindly furnished to us by her as part of a collabora-

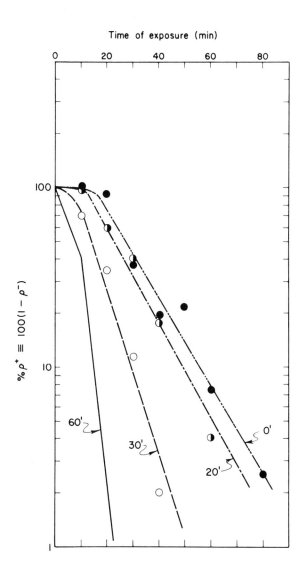

Figure 3. Kinetics of mutagenesis by EtdBr as a function of starvation in buffer. Cells of a commercial strain of *S. cerevisiae* (Fleischmann) were grown on 5% glucose to $A_{600}=0.4$, washed and resuspended at a cell concentration of 2×10^6/ml in 0.1M phosphate buffer, pH 6.5 and aerated at $30°C$ for the time shown. Aliquots were removed, made 10 μM in EtdBr and the extent of mutagenesis determined (Mahler and Perlman, 1972b) on continued incubation. The curve at 60 min represents the average of three separate runs.

tive effort. The mutant phenotype is characterized as particularly
and specifically susceptible to petite induction by UV, and thus
these mutants probably contain deficiencies in various steps of
mitochondrial repair system(s) for such lesions. Of these *uvs* *p5*
is a chromosomal mutant, exhibiting the normal, Mendelian pattern
of segregation upon meiosis and is believed by Moustacchi (private
communication) to be incision-defective. The synthesis of mtDNA
is as sensitive to EtdBr as is the wild type, but as can be seen
from Fig. 4 this *deficiency* affords considerable *protection* to
mutagenesis by this agent: hence incision, or an event depending
on this process, specified by a nuclear gene is *essential* for mutagenesis by EtdBr. On the other hand *uvs* *p72* exhibits a non-Mendelian
pattern of segregation, characteristic of cytoplasmic, and here
probably of mitochondrial, genes. Introduction of this mutation
makes the cell hypermutable by EtdBr as well as by other mutagens
and, under conditions of catabolite repression, also enhances its
spontaneous mutation frequency. As is seen in the Figure the enhancement of over-all rate by EtdBr is accounted for, at least in
part, by a decrease in the lag period - or the time required for
the saturation of this particular repair system. Similar results
are obtained with Berenil acting on either growing or nongrowing
cells, and with both mutagens under repressing or non-repressing
conditions. Thus, a deficiency in a second component of a UV
repair system is required for a more rapid or efficient fixation,
or consolidation, of the initial mutagenic lesion.

Modulations by the Inner Membrane

Following our discovery (Perlman and Mahler, 1971b) that mutagenesis by EtdBr could be modulated by simply incubating exposed
cells in buffer at 45°C, a variety of agents or treatments have
come to light which produce similar effects (for review see Mahler,
1973). Operationally we have defined (Mahler and Perlman, 1972b)
these modulations as a) *protection* (and its converse, *enhancement*),
b) *competition* and c) *cure* or *reversal*, depending on whether the
modulating agent or treatment is added a) prior to, b) simultaneously with or c) subsequent to the exposure to the mutagen proper. Of
the effective compounds the most interesting is probably Antimycin
A. This antibiotic is a highly effective and specific inhibitor
of respiration in yeast mitochondria (Mahler *et al.*, 1964; Butow
and Zeydel, 1968; Kovac *et al.*, 1970; Mahler and Perlman, 1971a).
It binds strongly and specifically, exclusively to a component of
the inner mitochondrial membrane and blocks its respiratory chain
between cytochrome b_T and cytochrome C_1 (Jagow and Klingenberg,
1972; Jagow *et al.*, 1973). As shown by Dr. M. Waring at Cambridge University (personal communication) it does *not* bind to covalently closed or relaxed circular DNA. Yet it is a most effective
modulator of mitochondrial mutagenesis by EtdBr (Krieger, 1972;

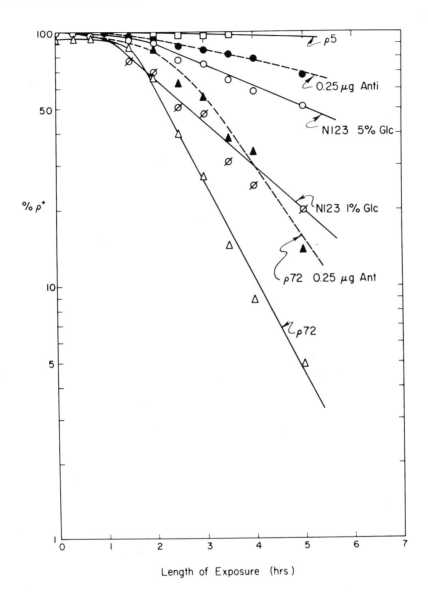

Figure 4. Kinetics of mutagenesis by EtdBr of strains defective in mitochondrial repair functions. Cells of the three strains, obtained from Dr. Moustacchi, were grown and treated as described in the legend to Fig. 3. One sample of the wild type was also grown on 1% instead of 5% glucose. Mutagenesis was performed after 60 min starvation with 5 µM EtdBr, in the presence of 0.25 µg/ml of Antimycin A where indicated.

Mahler and Perlman, 1972b), and can perform this task in all three ways described, even in repressed mitochondria, when respiration and the concentration of all possible interaction sites should be minimal. Fig. 5 shows results for the competition and cure by this agent. We have found that the effect can be titrated and that with most strains (Fig. 6) 0.25 µg of Antimycin added to $\sim$2 X 10^6 cells per ml affords almost complete protection of repressed cells in the competition assay. Extensive study of the molecular basis for this effect as well as for reversal has shown that Antimycin A does not prevent the nucleolytic attacks on mtDNA (Fig. 7). In fact, other experiments indicate that under conditions of protection or reversal from $\sim$1% ρ^+ to 50% ρ^- or better, it does not prevent the degradation of DNA to a point where the level of parental counts in the mtDNA region of CsCl gradients has dropped to $\sim$5%. We are therefore inclined to believe that "competition" or "cure" of the mutagenic event are misnomers in the sense that the effects responsible become manifest relatively late in the sequence leading to fixation of the mutagenic lesion, subsequent to the fragmentation of at least the bulk of the mtDNA. What *is* brought about by Antimycin - as well as by euflavine - the effects of which are similar at a concentration of $\geq$5 µM (Fig. 6) - appears to be the retention or reconstruction of *at least one* intact mitochondrial genome per cell, perhaps by a process akin to multiplicity reactivation and marker rescue in phage genetics. Perhaps the apparent reversal and other modulations of the action of EtdBr in other systems (*e.g.* Whittaker *et al.*, 1972; Luha *et al.*, 1971; Flechtner and Sager, 1973) can be accounted for in similar terms. However, because of the specificity of Antimycin A, this particular process almost certainly requires the participation of a peculiarly mitochondrial entity, its inner membrane. This membrane is also known to be capable of strong, hydrophobic interactions with EtdBr and acridines (Azzi and Santato, 1971). We recall the observation that the elaboration of an entity at or close to the binding site for Antimycin A, namely cytochrome b_T, appears itself to be dependent on mitochondrial protein synthesis. Since *uvs* ρ72 can still be protected or cured by Antimycin (Fig. 6) we have tentatively identified two mitochondrial components required for genetic activity of mtDNA, one of them, at least, closely linked to a specific inner membrane function.

ACKNOWLEDGMENTS

    This research was supported by Research Grant PHS R01 GM 12228 from the Institute of General Medical Sciences, National Institutes of Health, U.S. Public Health Service; the author holds a Research Career Award (K06 05060) from this institute.

    I wish to thank the various former and current members of the yeast biogenesis group cited in the text as well as my colleagues,

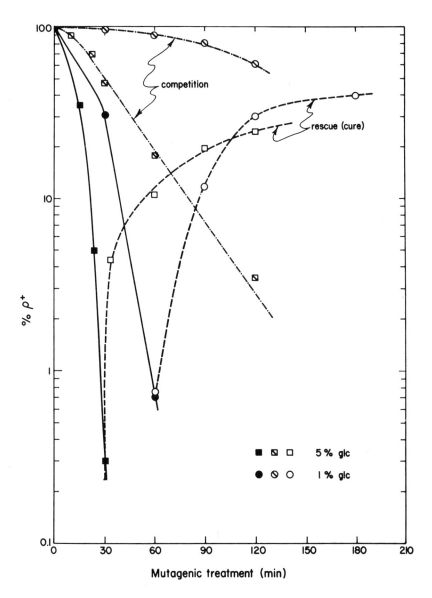

Figure 5. Influence of Antimycin A on kinetics of mutagenesis by
EtdBr. The strain and conditions used were identical to the ones
described in Fig. 3 except for the carbon source which was 1% or
5% glucose, as indicated. Starvation was for 60 min in buffer and
mutagenesis used 25 μM EtdBr, in the presence of 1 μg/ml Antimycin
A where indicated. Aliquots of the EtdBr sample were removed at
30 and 60 min, filtered, washed and resuspended in buffer containing 1 μg/ml Antimycin A and tested for rescue after further incubation as shown.

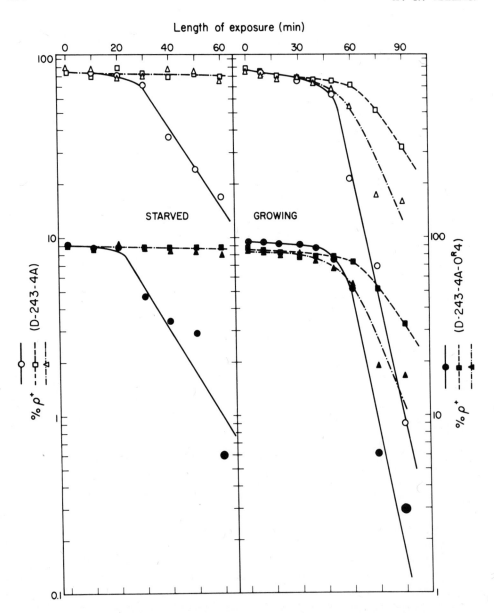

Figure 6. Influence of Antimycin A and euflavine on kinetics of mutagenesis of haploid cells. Cultures of two haploid strains, described by and obtained from Dr. R. Criddle (Shannon *et al.*, 1973), one wild type (D243-4A) and one carrying a mitochondrial marker for oligomycin resistance (D243-4A-O[R]4) were grown on 5% glucose, harvested and mutagenized with 5 μM EtdBr, either after starvation for 60 min (left), or after suspension in fresh medium at a cell concentration of 2 X 10[6]/ml (circles). Other aliquots

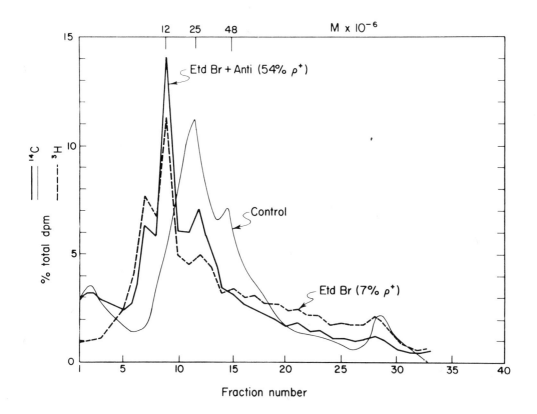

Figure 7. Antimycin A has no effect on registration induced by
EtdBr. The protocol used was similar to that described in the
legend to Fig. 2 except that mutagenesis was by 5 µM EtdBr on cells
resuspended in complete medium without prior starvation and incubated for 120 min in the presence ([^{14}C]) or absence ([^{3}H]) of
1 µg/ml Antimycin A. Controls, labeled with [^{3}H], and EtdBr-
treated cells, labeled with [^{14}C], were treated as above, isolated,
mixed and analyzed. Their patterns were identical to those shown
with the isotopes reversed and are not shown.

contained, in addition to EtdBr, either 0.25 µg/ml Antimycin A
(squares) or 10 µM euflavine (triangles).

Drs. G. Gimes of the Department of Zoology, Indiana University;
P. Perlman, Department of Genetics, Ohio State University; E.
Moustacchi of the Institut de Radium, 91 Orsay, France; P. Slonim-
ski of the Institut de Génétique Moléculaire, 91 Gif, France, and
M. Waring, Department of Pharmacology, University of Cambridge,
England, for their ideas, for their continued collaboration and
for permitting me to cite their unpublished observations. Ms. C.
Williams and K. Assimos provided devoted and competent technical
assistance.

REFERENCES

Allen, N. E. and A. M. MacQuillan. 1969. Target analysis of mitochondrial units in yeast. J. Bact. 97: 1142.

Ashwell, M. and T. S. Work. 1970. The biogenesis of mitochondria.
Ann. Rev. Biochem. 39: 251.

Azzi, A. and M. Santato. 1971. Interaction of ethidium with the
mitochondrial membrane: Cooperative binding and energy-linked
changes. Biochem. Biophys. Res. Comm. 44: 211.

Bernardi, G., F. Carnevali, A. Nicolaieff, G. Piperno and G. Tecce.
1968. Separation and characterization of a satellite DNA from a
yeast cytoplasmic "petite" mutant. J. Mol. Biol. 37: 493.

Bicknell, J. N. and H. C. Douglas. 1970. Nucleic acid homologies
among species of *Saccharomyces*. J. Bact. 101: 505.

Blamire, J., D. R. Cryer, D. B. Finkelstein and J. Marmur. 1972.
Sedimentation properties of yeast nuclear and mitochondrial DNA.
J. Mol. Biol. 67: 11.

Boardman, N. K., A. W. Linnane and R. M. Smillie. 1971. Autonomy
and Biogenesis of Mitochondria and Chloroplasts, North Holland,
Amsterdam, London.

Bolotin, M., D. Coen, J. Deutsch, B. Dujon, P. Netter, E. Petrochilo
and P. P. Slonimski. 1971. La recombinaison des mitochondries chez
Saccharomyces cerevisiae. Bull. de Inst. Past. 69: 215.

Borst, P. and L. A. Grivell. 1971. Mitochondrial ribosomes. FEBS
Lett. 13: 73.

Borst, P. 1972. Mitochondrial nucleic acids. Ann. Rev. Biochem.
41: 333.

Borst, P. and R. A. Flavell. 1972. Mitochondrial DNA: Structure, genes, replication. In (J. G. van den Bergh, P. Borst, L. L. M. van Deemen, J. C. Riemersma, E. C. Slater, and J. M. Tager, eds.) Mitochondria/Biomembranes. p. 1. North-Holland, Amsterdam.

Butow, R. A. and M. Zeydel. 1968. The isolation of an antimycin-resistant mutant of *Torulopsis utilis*. J. Biol. Chem. $\underline{243}$: 2545.

Christiansen, C., A. Leth Bak, A. Stenderup and G. Christiansen. 1971. Repetitive DNA in yeasts. Nature New Biol. $\underline{231}$: 176.

Cohen, M., J. Casey, M. Rabinowitz and G. S. Getz. 1972. Hybridization of mitochondrial transfer RNA and mitochondrial DNA in petite mutants of yeast. J. Mol. Biol. $\underline{63}$: 441.

Cohen, M. and M. Rabinowitz. 1973. Analysis of grande and petite yeast mitochondrial DNA by tRNA hybridization. Biochim. Biophys. Acta in press.

Dawid, I. B. 1972a. Mitochondrial RNA in *Xenopus laevis*. I. The expression of the mitochondrial genome. J. Mol. Biol. $\underline{63}$: 201.

Dawid, I. B. 1972b. Evolution of mitochondrial DNA sequences in *Xenopus*. Devel. Biol. $\underline{29}$: 139.

Dawidowicz, K. 1972. Studies on the mitochondrial protein synthesis system in *Saccharomyces cerevisiae*. Ph.D. Dissertation, Indiana University.

Dawidowicz, K. and H. R. Mahler. 1973. Synthesis of mitochondrial proteins. In (F. T. Kenny, B. A. Hamkalo, G. Favelukes and J. T. August, eds.) Gene Expression and Its Regulation. p. 503. Plenum Press, New York.

Flechtner, V. R. and R. Sager. 1973. Ethidium bromide induced selective and reversible loss of chloroplast DNA. Nature New Biol. $\underline{241}$: 277.

Freifelder, D. 1970. Molecular weights of coliphages and coliphage DNA. IV. Molecular weights of DNA from bacteriophages T4, T5 and T7 and the general problem of determination of M. J. Mol. Biol. $\underline{54}$: 567.

Galper, J. B. and J. E. Darnell. 1971. Mitochondrial protein synthesis in HeLa cells. J. Mol. Biol. $\underline{57}$: 363.

Goldring, E. S., L. I. Grossman, D. Krupnick, D. R. Cryer and J. Marmur. 1970. The petite mutation in yeast. Loss of mitochondrial deoxyribonucleic acid during induction of petites with ethidium bromide. J. Mol. Biol. $\underline{52}$: 323.

Goldring, E. S., L. I. Grossman and J. Marmur. 1971. Petite muta-tion in yeast. II. Isolation of mutants containing mitochondrial deoxyribonucleic acid of reduced size. J. Bact. 107: 377.

Hartwell, L. H., H. T. Hutchison, T. M. Holland and C. S. McLaughlin. 1970. The effect of cycloheximide upon polyribosome stability in two yeast mutants defective respectively in the initiation. Molec. Gen. Genetics 106: 347.

Hatefi, Y., W. G. Hanstein and K. A. Davis. 1973. Structure of electron transfer chain. Ann. N. Y. Acad. Sci. in press.

Hollenberg, C. P., P. Borst and E. F. J. van Bruggen. 1970. Mito-chondrial DNA. V. A 25μ closed circular duplex DNA molecule in wild type yeast mitochondria. Structure and genetic complexity. Biochim. Biophys. Acta 209:1.

Hollenberg, C. P., P. Borst and E. F. J. van Bruggen. 1972. Mito-chondrial DNA from cytoplasmic petite mutants of yeast. Biochim. Biophys. Acta 277: 35.

Hutchison, H. T., L. H. Hartwell and C. S. McLaughlin. 1969. Temperature-sensitive yeast mutant defective in ribonucleic acid production. J. Bact. 99: 807.

Jagow, von G. and M. Klingenberg. 1972. Close correlation between antimycin titer and cytochrome b$_T$ content in mitochondria of chlor-amphenicol treated Neurospora crassa. FEBS Lett. 24: 278.

Jagow, von G., H. Weiss and M. Klingenberg. 1973. Comparison of the respiratory chain of Neurospora crassa wild type and the mi-mutants mi-1 and mi-3. Eur. J. Biochem. 33: 140.

King, M. E., G. C. Godman and D. W. King. 1972. Respiratory enzymes and mitochondrial morphology of HeLa and L cells treated with chlor-amphenicol and ethidium bromide. J. Cell Biol. 53: 127.

Koch, J. 1973. Introduction of "nicks" and "chops" into human mitochondrial DNA in vivo and in vitro. Eur. J. Biochem. 33: 98.

Kovac, L., P. Smigan, E. Hrusovska and B. Hess. 1970. Interactions of uncoupling agents and of antimycin a with cytochrome b in yeast and heart muscle preparation under anaerobic conditions. Arch. Biochem. Biophys. 139: 370.

Kraml, J. and H. R. Mahler. 1967. Biochemical correlates of respi-ratory deficiency. VIII. A precipitating antiserum against cyto-chrome oxidase of yeast and its use in the study of respiratory deficiency. Immunochemistry 4: 213.

Krieger, N. 1972. Effects of antimycin a on mutagenesis by
ethidium bromide. Senior Thesis, Department of Chemistry, Indiana
University.

Kroon, A. M., E. Agsteribbe and H. de Vries. 1972. Protein syn-
thesis in mitochondria and chloroplasts. In (L. Bosch, ed.) The
Mechanism of Protein Synthesis and Its Regulation. p. 539. North-
Holland, Amsterdam.

Linnane, A. W. and J. M. Haslam. 1970. The biogenesis of yeast
mitochondria. Current Topics in Cellular Regulation 2: 101.

Linnane, A. W., J. M. Haslam, H. B. Lukins and P. Nagley. 1972.
The biogenesis of mitochondria in microorganisms. Ann. Rev.
Microbiol. 26: 163.

Luha, A. A., L. E. Sarcoe and P. A. Whittaker. 1971. Biosynthesis
of yeast mitochondria. Drug effects on the petite negative yeast
Kluyveromyces lactis. Biochem. Biophys. Res. Comm. 44: 396.

Mahler, H. R., B. Mackler, S. Grandchamp and P. P. Slonimski. 1964.
Biochemical correlates of respiratory deficiency. I. The isolation
of a respiratory particle. Biochemistry 3: 668.

Mahler, H. R. and P. S. Perlman. 1971. Mitochondriogenesis analyzed by blocks on mitochondrial translation and transcription. Biochemistry 10: 2979.

Mahler, H. R., B. D. Mehrotra and P. S. Perlman. 1971a. Formation
of yeast mitochondria. V. Ethidium bromide as a probe for the
functions of mitochondrial DNA. Prog. in Molec. and Subcell.
Biol. 2: 274.

Mahler, H. R., P. Perlman and B. D. Mehrotra. 1971b. Formation of
yeast mitochondria. IV. Mitochondrial specification of the
respiratory chain. In (N. K. Boardman, A. W. Linnane and R. M.
Smillie, eds.) Autonomy and Biogenesis of Mitochondria and Chloroplast. p. 492. North-Holland, Amsterdam.

Mahler, H. R., P. S. Perlman, P. Slonimski, M. J. Deutsch, H.
Fukuhara and C. Faye. 1971c. Information content of mitochondrial
DNA. Fed. Proc. 30: 1149.

Mahler, H. R. and P. S. Perlman. 1972a. Effects of mutagenic
treatment by ethidium bromide on cellular and mitochondrial phenotype. Arch. Biochem. Biophys. 148: 115.

Mahler, H. R. and P. S. Perlman. 1972b. Mitochondrial membranes
and mutagenesis by ethidium bromide. J. Supramol. Structure 1: 105.

Mahler, H. R., K. Dawidowicz and F. Feldman. 1972. Formate as a specific label for mitochondrial translational products. J. Biol. Chem. 247: 7439.

Mahler, H. R. 1973a. Biogenetic autonomy of mitochondria. CRC Critical Reviews in Biochemistry in press.

Mahler, H. R. 1973b. Structural requirements for mitochondrial mutagenesis. J. Supramol. Structure in press.

Mahler, H. R. and K. Dawidowicz. 1973. Autonomy of mitochondria of *Saccharomyces cerevisiae* in their production of messenger RNA. Proc. Nat. Acad. Sci. 70: 111.

Mahler, H. R. and P. S. Perlman. 1973. Induction of respiration deficient mutants in *Saccharomyces cerevisiae* by berenil. I. Berenil, a novel non-intercalating mutagen. Molec. Gen. Genetics 121: 285.

Mason, T., E. Ebner, R. O. Poyton, J. Saltzgaber, D. C. Wharton, L. Mennucci and G. Schatz. 1972. The participation of mitochondrial and cytoplasmic protein synthesis in mitochondrial formation. In (G. S. van den Bergh, P. Borst, and E. C. Slater, eds.) Mitochondria, Biogenesis and Bioenergetics. 8th Meeting Fed. Europ. Biochem. Soc. in press. North-Holland, Amsterdam.

Mehrotra, B. D. and H. R. Mahler. 1968. Characterization of some unusual DNAs from the mitochondria from certain "petite" strains of *Saccharomyces cerevisiae*. Arch. Biochem. Biophys. 128: 685.

Moustacchi, E. 1969. Cytoplasmic and nuclear genetic events induced by UV light in strains of *Saccharomyces cerevisiae* with different UV sensitivities. Mutation Res. 7: 171.

Moustacchi, E. 1971. Evidence for nucleus independent steps in control of repair of mitochondrial damage. IV. UV-induction of the cytoplasmic "petite" mutation in UV-sensitive nuclear mutants of *Saccharomyces cerevisiae*. Molec. Gen. Genetics 114: 50.

Nagley, P. and A. W. Linnane. 1972. Biogenesis of mitochondria. XXI. Studies on the nature of the mitochondrial genome in yeast: The degenerative effects of ethidium bromide on mitochondrial genetic information in a respiratory competent strain. J. Mol. Biol. 66: 181.

Nass, M. M. K. 1970. Abnormal DNA patterns in animal mitochondria: Ethidium bromide-induced breakdown of closed circular DNA and conditions leading to oligomer accumulation. Proc. Nat. Acad. Sci. 67: 1926.

Parsons, P. and M. V. Simpson. 1973. Deoxyribonucleic acid bio-synthesis in mitochondria. J. Biol. Chem. 248: 1912.

Perlman, P. S. and H. R. Mahler. 1971a. Molecular consequences of ethidium bromide mutagenesis. Nature New Biol. 231: 12.

Perlman, P. S. and H. R. Mahler. 1971b. A premutational state induced in yeast by ethidium bromide. Biochem. Biophys. Res. Comm. 44: 261.

Perlman, P. S. and H. R. Mahler. 1973. Induction of respiration deficient mutants in *Saccharomyces cerevisiae* by berenil. II. Characteristics of the process. Molec. Gen. Genetics 121: 295.

Perlman, P. S., H. T. Abelson and S. Penman. 1973. Mitochondrial protein synthesis: RNA with the properties of eukaryotic messenger RNA. Proc. Nat. Acad. Sci. 70: 350.

Preer, J. R., Jr. 1971. Extrachromosomal Inheritance: Hereditary Symbionts, Mitochondria, Chloroplasts. Ann. Rev. Gen. 5: 361.

Rabinowitz, M. and H. Swift. 1970. Mitochondrial nucleic acids and their relation to the biogenesis of mitochondria. Physiol. Rev. 50: 376.

Reijnders, L., C. M. Kleisen, L. A. Grivell and P. Borst. 1972. Hybridization studies with yeast mitochondrial RNAs. Biochim. Biophys. Acta 272: 396.

Sager, R. 1972. Cytoplasmic Genes and Organelles. Academic Press, New York.

Sanders, J. P. M., R. A. Flavell, P. Borst and J. N. M. Mol. 1973. Nature of the base sequence conserved in the mitochondrial DNA of a low-density petite. Biochim. Biophys. Acta in press.

Saunders, G. W., E. B. Gingold, M. K. Trembath, H. B. Lukins and A. W. Linnane. 1971. Mitochondrial genetics in yeast: Segregation of a cytoplasmic determinant in crosses and its loss or retention in the petite. In (N. K. Boardman, A. W. Linnane, and R. M. Smillie, eds.) Autonomy and Biogenesis of Mitochondria and Chloroplasts. p. 185. North-Holland, London.

Schatz, G. 1970. Biogenesis of mitochondria. In (E. Racker, ed.) Membranes of Mitochondria and Chloroplasts. p. 251. Van Nostrand Reinhold, New York.

Schweizer, E. and H. O. Halvorson. 1969. On the regulation of ribosomal RNA synthesis in yeast. Exp. Cell Res. 56: 239.

Shakespeare, P. G. and H. R. Mahler. 1972. Properties and use of an antiserum to cytochrome oxidase from baker's yeast. Arch. Biochem. Biophys. 151: 496.

Shankel, D. M. and B. Molholt. 1973. Ethidium bromide inhibition of dark repair processes in ultraviolet irradiated T1 bacteriophage and bacteria. Studia Biophysica (Berlin) in press.

Shannon, C., R. Enns, L. Short, K. Burchiel and R. S. Criddle. 1973. Alterations in mitochondrial ATPase activity resulting from mutation of mitochondrial DNA. J. Biol. Chem. in press.

Slonimski, P. P., G. Perrodin and J. H. Croft. 1968. Ethidium bromide induced mutation of yeast mitochondria: Complete transformation of cells into respiratory deficient nonchromosomal "petites". Biochem. Biophys. Res. Comm. 30: 232.

Smith, A. E. and K. A. Marcker. 1970. Cytoplasmic methionine transfer RNAs from eukaryotes. Nature 226: 607.

Tzagoloff, A. and A. Akai. 1972. Assembly of the mitochondrial membrane system. VIII. Properties of the products of mitochondrial protein synthesis in yeast. J. Biol. Chem. 247: 6517.

Tzagoloff, A., A. Akai and M. F. Sierra. 1972. Assembly of the mitochondrial membrane system. VII. Synthesis and integration of F_1 subunits into the rutamycin-sensitive adenosine triphosphatase. J. Biol. Chem. 247: 6511.

Waring, M. 1970. Variation of the supercoils in closed circular DNA by binding of antibiotics and drugs: Evidence for molecular models involving intercalation. J. Mol. Biol. 54: 247.

Weiss, H. 1972. Cytochrome b on *Neurospora crassa* mitochondria. A membrane protein containing subunits of cytoplasmic and mitochondrial origin. Eur. J. Biochem. 30: 469.

Whittaker, P. A., R. C. Hammond and A. A. Luha. 1972. Mechanism of mitochondrial mutation in yeast. Nature New Biol. 238: 206.

Williamson, D. H. 1970. The effect of environmental and genetic factors on the replication of mitochondrial DNA in yeast. Control of Organelle Development 23: 247.

16. INVOLVEMENT OF RNA IN THE PROCESS OF PUFF INDUCTION IN POLYTENE CHROMOSOMES

A. Graessmann*, M. Graessmann* and F. J. S. Lara[†]

*Institut für Molekularbiologie und Biochemie, Freie Universität, Arnimallee 22, 1 Berlin 33 and [†]Department of Biochemistry, Institute of Chemistry, C.P. 20780, São Paulo, Brasil

A variety of agents can induce puffs in the polytene chromosomes of dipteran salivary glands. Ecdysone and its analogues and temperature shocks are best suited for studies on the mechanism of puff induction because the puffs they produce are the same as those which occur during normal development (for review, Berendes, 1972, 1973). From these studies it appears that an interaction between the puff-inducing agents and cytoplasmic factors is necessary for puff induction and that the involvement of RNA in this process is likely.

We have studied the role of RNA in puff induction on chromosomes of *Rhynchosciara* salivary gland cells. At defined periods in larval development, the so-called DNA puffs appear in the chromosomes (Breuer and Pavan, 1955) and it appears that gene amplification occurs in these puffs (Breuer and Pavan, 1955; Ficq and Pavan, 1957; Rudkin and Corlette, 1957; Meneghini *et al.*, 1971). Although RNA synthesis occurs in these puffs, the nature of RNA transcribed remains to be established. Recent results (Balsamo *et al.*, 1973) suggest that the RNA transcribed in the amplified regions of the genome is restricted to the nucleus.

Our experimental design consisted of injecting into the cytoplasm of salivary gland cells RNA preparations obtained from glands of larvae of distinct developmental stage. In one of these the giant DNA puffs are present (period IV of the 4th instar) and in the other they are absent (period II of the 4th instar). The recipient cells were from salivary glands in period II of the 4th instar, lacking the giant DNA puffs in their chromosomes. The division of the 4th instar of developing *Rhynchosciara* larva was originally proposed by Guaraciaba and Toledo (1967) and later modified by Terra *et al.* (1973a).

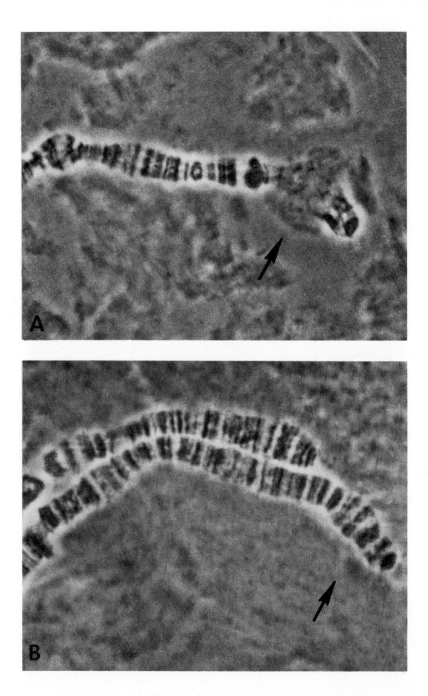

Figure 1. (A) Puff B-2 (arrow) in chromosome B of a salivary gland cell from a period II 4th instar larva induced by intracytoplasmic injection of an RNA preparation from glands in period IV of the 4th

Injections were made with glass microneedles using a Leitz micromanipulator according to the technique developed for mammalian cells by Graessmann (1970) and Graessmann and Graessmann (1971). Recipient glands were extirpated from the larvae and 10^{-10} ml of a RNA solution containing 2-3 mg/ml was injected into each of the 10-15 cells in one side of the proximal extremity of the salivary gland. The organ was then incubated for 3 hours at 23°C in the medium developed by Terra *et al.* (1973b) supplemented with 10% bovine serum. At the end of the incubation the glands were squashed using the technique of Sauaia *et al.* (1971) and preparations were examined by phase contrast microscopy.

RNA was prepared by the SDS - Pronase method of Daneholt (1972), extracted with phenol, precipitated with alcohol in the presence of 200 mM NaCl, and dissolved in 10 mM Tris, 100 mM NaCl, pH 7.4. For control experiments, aimed at verifying the nature of the active molecules, the preparations were further treated with either RNase (90 µg/ml, 25°C, 30 min) and then SDS - Pronase digested (25°C, 30 min), phenol-extracted and precipitated with alcohol in the presence of yeast tRNA or DNase (30 µg/ml in the usual suspension buffer containing 5 mM $MgCl_2$, 25°C, 30 min), followed by phenol treatment and ethanol precipitation.

Our results (Figs. 1 and 2) show that the RNA, extracted from salivary glands of period IV which show giant DNA puffs B-2 and C-3 (Breuer and Pavan, 1955; Guevara, 1971), when injected in younger host gland cells (period II) induce formation of puffs B-2 and C-5 within three hours. At least in the case of DNA-puff B-2 the response is specific to RNA-donor stage. On the other hand even in the experimental donor, puff C-5 would have appeared at a still later stage. Control experiments in which the RNA preparation was obtained from salivary gland cells in the same period of development as the recipient cells (period II) showed no puff induction nor any other detectable effect on chromosome morphology. Puff-inducing activity of the RNA preparations was destroyed by treatment with RNase but not after treatment with DNase. Injection into the recipient cells of the solvent in which the RNA was dissolved did not induce any puffs.

---

instar when puff B-2 normally forms. Normally puff B-2 would appear in the recipient cells 10 days later in the course of development. (B) Chromosome B (arrow) at region B-2 and chromosome A from a cell of a gland in period II of the 4th instar injected with an RNA preparation from cells of the same developmental period. Note the absence of a puff in region B-2, normal for this period of development (X1600).

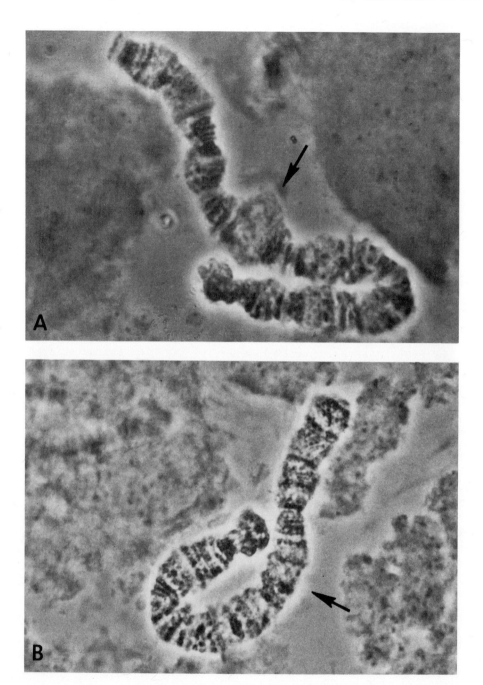

Figure 2. (A) Chromosome C with a puff in region C-5 (arrow) induced by RNA injection as in Fig. 1A. (B) Chromosome C without a puff
from a cell treated in the same way as in Fig. 1B. (X1600).

Models that include the participation of RNA molecules in gene control mechanisms have been proposed by Frenster (1965a) and by Britten and Davidson (1969). Experimental evidence for the participation of RNA in such processes have been presented by Frenster (1965b) and Bonner and associates (for review, Huang and Smith, 1972) have obtained a unique protein bound RNA from chromatin preparations that may play a role in the control of transcription in eukaryotes. Experiments indicative of the participation of RNA molecules in puff formation were carried out recently by Holt, van der Velden and Berendes (quoted in Berendes, 1972); RNase injected into nuclei of salivary gland cells of *Drosophila* inhibited puff induction by temperature shock.

The present results constitute more direct evidence for the role of RNA in puff formation. It is especially noteworthy that the induction of puffs occuring in the normal development of *Rhynchosciara* can be brought about by RNA preparations obtained from the specific stage of development in which these puffs occur. These results clearly indicate the prospects of this kind of experimentation in the study of gene action.

ACKNOWLEDGMENTS

This work was supported by funds from the Project BIOQ/FAPESP (quimicas 70/1461). A.G. is a visiting professor at the University of São Paulo under this Project. We acknowledge the help of Dr. L. C. Simões and J. M. Amabis in the preparations of the photographs and thank them for a critical reading of the manuscript. We are especially grateful to Dr. S. P. Modak for many discussions and for help in the preparation of the manuscript.

REFERENCES

Balsamo, J., J. M. Hierro and F. J. S. Lara. 1973. Transcription of repetitive DNA sequences in *Rhynchosciara* salivary glands. Cell Differentiation 2: 119.

Berendes, H. D. 1972. The control of puffing in *Drosophila hydei*. Results and Problems in Cell Differentiation 4: 181.

Berendes, H. D. 1973. Synthetic activity of polytene chromosomes. Int. Rev. Cytol. in press.

Breuer, M. E. and C. Pavan. 1955. Behaviour of polytene chromosomes of *Rhynchosciara angelae* at different stages of larval development. Chromosoma 7: 371.

Britten, R. J. and E. H. Davidson. 1969. Gene regulation for higher cells: a theory. Science 165: 349.

Daneholt, B. 1972. Giant RNA-transcript in a Balbiani ring. Nature New Biol. 240: 229.

Ficq, A. and C. Pavan. 1957. Autoradiography of polytene chromosomes of Rhynchosciara angelae at different stages of larval development. Nature 180: 983.

Frenster, J. H. 1965a. A model of specific derepression within interphase chromatin. Nature 206: 1269.

Frenster, J. H. 1965b. Nuclear polyanions as derepressors of synthesis of ribonucleic acid. Nature 206: 680.

Graessmann, A. 1970. Mikrochirurgische Zellkerntransplantation bei Säugetierzellen. Exp. Cell Res. 60: 373.

Graessmann, A. and M. Graessmann. 1971. Über die Bildung von Melanin in Müskelzellen nach der direkten übertragung von RNA aus Harding-Passey-Melanomzellen. Hoppe-Seyler's Zeit. Physiol. Chem. 352: 527.

Guaraciaba, H. L. B. and L. F. A. Toledo. 1967. Age determination of Rhynchosciara angelae larvae. Rev. Brasil. Biol. 27: 321.

Huang, R. C. C. and M. M. Smith. 1972. Nucleic acid hybridization and the nature of protein bound RNA. Results and Problems in Cell Differentiation 3: 65.

Meneghini, R., H. A. Armelin, H. J. Balsamo and F. J. S. Lara. 1971. Indication of gene amplification in Rhynchosciara by RNA-DNA hybridization. J. Cell Biol. 49: 421.

Paulo, M. P. 1971. Estudo citológico da fisiologia e diferenciacão cromossômica durante o desenvolvimento larval de Rhynchosciara angelae. Thesis, University of São Paulo, São Paulo, Brasil.

Rudkin, G. T. and S. L. Corlette. 1957. Disproportionate synthesis of DNA in a polytene chromosome region. Proc. Nat. Acad. Sci. 43: 964.

Sauaia, H., E. M. Laicine and M. A. R. Alves. 1971. Hydroxyurea induced inhibition of DNA puff development in the salivary gland chromosomes of Bradysia hygida. Chromosoma 34: 129.

Terra, W. R., A. G. de Bianchi, A. G. Gambarini and F. J. S. Lara. 1973a. Haemolymph amino acids, related compounds and their relationship to cocoon production by *Rhynchosciara americana* (Dipera) larvae. J. Insect. Physiol. in press.

Terra, W. R., A. G. de Bianchi, A. G. Gambarini and F. J. S. Lara. 1973b. Culture medium for maintenance of *Rhynchosciara* (Diptera) larvae. In Vitro in press.

17. STIMULATION OF RNA POLYMERASE III BY HISTONES AND OTHER

POLYCATIONS

B. D. Hall, M. Brzezinska, C. P. Hollenberg and
L. D. Schultz

*Departments of Genetics and Biochemistry, University of
Washington, Seattle, Washington*

Three major RNA polymerases are obtained by extracting either whole yeast cells (Adman *et al.*, 1972) or nuclei (Brogt and Planta, 1972) by the procedure of Roeder and Rutter (1969). Each of the components found in yeast (Fig. 1) corresponds to one of the RNA polymerases I, II, and III found in sea urchins or rat liver nuclei (Blatti *et al.*, 1970). The relative activity on different templates and activity versus salt relationships are remarkably similar for each pair of corresponding animal and yeast enzymes (Adman *et al.*, 1972).

An RNA polymerase stimulatory factor can be obtained from yeast by high-salt extraction of complexes of RNA polymerase and DNA from the crude lysate. This factor, π-factor (Di Mauro *et al.*, 1972) is a small, heat-stable protein. Like histones, π-factor binds to DNA and has a tendency to aggregate but can be solubilized by high salt or urea. Of the three yeast RNA polymerases, enzyme III is most strongly stimulated by π.

More detailed studies of enzyme III have shown that the activity of this enzyme does not vary linearly with concentration, but instead shows a cooperative curve (Fig. 2, lower curve). By adding to enzyme III either π or histones (sea urchin), activity becomes proportional to enzyme concentration. A possible interpretation of these results is that the cooperativity is simply a consequence of enzyme denaturation in the lower range of total protein concentration. The possibility that histones and π merely protect enzyme III non-specifically is ruled out by the failure of either serum albumin (Fig. 2) or lysozyme (Fig. 3) to stimulate at low enzyme concentration. Furthermore, π can activate enzyme III even after

217

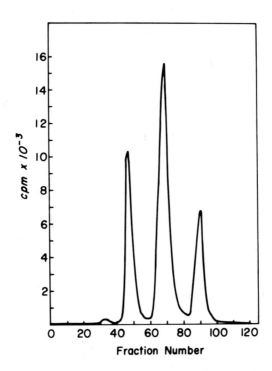

Figure 1.   Resolution of yeast DNA-dependent RNA polymerase activities by DEAE-Sephadex chromatography.   Extraction and chromatography
were performed by a modification of the procedure of Adman *et al.*
(1972) with the exception that the extraction buffer contained 0.6
mg phenylmethylsulfonyl fluoride per ml and 10% ethanol.   To 5.0 gm
of wet packed yeast cells (strain A364A) were added 5.0 ml H_2O,
10.0 ml extraction buffer and 10.0 gm 0.45 mm glass beads.   The
cells were disrupted and the resulting homogenate sonicated and
centrifuged as described previously (Adman *et al.*, 1972).   Eleven
ml of the resulting crude extract was diluted with 77 ml TGED buffer
(0.05M TrisCl, pH 7.9;   25% v/v glycerol;   0.5M EDTA and 0.5 mM
dithiothreitol) containing 0.3 mg/ml phenylmethylsulfonyl fluoride
and 5% ethanol.   This was applied to a 2.6 X 12 cm DEAE-Sephadex
A-25 column equilibrated with 0.05M $(NH_4)_2SO_4$ in TGED buffer.
Washing, column elution and RNA polymerase assay were as described
previously (Adman *et al.*, 1972).

the enzyme [at low (inactive) concentration] has been incubated for
30 minutes in complete reaction mix (Fig. 4).   This shows that the
enzyme is not inactivated during incubation without π;   it merely
fails to make RNA.

To study the structural basis for stimulation by histones, we
have tested other polycations for ability to stimulate RNA poly-

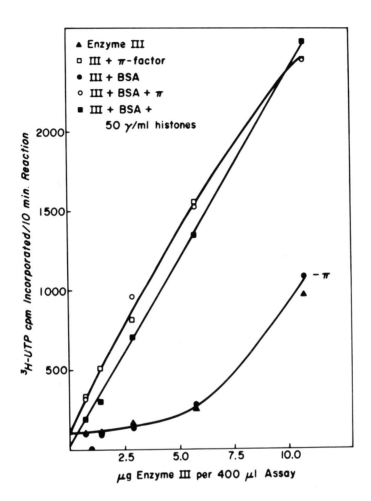

Figure 2. Effect of π-factor, bovine serum albumin and sea urchin histones upon [³H]UMP incorporation by RNA polymerase III. Reactions (400 µl) contained 50 mM TrisCl (pH 7.9), 1.6 mM MnCl₂, 0.1 mM EDTA, 0.1 mM dithiothreitol, 0.1 M (NH₄)₂SO₄, 0.5 mM ATP, CTP and GTP, and 0.05 mM [³H]UTP, 300 Ci/mol). The template was calf thymus DNA (100 µg/ml). Reactions were run for 10 min at 30°C after which 20 µl aliquots were spotted on paper filters which were tri-chloroacetic acid-washed. π-factor, prepared as previously described (Di Mauro *et al.*, 1972) was added to 90 µg/ml final concentration. Histones were acid-extracted from early blastula nuclei of *Strongylocentrotus purpuratus* by Byron Gallis. Yeast RNA polymerase III was prepared by the procedure of Adman *et al.* (1972).

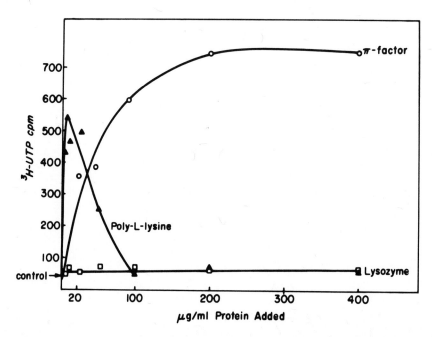

Figure 3. Stimulation of enzyme III by π-factor and poly(L-lysine) (Miles-Yeda Ltd., M.W. = 5,000-8,000). Conditions of reaction, including π-factor concentration, as in Fig. 2. Enzyme III concentration was 7 µg/ml; lysozyme utilized was 3X recrystallized egg-white lysozyme (Sigma).

merase III. Low concentrations of polylysine cause a large stimulation; higher concentrations block transcription (Fig. 3) and also precipitate the DNA template. Effective stimulation of polymerase III has also been obtained with spermine (Fig. 5) (a tetramine), spermidine (a triamine), but not with the diamine putrescine.

One feature common to all these stimulating molecules is the ability to bind strongly to double-stranded DNA. Structural models for such complexes involving a regular juxtaposition of amino groups opposite DNA phosphate groups have been proposed for complexes of DNA with spermine or spermidine (Liquori *et al.*, 1967), with poly-lysine (Tsuboi *et al.*, 1966) and with histones 1 and 4 (Olins, 1969; Sung and Dixon, 1970).

From the data we have on stimulation of eukaryotic RNA polymerase III by these polycations, it is not possible to determine with certainty whether stimulation acts at the level of initiation, continuation of chain growth, or release of arrested RNA polymerase followed by reinitiation. Stimulation of bacterial RNA polymerase by polyamines (Fox and Weiss, 1964; Krakow, 1963) is thought to

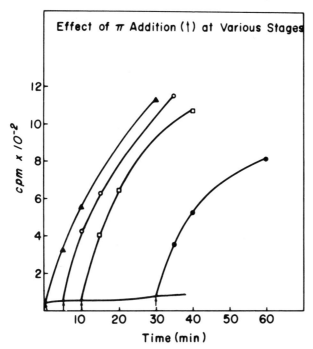

Figure 4. Stimulation of enzyme III by π addition after incubation at 30°C. Incubation conditions were those in Figs. 1-3 except that 200 μg/ml bovine serum albumin was present. Final concentrations were: π, 90 μg/ml; RNA polymerase III, 7 μg/ml. π-factor was added at the indicated times and synthesis was measured during the following period. Filled circles, π added at 30 min; solid line, RNA synthesis without addition of π.

result from either increased chain growth or reinitiation. While this type of "polyamine effect" may be involved in the stimulation we have observed, there is also evidence for an effect of π-factor and histones upon binding of RNA polymerase to DNA. By using the RNA polymerase inhibitor rifamycin AF/013 (Meilhac *et al.*, 1972) we have assayed for the ability of π and histone to mediate the formation of preinitiation complexes between RNA polymerase III and DNA. Our assay for preinitiation complexes is like that employing rifampicin to assay for the binding of E. *coli* RNA polymerase to promoter regions of DNA (Bautz and Bautz, 1970; Hinkle *et al.*, 1972). Although these two inhibitors may differ in detailed mode of action, we have found this drug useful for studying binding of enzyme III to DNA. No rifamycin AF/013-resistant complexes are formed when RNA polymerase III is incubated with DNA at 30°C. However, a prior incubation of enzyme and DNA in the presence of π, histone, or polyamine will protect a substantial fraction of the RNA polymerase molecules from subsequent inhibition by the rifamycin.

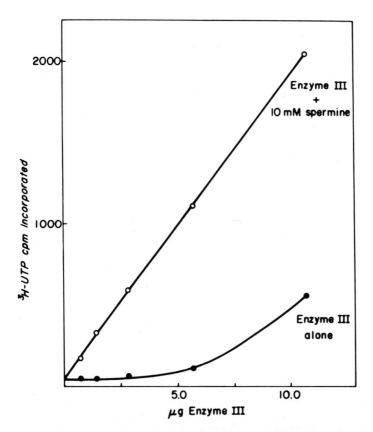

Figure 5. Stimulation of enzyme III by spermine. Conditions for the reaction as in Fig. 2. Spermine tetrahydrochloride (Calbiochem) was utilized.

The observation presented here, that histones *stimulate* transcription, seem to contradict a major conclusion of many chromatin transcription experiments: that binding of histones *represses* gene transcription (Bonner *et al.*, 1968a). To explain why we have observed stimulation rather than repression, it is useful to compare the conditions of our experiment with those used by the Bonner group and by other workers who have transcribed chromatin.

(1) The ratio by weight of histone to DNA we have used (0.5; Fig. 2) is less than that in chromatin (0.8 to 1.35; Bonner *et al.*, 1968b); but similar to that in partially dehistonized chromatin (Smart and Bonner, 1971), which is still a relatively inactive template.

(2) We have used a eukaryotic RNA polymerase, yeast RNA polymerase III, to transcribe histone·DNA complexes whereas, in the majority of *in vitro* chromatin transcription experiments, bacterial RNA polymerase has been used.

(3) Our transcription experiments were done in a medium of much higher salt concentration than that prescribed for measuring chromatin template activity with bacterial RNA polymerase (Bonner *et al.*, 1968b). In experiments measuring the effects of π on transcription by yeast polymerases I and II (C. P. Hollenberg, unpublished), it was clear that inhibitory effects of basic proteins overshadow stimulatory effects when the salt concentration is low. Because we used in this work an enzyme (yeast polymerase III) that is active under high salt conditions, we have been able to notice stimulatory effects of histones that would be masked by inhibitory effects at lower salt concentrations. In order to evaluate the relative physiological significance of histone stimulation, as compared to histone inhibition, it thus becomes important to know more about the ionic environment within the cell nucleus.

Concerning the mechanism by which π, histones and polyamines stimulate transcription, it is difficult to make a specific proposal on the basis of our rather limited data. However, by comparing the effects of π in our system with those produced by a similarly heat-stable bacterial transcription factor, certain interesting possibilities become apparent. D factor (Ghosh and Echols, 1972), H factor (Cukier-Kahn *et al.*, 1972) and π all stimulate under conditions of template excess. Under these conditions, a considerable amount of binding and initiation of *E. coli* polymerase on λ phage DNA occurs away from the "proper" promoters P_L and P_R. The experiments of Ghosh and Echols show that D protein causes a greater fraction of the binding/initiation events to occur at P_L and P_R rather than elsewhere.

The ability of π-factor to mediate the formation of pre-initiation complexes (see above) suggest that π and D factors may act in a similar manner. Efficient and accurate transcription requires that RNA polymerase molecules ignore the large number of potential binding sites represented by most of the DNA and bind instead at the much smaller number of sites represented by promoter regions.* In

---

* The term "promoter region" is used in this discussion in a broad sense: meaning a region of DNA in which, once RNA polymerase is bound, the likelihood of RNA chain initiation is very high. No distinction is made between *in vivo* and *in vitro* promoter regions; of course this does not imply that they are necessarily the same.

a simplified transcription system, containing only RNA polymerase and DNA, it is apparent that binding to nonpromoter regions significantly decreases the number of RNA polymerase molecules available to bind at promoters (Hinkle and Chamberlin, 1972). Since upon binding to DNA, RNA polymerase molecules distribute themselves between inactive and active binding sites (promoters), the possibility exists that chromosomal proteins may stimulate transcription by affecting DNA conformation. If the binding of histones serves to increase the "contrast" between promoter and nonpromoter regions insofar as RNA polymerase binding is concerned, then histone would act to stimulate transcription, particularly when RNA polymerase is limiting. It will be of great interest to know whether the mechanism whereby DNA-bound histones stimulate transcription is direct or indirect. Crick (1971) has suggested that chromosomal proteins bound near promoter regions of DNA may act to increase the affinity or rate with which promoter regions bind RNA polymerase. Alternatively, DNA-bound polycations might stimulate transcription primarily by decreasing the polymerase binding affinity of nonpromoter regions. The stimulation results from an increase in the number of RNA polymerase molecules available to bind to promoter regions.

ACKNOWLEDGMENT

This research was supported by grant GM 11895 from the NIH.

REFERENCES

Adman, R., L. D. Schultz and B. D. Hall. 1972. Transcription in yeast: separation and properties of multiple RNA polymerases. Proc. Nat. Acad. Sci. 69: 1702.

Bautz, E. K. F. and F. A. Bautz. 1970. Studies on the function of the RNA polymerase σ factor in promoter selection. Cold Spring Harbor Symp. Quant. Biol. 35: 227.

Blatti, S. P., C. J. Ingles, T. J. Lindell, P. W. Morris, R. F. Weaver, F. Weinberg and W. J. Rutter. 1970. Structure and regulatory properties of eukaryotic RNA polymerase. Cold Spring Harbor Symp. Quant. Biol. 35: 649.

Bonner, J., M. E. Dahmus, D. Fambrough, R. C. Huang, K. Marushige and D. Tuan. 1968a. The biology of isolated chromatin. Science 159: 47.

Bonner, J., G. R. Chalkley, M. Dahmus, D. Fambrough, F. Fujimura, R. C. Huang, J. Huberman, R. Jensen, K. Marushige, H. Olenbusch,

B. Olivera and J. Widholm. 1968b. Isolation and characterization of chromosomal nucleoproteins. Methods in Enzymol. 12: 57.

Brogt, Th. M. and R. J. Planta. 1972. Characteristics of DNA-dependent RNA polymerase activity from isolated yeast nuclei. FEBS Lett. 20: 47.

Cukier-Kahn, R., M. Jacquet and F. Gros. 1972. Two heat-resistant, low molecular weight proteins from *Escherichia coli* that stimulate DNA-directed RNA synthesis. Proc. Nat. Acad. Sci. 69: 3643.

Crick, F. 1971. General model for the chromosomes of higher organisms. Nature 234: 25.

Di Mauro, E., C. P. Hollenberg and B. D. Hall. 1972. Transcription in yeast: a factor that stimulates yeast RNA polymerases. Proc. Nat. Acad. Sci. 69: 2818.

Fox, C. F. and S. B. Weiss. 1964. Enzymatic synthesis of ribonucleic acid: II. Properties of the DNA-primed reaction with *Micrococcus lysodeikticus* ribonucleic acid polymerase. J. Biol. Chem. 239: 175.

Ghosh, S. and H. Echols. 1972. Purification and properties of D protein: a transcription factor of *Escherichia coli*. Proc. Nat. Acad. Sci. 69: 3660.

Hinkle, D. C. and M. Chamberlin. 1972. Studies of the binding of *Escherichia coli* RNA polymerase to DNA II. The kinetics of the binding reaction. J. Mol. Biol. 70: 187.

Hinkle, D. C., W. F. Mangel and M. J. Chamberlin. 1972. Studies of the binding of *Escherichia coli* RNA polymerase to DNA: IV. The effect of rifampicin on binding and on RNA chain initiation. J. Mol. Biol. 70: 209.

Huang, R. C. and J. Bonner. 1962. Histone, a suppressor of chromosomal RNA synthesis. Proc. Nat. Acad. Sci. 48: 1216.

Krakow, J. S. 1963. Ribonucleic acid polymerase of *Azotobacter vinelandii*: III. Effect of polyamines. Biochim. Biophys. Acta 72: 566.

Liquori, A. M., L. Constantino, V. Crescenzi, V. Elia, E. Giglio, R. Pulti, M. de Santis Savino and V. Vitagliano. 1967. Complexes between DNA and polyamines: a molecular model. J. Mol. Biol. 24: 113.

Meilhac, M., Z. Tysper and P. Chambon. 1972. Animal DNA-dependent RNA polymerases. 4. Studies on inhibition by rifamycin derivatives. Eur. J. Biochem. 28: 291.

Olins, D. E. 1969. Interaction of lysine-rich histones and DNA. J. Mol. Biol. 43: 439.

Roeder, R. G. and W. J. Rutter. 1969. Multiple forms of DNA-dependent RNA polymerase in eukaryotic organisms. Nature 224: 234.

Smart, J. E. and J. Bonner. 1971. Studies on the role of histones in relation to the template activity and precipitability of chromatin at physiological ionic strengths. J. Mol. Biol. 58: 675.

Sung, M. and G. H. Dixon. 1970. Modification of histones during spermiogenesis in trout: A molecular mechanism for altering histone binding to DNA. Proc. Nat. Acad. Sci. 67: 1616.

Tsuboi, M., K. Matsuo and P. O. P. Ts'o. 1966. Interaction of poly-L-lysine and nucleic acids. J. Mol. Biol. 15: 256.

18. A TRANSCRIPTION COMPLEX FROM CHLOROPLASTS OF *EUGLENA GRACILIS*

Richard B. Hallick* and William J. Rutter

Department of Biochemistry and Biophysics, University of California, San Francisco, San Francisco, California

Studies on RNA synthesis and the regulation of gene expression in nuclei are hampered by the complexity of the template. Another eukaryotic transcription system is that of the cellular organelles (mitochondria and chloroplasts), whose genomes are small and well defined. We have focused our attention on the transcription of these genomes.

In the course of our purification of RNA polymerase from *Euglena gracilis* chloroplasts, we found that the enzyme remains associated with the chloroplast DNA. In contrast to the strategy often used in studying transcription, of resolving and purifying the RNA polymerase for reconstitution with a purified DNA template, we have chosen to isolate the genome as a transcription complex composed of the DNA plus the RNA polymerase and any regulatory elements that may fortuitously remain with the DNA.

Chloroplasts were isolated from *E. gracilis* Z (Manning *et al.*, 1971) and lysed in a buffer containing Triton X-100. This lysate was further purified by differential centrifugation and gel filtration chromatography on Agarose A-5M (Fig. 1). The RNA polymerase eluted with the chloroplast DNA as a sharp band excluded by the column. More than 99% of the protein and all the pigment was retained by the column, and hence removed by this procedure. A 600-fold purification of RNA polymerase from purified organelles was obtained.

---

* Present address: Department of Chemistry, University of Colorado, Boulder, Colorado.

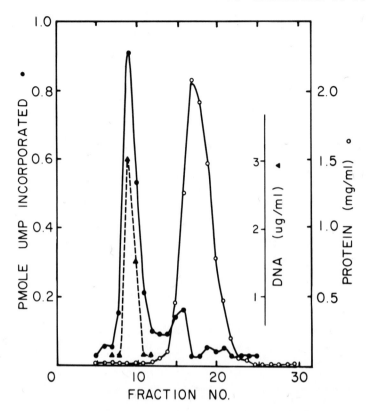

Figure 1. Purification of *Euglena* chloroplast transcription complex
by gel filtration chromatography on Agarose A-5M. Details of the
purification procedure are described elsewhere (Hallick, Richards
and Rutter, in preparation). Protein was estimated as previously
described (Rutter, 1967). DNA was determined by the diphenylamine
method (Burton, 1956). The RNA polymerase reaction contained 0.05M
TrisHCl, pH 7.9; 0.02M $MgCl_2$; 0.04M $(NH_4)_2SO_4$; 0.6 mM ATP, CTP and
GTP and 0.01 mM $[5,6-^3H]$UTP. After 10 min incubation at 30°C, reactions were stopped by pipetting 0.04 ml of the reaction mixture
onto Whatman DE-81 filter discs as previously described (Blatti *et
al.*, 1970).

The specific activity of the enzyme in the transcription complex, 18 nmoles UMP incorporated/mg protein in 10 min, is about 5%
of the specific activity of the purified eukaryotic nuclear enzymes.
This specific activity is based on the transcription of endogenous
DNA, which is present at a concentration of 1 µg/ml in the RNA polymerase assay, a concentration about 1% of that needed to saturate
purified nuclear enzymes. Addition of a ten-fold excess of exogenous chloroplast DNA did not influence the reaction, suggesting that

a specific complex exists between the RNA polymerase and chloroplast DNA. The endogenous DNA has been characterized by sedimentation to equilibrium in neutral CsCl gradients. Its buoyant density (1.685 g/cm^3) was identical to that of *Euglena* chloroplast DNA. No nuclear DNA contamination (ρ = 1.707 g/cm^3) was evident.

RNA synthesis by the transcription complex continues for at least two hours *in vitro* (Fig. 2). Maximal RNA synthesis requires the four ribonucleotide triphosphates and a divalent cation (Mg^{++} or Mn^{++}). When GTP is left out of the reaction, a 75% inhbition is observed (Fig. 2). Similar results are obtained when either ATP or CTP is omitted. Magnesium is the preferred divalent metal ion. The

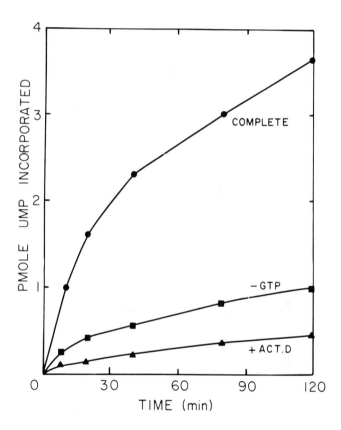

Figure 2. Kinetics of RNA synthesis by the chloroplast transcription complex. RNA synthesis was measured *in vitro* as described in Fig. 1. Circles, complete reactions mixture; triangles, complete reaction mixture plus 50 µg/ml actinomycin D; squares, reaction mixture minus GTP.

considerable preference for Mg^{++} (Mg^{++}/Mn^{++} activity ratio = 5.6) is noteworthy, since most isolated eukaryotic RNA polymerases utilize Mn^{++} at least as well as Mg^{++}. Activity is inhibited by increasing ionic strength, and is maximal at the lowest ionic strength tested, 0.04 M $(NH_4)_2SO_4$.

As would be expected for a DNA-dependent reaction, RNA synthesis is 90% inhibited by actinomycin D (50 μg/ml). In contrast, rifampicin at a concentration of 100 μg/ml has no effect on the kinetics of the reaction. It has previously been reported that *Euglena* chloroplast RNA transcription is of a prokaryotic nature because rifampicin blocks the accumulation of chloroplast rRNA *in vivo* (Brown *et al.*, 1969). Since rifampicin is an inhibitor of initiation of transcription, it is possible that the complex is not initiating *in vitro*, but only completing RNA strands. Alternatively, the enzyme present in this complex is not sensitive.

The *in vitro* RNA transcript has been purified by phenol extraction and chromatography on Sephadex G-25. All four ribonucleotide triphosphates are incorporated. The product is base-labile, and is sensitive to ribonuclease T_2. The base composition of the RNA product is substantially different from that of the chloroplast DNA, indicating that the *in vitro* RNA does not represent a simple symmetric transcript of both strands of the chloroplast DNA.

In collaboration with Dr. O. C. Richards we have begun to characterize this transcript by hybridization with isolated heavy, light and satellite single-stranded DNA from *Euglena* chloroplasts. In a reaction carried out with DNA excess, 60% of the RNA hybridized to the light single strand population, 53% to the heavy and 13% to the satellite DNA (based on S1 nuclease digestion as a measure of hybridization, Sutton, 1971; Leong *et al.*, 1972). Therefore the RNA product is complementary to the chloroplast DNA.

In conclusion, we have obtained a highly purified complex of chloroplast DNA and its attendant RNA polymerase. This material has the properties of a transcription complex: 1) it transcribes at very low levels of DNA; 2) it is indifferent to exogenous DNA; 3) the RNA product is complementary to the organelle DNA, but is not a simple symmetric copy of it.

ACKNOWLEDGMENTS

The authors thank Dr. Oliver C. Richards for purified *Euglena* chloroplasts and Graeme Bell for buoyant density analysis of DNA samples. This work was supported by USPHS, NIH grants HD 04617; NSF grant #3-5256 and American Cancer Society Postdoctoral Fellowship PF-794.

REFERENCES

Blatti, S. P., C. J. Ingles, T. J. Lindell, P. W. Morris, R. F. Weaver, F. Weinberg and W. J. Rutter. 1970. Structure and regulatory properties of eucaryotic RNA polymerase. Cold Spring Harbor Symp. Quant. Biol. 35: 649.

Brown, R. D., D. Bastia and R. Haselkorn. 1969. Effect of rifampicin on transcription in chloroplasts of *Euglena*. Lepetit Colloq. Biol. Med. 1: 309.

Burton, K. 1956. A study of the conditions and mechanism of the diphenylamine reaction for the colorimetric estimation of DNA. Biochem. J. 62: 315.

Leong, J., A. Garapin, N. Jackson, L. Fanshier, W. Levinson and J. M. Bishop. 1972. Virus-specific ribonucleic acid in cells producing Rous Sarcoma virus: detection and characterization. J. Virol. 9: 891.

Manning, J. E., D. R. Wolstenholme, R. S. Ryan, J. A. Hunter and O. C. Richards. 1971. Circular chloroplast DNA from *Euglena gracilis*. Proc. Nat. Acad. Sci. 68: 1169.

Rutter, W. J. 1967. Protein determination in embryos. In (F. H. Wilt and N. K. Wessels, eds.) Methods in Developmental Biology. p. 671. T. Y. Crowell Co., New York.

Sutton, W. D. 1971. A crude nuclease preparation suitable for use in DNA reassociation experiments. Biochim. Biophys. Acta 240: 522.

19. STUDIES ON THE REPLICATION OF DNA

Bruce Alberts

Department of Biochemical Sciences, Princeton University, Princeton, New Jersey

The goal of our work is to understand the basic mechanism of DNA replication, with special emphasis on the protein and nucleic acid interactions involved. It appears that replication is carried out by a complex of several proteins (Barry and Alberts, 1972; Schekman *et al.*, 1972; reviewed in Klein and Bonhoeffer, 1972), quite possibly interwoven with the DNA to create a particle with a unique three-dimensional conformation (Alberts, 1971). However, attempts to purify intact DNA replication forks with these proteins attached have thus far failed, apparently reflecting a basic lability of the entire structure (Fuchs and Hanawalt, 1970; Miller and Buckley, 1970; C. Manoil, R. Peniston and B. Alberts, in preparation). This lability of the "replication apparatus" greatly complicates *in vitro* studies of replication mechanisms (see, for example, Schaller *et al.*, 1972). In this context, it is relevant to note how the comparative stability of ribosome and RNA polymerase protein complexes has enabled striking advances in our knowledge of the biochemistry of translation and transcription.

Inspired by the reconstitution of functional ribosomal particles from their individual components (Traub and Nomura, 1968), we have decided to approach the replication problem by individually isolating each of the proteins of one DNA-replication apparatus, trusting that we can eventually get this structure to self-assemble *in vitro* by incubating intracellular concentrations of these proteins with DNA. With this goal in mind, we have focused our attention on the T4 bacteriophage replication system. Its major advantage is that the genetics of T4 replication have been well worked out, beginning with the isolation and characterization of conditional-lethal mutants by Epstein and Edgar and their colleagues (Epstein *et al.*,

1963). In addition, about 60 replication forks are established in each infected cell (Werner, 1968); this makes the T4 system a relatively rich source for biochemical isolation of replication proteins, especially with the recent discovery of a T4 mutant which overproduces some of these gene products (J. S. Wiberg *et al.*, manuscript submitted; J. Karam, personal communication).

E. coli cells infected with T4 bacteriophage carrying an amber mutation in gene 32, 41, 43, 45, 44, or 62 synthesize little or no DNA, even though all four deoxyribonucleotide triphosphates are present (Epstein *et al.*, 1963; Warner and Hobbs, 1967; Kozinski and Felgenhauer, 1967; Mathews, 1972). In addition, temperature-sensitive mutants have been isolated for the products of genes 32, 41, 43 and 45, which cause T4 DNA replication to cease within one minute after a shift from a permissive temperature (25°C) to a non-permissive temperature (42°C) (Riva *et al.*, 1970). In fact, replication forks stop completely before moving even one-fifth the length of one mature T4 genome following the shift to 42°C (M. Curtis and B. Alberts, in preparation). Each of these four proteins therefore appears to be involved directly in the DNA polymerization process. The other two gene products (genes 44 and 62) appear to function as a single tight complex of two polypeptide chains (Barry and Alberts, 1972). Phages carrying temperature-sensitive mutations in gene 44 replicate their DNA normally at 42°C if allowed 10 minutes of prior infection at 30°C (Riva *et al.*, 1970; J. Karam, personal communication). It is thus possible that these two gene products function only in the initial stages of T4 DNA synthesis. However, no firm conclusion can be drawn in this respect, especially since the altered polypeptide may be stabilized to heat inactivation as soon as the 44-62 complex forms.

Two of the T4 replication gene products have been extensively characterized. The product of gene 43 is T4 DNA polymerase (De-Waard *et al.*, 1965; Warner and Barnes, 1966) and the product of gene 32 is a DNA-unwinding protein, "32-protein" (Alberts and Frey, 1970; Delius *et al.*, 1972). The gene for DNA polymerase maps in a cluster of replication genes (41, 43, 62, 44, and 45) which surround the T4 replication origin as defined by Mosig and coworkers (Marsh *et al.*, 1971; but see Delius *et al.*, 1971). This tight clustering suggests that these gene products interact with each other (Stahl, 1967); likewise, their close linkage to the replication origin suggests that at least one of these proteins acts with sequence specificity in the initiation of replication forks.

Before proceeding with a discussion of our current work on the protein products of T4 genes 41 and 45 and the 44-62 complex, several properties of DNA polymerases and DNA-unwinding proteins will be reviewed. When combined with data from *in vivo* studies, these properties enable a general view of DNA replication to be de-

rived; this will be useful when considering possible functions for
these other proteins, whose mode of action is as yet unknown.

PROPERTIES OF T4 DNA POLYMERASE

The T4 DNA polymerase consists of a single polypeptide chain
of 110,000 daltons; its functional properties (Aposhian and Kornberg, 1962; Goulian *et al.*, 1968) are essentially identical to
those of the replicative polymerase in uninfected cells, *E. coli*
DNA polymerase III (Kornberg and Gefter, 1972). *In vitro* DNA synthesis by these polymerases requires a single-stranded DNA template
chain which is paired along part of its length with a shorter complementary chain of DNA (or RNA); the free 3'-OH terminus of this
second chain then acts as "primer" (Bollum, 1964). An example of
one such template is shown in Fig. 1A.

Three important *in vitro* properties of polymerase which we
shall stress when analyzing its *in vivo* function follow. 1) All
chain growth is in the 5' to 3' chain-direction only. Each polymerization step involves attack of a 3'-OH of a polymer chain end
on the activated 5' end of an incoming deoxyribonucleotide 5' triphosphate monomer. The β and γ phosphates of the monomer are released as pyrophosphate with formation of the new phosphodiester
bond. 2) The polymerase cannot start a new DNA chain, since it
cannot join two monomers together. DNA polymerases always begin
by extending a pre-existing "primer" chain. 3) The T4 DNA polymerase will not utilize double-helical templates. In addition to
a primer chain, the polymerase has an absolute requirement for a
template DNA strand and the segment to be copied must be single-
stranded.

A crucial further requirement for *in vitro* polymerization was
discovered recently by Brutlag and Kornberg (1972), who showed that,
for polymerization, both T4 and *E. coli* polymerases have an absolute requirement for a Watson-Crick base-paired residue at the 3'OH
primer terminus. When confronted with a template with a terminal
mismatch (Fig. 1B), these polymerases make use of their built-in
3' → 5' exonuclease activities to clip off unpaired primer residues
by hydrolysis; this continues until enough nucleotides are removed
to generate an active template (*i.e.*, to convert the template in
Fig. 1B to that in Fig. 1A; see also Englund, 1971). As a result,
these polymerases will efficiently remove their own polymerization
errors. The apparent consequence is fantastic accuracy: one mistake in approximately 10^{10} base-pair replications in *E. coli* (Drake,
1969). Since the self-correcting feature allows polymerase to select for proper template pairing by each added nucleoside triphosphate in two separate reactions - forward and backwards, the mistake
frequency at each step could be as large as 1 in 10^5 in this example

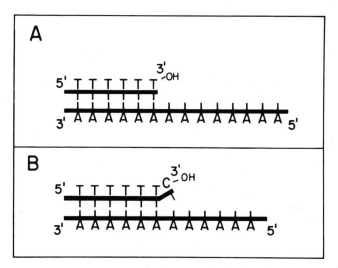

Figure 1.   Active and inactive synthetic polynucleotide templates
for DNA polymerases. A. Template with base-paired primer terminus
(active).   B. Template with mismatched primer terminus (inactive)
(from Brutlag and Kornberg, 1972).

$(10^{-5} \times 10^{-5} = 10^{-10})$. Note that whereas an error frequency of
10^{-10} would require 14 Kcal/mole in discrimination energy if it
had to be attained in the polymerization step alone, as little as
7 Kcal/mole would be needed in a two-step mechanism.[1]

I would like to propose that development of such a two-step
base-selection mechanism was essential to provide an error frequency
in replication low enough to allow any organism with a large number
of essential genes to survive (for arguments concerning maximum mutation load, see Crow and Kimura, 1970).[2] Accepting this hypothesis,

---

[1] This is calculated from the standard relationship $W_1/W_2 =$
$\exp(-\Delta G/RT)$, where ΔG is the difference in free energy between
$state_1$ and $state_2$ ("discrimination energy"), and W_1 and W_2 are their
relative probabilities.

[2] The self-correcting feature of DNA polymerase clearly requires
that it reject templates with a mismatched primer terminus (as in
Fig. 1B). However, the built-in $3' \rightarrow 5'$ exonuclease activity of the
prokaryotic polymerases is not essential, since other enzymes could
remove the terminal mismatched nucleotide after the polymerase is
released. In fact, this exonuclease activity appears to be greatly
reduced or missing in several eukaryotic DNA polymerases examined
(Chang and Bollum, 1973).

it becomes clear why no DNA polymerase is able to start a new polynucleotide chain *de novo,* whereas DNA-dependent RNA polymerases can
do so: The necessity to be self-correcting gives DNA polymerase a
catholic requirement for a perfectly base-paired primer terminus;
to ask this enzyme to start synthesis in the complete absence of
primer, without losing any of its discrimination between the two
templates in Fig. 1, seems contradictory. In contrast, the RNA
polymerases need not be self-correcting, inasmuch as relatively
high error rates can be tolerated during transcription.

   This line of reasoning likewise suggests an explanation for
the failure to find a second DNA polymerase which adds deoxyribonucleotide 5' triphosphates in such a way as to cause chains to grow
in the 3' → 5' direction. Despite the relatively simple type of
replication fork mechanism that this would allow for such a 3' →
5' polymerase, the growing 5' chain end (rather than the incoming
mononucleotide) carries the triphosphate activation. Thus, mistakes
in polymerization cannot be hydrolyzed away without a special enzymatic system for reactivating the bare 5' chain end thus created.

PROPERTIES OF T4 DNA-UNWINDING PROTEIN

   The T4 gene 32 protein (Alberts and Frey, 1970) has a monomer
molecular weight of 35,000 daltons, and at high concentrations it
can self-aggregate to form large multimeric complexes (Huberman
et al., 1971; Carroll *et al.,* 1972). It closely resembles a
22,000 dalton DNA-unwinding protein isolated from uninfected E. *coli*
(Sigal *et al.,* 1972) and has properties which are similar, but not
identical, to the gene 5 protein of filamentous bacteriophage
(Alberts *et al.,* 1972; Oey and Knippers, 1972) and to helix-unwinding proteins isolated from calf thymus (Herrick and Alberts, 1973
and in preparation).

   1) The gene 32-protein binds tightly to single-stranded DNA,
but only weakly, if at all, to double-stranded DNA or to RNA. At
saturation, one protein monomer of 35,000 daltons is bound per
every 10 DNA nucleotides (a weight ratio of protein to DNA of 12:1);
this holds the DNA strand in an extended conformation with a 4.6 Å
translation distance per nucleotide (Delius *et al.,* 1972). A schematic diagram of this complex is shown in Fig. 2A; as indicated,
the protein monomers must be in contact to account for the highly
cooperative nature of their binding. The nucleotide bases in the
complex appear to be left uncovered and exposed, with little (if
any) base specificity in the binding.

   2) Because of its specific affinity for single-stranded DNA,
32-protein catalyzes DNA denaturation. This process is schematically illustrated in Fig. 2B; by virtue of the coupled equilibria
shown, the denaturation reaction is driven to the right, thus lower-
ing the midpoint (T_m) of the helix-coil transition by about 40°C.

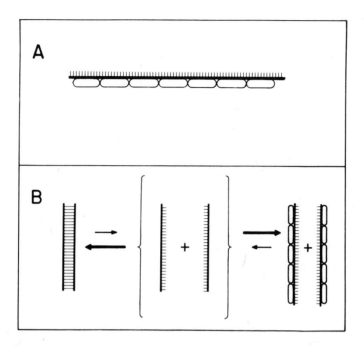

Figure 2.   Schematic representation of DNA-unwinding protein interactions with DNA.   A.   Complex with single-stranded DNA.   B. Shift
in helix-melting equilibrium caused by DNA-binding specificity.

        Since the T_m of T4 DNA under physiological salt conditions
in vitro is about 85°C (Marmur and Doty, 1962), we would estimate
that, with unwinding protein present, helical regions of T4 DNA
should melt inside the cell at about 45°C.   Thus, while regions of
perfect helix should be transiently invaded by 32-protein *in vivo*,
the reverse reaction will be faster than the forward reaction, so
that an opened helical region rapidly reforms (Fig. 3A).   On the
other hand, single-stranded DNA is highly folded *in vitro* due to
the formation of many short intrastrand "hairpin" helices (Doty *et
al.*, 1960; Studier, 1969).   Because these helices are weak (due
to imperfect base-pairing), they are easy targets for 32-protein
induced denaturation, and should be kept permanently open within
the cell (Fig. 3B).

        3) Using a DNA template like that shown in Fig. 1A, but pro-
duced from a natural DNA by limited exonuclease-III degradation,
marked stimulations of T4 DNA polymerase by T4 32-protein and of
E. coli DNA polymerase II by the 22,000 dalton *E. coli* DNA-unwinding
protein were obtained.   However, there was no noticeable effect of
E. coli unwinding protein on the T4 polymerase, nor of T4 unwinding
protein on the *E. coli* polymerase (Sigal *et al.*, 1972).   This speci-

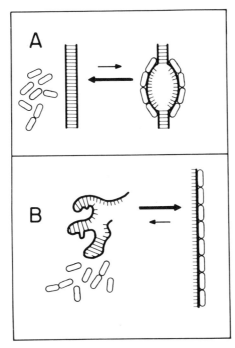

Figure 3.   Helix-melting equilibria in the presence of T4 gene 32-protein under physiological conditions.   A. Perfect double-helices. B. The imperfectly base-paired helices of single-stranded DNA.

ficity may arise from the fact that the two DNA-unwinding proteins hold the DNA template single-strands in quite different conformations; at any rate, it strongly implies that polymerase and unwinding protein function together *in vivo*, as well as *in vitro*.

MODELS FOR *IN VIVO* POLYMERIZATION AT THE REPLICATION FORK

In view of the strong genetic evidence that both the T4 DNA polymerase and DNA-unwinding protein are essential for the polymerization process, it is instructive to ask how these two proteins might work together in T4 replication forks. Our current view of a replication fork is based upon work in many laboratories, and is schematically illustrated in Fig. 4. Because of the antiparallel orientation of strands in the DNA double-helix, a discontinuous mode of DNA synthesis is necessary on one template strand if all of the DNA is to be made with a self-correcting, 5' → 3' DNA polymerase. Both biochemical analysis of initial DNA products (Sugino and Okazaki, 1972) and electron microscopy of forks (Inman and Schnos, 1971; Wolfson and Dressler, 1972) indicate a length of about 10^3 nucleo-

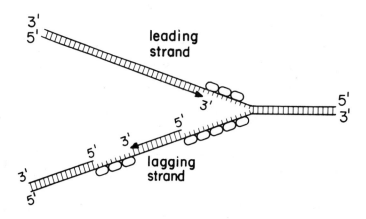

Figure 4.   Schematic representation of possible DNA polymerase and
unwinding protein cooperation in the T4 DNA replication fork.

tides between adjacent polymerase starts on the "lagging side" of
the fork. On the "leading side" of the fork, synthesis can be
either continuous (as indicated in Fig. 4) or discontinuous, perhaps
depending on physiological conditions. However, the discontinuous
synthesis on the leading side is best viewed as a competition between polymerase continuation and polymerase restart mechanisms
(Olivera and Bonhoeffer, 1972); since such restarts do not appear
to lead to gap formation in the daughter strand, this synthesis
can be treated for our purposes as continuous.

A replication fork such as that in Fig. 4 necessarily contains
substantial lengths of single-stranded DNA on its lagging side; as
indicated, such DNA is almost certain to be covered with tightly
bound DNA unwinding-protein. While it is possible that the role of
the 32-protein in T4 DNA replication is solely to keep these single-
stranded template strands aligned, it seems more likely that it
also has a helix-opening role in leading strand synthesis. Some
such destabilization of the helix ahead of the fork seems essential,
in view of the fact that double-helical templates cannot be copied
by the T4 DNA polymerase. An obvious objection to our proposal is
that 32-protein should invade double-helical regions only with
great difficulty inside the cell (see above). However, the pre-fork
region may be much easier to open than intact helices, due to the
fact that cooperative 32-protein binding can be nucleated on both
the lagging strand 32-protein complexes (Fig. 4), and on the leading
strand molecule of DNA polymerase (for which 32-protein has substantial affinity: Huberman *et al.*, 1971).

The model in Fig. 4 assumes that two DNA polymerase molecules
are working at any one time in the fork; in such a model, synthesis

on the two sides of the fork could be tightly coupled by some physical linkage between the two polymerase sites. If so, the 32-protein
molecules leaving the single-stranded template strand on the lagging
side (as the polymerase passes) might be directly recirculated
through the fork without mixing with cellular pools. Less specula-
tively, kinetic arguments can be made for direct reutilization of
any 32-protein molecules used to unwind the helix ahead of the fork;
in the model shown in Fig. 4, this is perhaps most readily accomplished if these protein molecules can slide, pushed by the polymerization
behind (for alternative schemes, see Alberts, 1971).

What evidence is available to support this role for 32-protein
at replication forks? Note that the model in Fig. 4 generates a
total of one Okazaki-piece length (about 10^3 nucleotides) of single-
stranded DNA on the lagging side of each fork. Since each 32-
protein monomer binds 10 nucleotides, 100 molecules of 32-protein
would be required per fork just to cover this DNA. Genetic experiments, in which 32-protein levels are varied by mixed infections,
suggest that 100-200 molecules of 32-protein are indeed necessary
to establish each T4 replication fork, in marked contrast to the
much smaller amounts of all of the other replication gene products
required (Snustad, 1968; Sinha and Snustad, 1971; reviewed by
Alberts, 1971). Recent biochemical measurements on DNA-protein
complexes isolated from T4-infected cells confirm these estimates;
in addition, they demonstrate that the bound 32-protein molecules
are present in long clusters, as predicted (C. Manoil, R. Peniston
and B. Alberts, in preparation).

The model in Fig. 4 accounts for all of the properties of T4
DNA polymerase discussed earlier, except for its inability to
start chains *de novo*. Okazaki and his coworkers have recently
shown that in *E. coli* discontinuous synthesis is primed by a special
piece of RNA (Sugino *et al.*, 1972; Sugino and Okazaki, 1973).
This RNA chain is estimated to be 50-100 nucleotides long, and it
appears to be synthesized *de novo* by a special, rifampicin-resistant
enzyme. After it serves as a primer for DNA-polymerase, the RNA
is erased and replaced by DNA; the specificity of the *E. coli*
ligase for a DNA-DNA junction could prevent nick sealing until
the last ribonucleotide is removed (Westergaard *et al.*, 1973).
Such a cycle of RNA synthesis and degradation is schematically
illustrated in Fig. 5.

Why does nature use such an elaborate mechanism to prime DNA
polymerase, when a DNA primer would seem more economical? A likely
answer follows directly from our previous discussions. The earlier
argument that a self-correcting polymerase cannot start chains *de*
novo also implies its converse: than an enzyme which starts chains
de novo cannot do a good job of self-correcting. Thus, any enzyme
which primes discontinuous synthesis will of necessity make a relatively inaccurate copy (*e.g.*, one error in 10^5?). Even if the

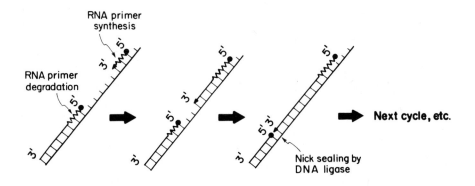

Figure 5. Lagging strand synthesis: a cycle of synthesis and degradation of the RNA primer needed to start Okazaki pieces (after
Sugino and Okazaki, 1972). Enzymes likely to function in RNA removal included RNase H (Keller, 1972) and the 5' → 3' exonuclease
activity of DNA polymerase I (Westergaard *et al.*, 1973).

amount of this copy which was retained in the final product constituted 1% or less of the total genome (10 nucleotides or less per
Okazaki fragment), the resulting increase in overall mutation rate
could be enormous. Thus, it seems reasonable to suggest that the
use of ribonucleotides to synthesize primer was of great evolutionary
advantage, since it automatically marked these sequences as "bad
copy" to be removed.

In conclusion, it seems likely that the mechanism of DNA replication sketched earlier (Figs. 4 and 5), sometimes views as the
whimsical result of historical accident, was specially selected to
ensure that the *entire* DNA sequence is very accurately copied (*i.e.*
copied by a self-correcting type of DNA polymerase).

MODELS FOR INITIATION OF NEW REPLICATION FORKS

We have seen that in *E. coli* the priming of Okazaki pieces is
an event which occurs about once per second on each DNA strand (*i.
e.* once per 10^3 nucleotides polymerized at 37°C), and that it appears to involve a special rifampicin-resistant RNA polymerase
which functions only at replication forks. This frequent priming
reaction should be clearly distinguished from a second process which
also may involve RNA: the *initiation* of chromosomal DNA replication. In bacteria, this latter process is carefully regulated since
it occurs only once per generation at a special DNA sequence which
specifies the replication origin (Yoshikawa and Sueoka, 1963; re-

viewed in Lark, 1969). For several genomes, chromosomal initiation appears to require rifampicin-*sensitive* RNA synthesis at this origin (Brutlag *et al.*, 1971; Lark, 1972; Dove *et al.*, 1971; Hayes and Szybalski, this Symposium).

The work of several laboratories has led to the idea that initiation of chromosome replication in bacteria (and thereby the entire cell cycle) is regulated by the accumulation of a special "initiator protein" (reviewed in Helmstetter, 1969). Work with inhibitors suggests that this protein is stable. Since initiation seems to be triggered only when the number of initiator protein molecules *per origin* (X) reaches some threshold level (Helmstetter *et al.*, 1968; Donachie, 1968; Maaløe and Kjeldgaard, 1966), this protein appears to be directly titrated against (and thereby measured by) chromosome origins. Consideration of the statistical fluctuations expected in such a system leads to the conclusion that X is large (Alberts, 1970); a recent quantitative treatment suggests that in fact X must represent 200 initiator molecules per origin or more (Sompayrac and Maaløe, 1973).

In the simplest view, the initiator might be a protein which binds non-cooperatively to the DNA at chromosome origins, and which is needed in at least 200 copies per origin to open the double-helix and establish replication forks there. Since RNA synthesis at the origin is apparently needed for initiation as well, one model for this process is that sketched in Fig. 6. Here an RNA polymerase and a DNA-unwinding type protein are imagined to work in concert in helix opening. The resulting structure resembles the D-loop intermediate visualized in mitochondrial DNA synthesis (Robberson *et al.*, 1972). As indicated, this loop might need to reach a minimum size before subsequent steps can proceed (*e.g.*, in order to expose start sites on the protein-covered strand). In this case, the number of molecules of the unwinding protein could be carefully measured in relation to the number of DNA origins, and this protein thereby becomes a suitable candidate for the "initiator." In this context, it is interesting to note that the gene 32-protein is required in 100-200 copies per T4 fork, and that it is the only replication protein not made in excess in the T4 system (Snustad, 1968). Thus its availability presumably controls the number of T4 replication forks made at early times after infection, when the number of these forks per cell is increasing (Werner, 1968; reviewed in Alberts, 1971).

ATTEMPTS TO ASSEMBLE THE T4 REPLICATION APPARATUS *IN VITRO*

To assemble a replication apparatus *in vitro*, all of its essential protein and nucleic acid components must be available in active form. At a minimum, this means that (in addition to polymerase and unwinding protein) the protein products of T4 genes 41,

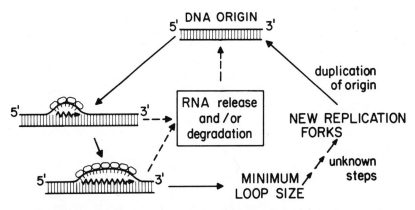

Figure 6.   General model for initiator protein-triggering of chromosomal DNA replication.   For most genomes the entire initiation
process appears to occur without breakage of the parental DNA
strands (Jaenisch *et al.*, 1971;   Robberson *et al.*, 1972;   Inman
and Schnos, 1971;   Delius *et al.*, 1971;   Wolfson and Dressler,
1972).   The "initiator" is visualized here as a DNA-unwinding type
of protein.   By binding tightly to single-stranded DNA, it stabil-
izes a DNA·RNA hybrid formed at the replication origin by an RNA
polymerase.   With only low levels of initiator present, the RNA
made would be quickly released by strand displacement, and the short
cycle indicated by dotted arrows would obtain (see Hayes and
Szybalski, this Symposium;   Buckley *et al.*, 1972).   Eventually
enough initiator accumulates per origin to achieve the "minimum
loop size" needed to establish replication forks there and a round
of DNA replication is triggered.   Since such an initiator-binding
loop must form only at the DNA origin, some protein component or
nucleic acid structure in it must be sequence-specific.

44, 45, and 62 must be purified to the point where they are free of
deleterious contaminants (*e.g.* nucleases).   Some monitoring for
retention of the functional integrity of each gene product seems
essential during the purification.   For this purpose, we have developed a crude *in vitro* synthesizing system which requires all of
these T4-induced proteins for maximal synthesis.   This system thereby provides a measure of the activity of these proteins, despite
the fact that their function in replication is unknown.

    Using such an "*in vitro* complementation" system as an assay,
T4 gene 45 protein and a complex of gene 44 and 62 proteins have
been purified to electrophoretic homogeneity in active form (Barry
and Alberts, 1972;   Barry *et al.*, 1973).   More recently, active
gene 41 protein has been highly purified as well (L. Moran, unpublished data).   In all cases, double-label radioisotope techniques
(with mixed phage amber-mutant lysates) have been used to confirm
the identity of the isolated proteins.

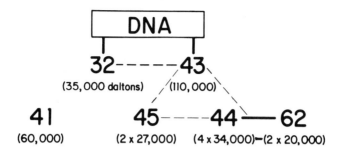

Figure 7.   Schematic diagram of some interactions of purified T4
replication proteins with each other and with DNA.   Bold numerals
are used to denote the gene number of each protein;   the subunit
molecular weights listed beneath were determined by sodium dodecyl
sulfate polyacrylamide gel electrophoresis.

        Fig. 7 presents a preliminary diagram that summarizes our
current knowledge of the physical properties of the known T4 replication proteins and their interactions with each other and with
DNA.   A solid connecting-line is used to denote a strong interaction,
while a dotted line signifies a weaker affinity.   The absence of a
particular interaction in the diagram is not necessarily meaningful,
since not all possibilities have been tested.   Moreover, while none
of the new T4 proteins appear to bind to DNA-cellulose columns
under our conditions, some of them might do so if these conditions
were changed.

        The only evidence for the suggested interactions involving 44-
62 and 45 proteins comes from their strongly synergistic effect in
stimulating T4 DNA polymerase reactions on single-stranded DNA templates *in vitro* (D. Mace and J. Goldberg, unpublished data);   the
exact mode of action of these proteins in this stimulation is currently under investigation.

        We have not yet been able to demonstrate catalysis of RNA
primer synthesis by the T4-induced proteins, nor have we been able
to obtain significant replication of a double-stranded T4 DNA template with them.   It is possible that we have not yet found the
proper *in vitro* conditions for their reassembly (see, for example,
Lieberman and Oishi, 1973).   Alternatively, we may still be missing
some essential protein components.   Likely candidates in this case
include some T4-induced proteins [*e.g.*, the products of genes 42
or 1 (Collinsworth and Matthews, 1973;   Chiu and Greenberg, 1968;
R. Greenberg, personal communication), gene y (Smith and Symonds,
1973), or the DNA-delay genes (Yegian *et al.*, 1971)].   Although
none of the 5 mutationally-defined *E. coli* replication gene products
appear to be essential for T4 DNA replication (Gross, 1972;   but

see Mosig *et al.*, 1972), a requirement for other host proteins is certainly possible (*e.g.*, the DNA-dependent RNA-polymerase).

It is our hope that the number of additional proteins needed for reconstitution of the T4 DNA-replication apparatus will be small, and that they can therefore be purified from crude extracts with the aid of appropriate assays. Progress along similar lines is being made in both the *E. coli* (Schekman *et al.*, 1972; Nusslein *et al.*, 1973; Wickner *et al.*, 1972) and T7 bacteriophage (Hinkle, 1973) replication systems. Through the combined efforts of all of these groups, a complete picture of the enzymology of DNA replication should emerge in the not too distant future.

ACKNOWLEDGMENT

I am indebted to my colleagues and students at Princeton for discussions and advice on this manuscript and to the National Institutes of Health and the American Cancer Society for grant support.

REFERENCES

Alberts, B. 1970. Function of gene 32-protein, a new protein essential for the genetic recombination and replication of T4 bacteriophage DNA. Fed. Proc. $\underline{29}$: 1154.

Alberts, B. 1971. On the structure of the replication apparatus. In (D. W. Ribbons, J. F. Woessner and J. Schultz, eds.) Nucleic Acid-Protein Interactions. p. 128. North Holland, Amsterdam.

Alberts, B. and L. Frey. 1970. T4 bacteriophage gene 32: a structural protein in the replication and recombination of DNA. Nature $\underline{227}$: 1313.

Alberts, B., L. Frey and H. Delius. 1972. Isolation and characterization of gene 5-protein of filamentous bacterial viruses. J. Mol. Biol. $\underline{68}$: 139.

Aposhian, H. V. and A. Kornberg. 1962. Enzymatic synthesis of deoxyribonucleic acid. IX. The polymerase formed after T2 bacteriophage infection of *E. coli*: a new enzyme. J. Biol. Chem. $\underline{237}$: 519.

Barry, J. and B. Alberts. 1972. *In vitro* complementation as an assay for new proteins required for bacteriophage T4 DNA replication: purification of the complex specified by T4 genes 44 and 62. Proc. Nat. Acad. Sci. $\underline{69}$: 2717.

Barry, J., H. Hama-Inaba, L. Moran, J. Wiberg and B. Alberts. 1973. Proteins of the T4 bacteriophage replication apparatus. In (R. D.

Wells and R. B. Inman, eds.) DNA Synthesis *In Vitro*. University Park Press, Baltimore. In press.

Bollum, F. J. 1964. Chemically defined templates and initiators for deoxyribopolynucleotide synthesis. Science 144: 560.

Brutlag, D. and A. Kornberg. 1972. Enzymatic synthesis of DNA. XXXVI. A proofreading function for the 3' → 5' exonuclease activity in DNA polymerases. J. Biol. Chem. 247: 241.

Brutlag, D., R. Schekman and A. Kornberg. 1971. A possible role for RNA polymerase in the initiation of M13 DNA synthesis. Proc. Nat. Acad. Sci. 68: 2826.

Buckley, P. J., L. Kosturko and A. W. Kozinski. 1972. *In vivo* production of an RNA-DNA copolymer after infection of *E. coli* by bacteriophage T4. Proc. Nat. Acad. Sci. 69: 3165.

Carroll, R. B., K. E. Neet and D. Goldthwait. 1972. Self-association of gene-32 protein of bacteriophage T4. Proc. Nat. Acad. Sci. 69: 2741.

Chang, L. M. S. and F. J. Bollum. 1973. A comparison of associated enzyme activities in various DNA polymerases. J. Biol. Chem. 248: 3398.

Chiu, C. S. and G. R. Greenberg. 1968. Evidence for a possible direct role of dCMP hydroxymethylase in T4 page DNA synthesis. Cold Spring Harbor Symp. Quant. Biol. 33: 351.

Collinsworth, W. L. and C. K. Matthews. 1973. DNA synthesis in plasmolyzed T4-infected cells. Fed. Proc. 32: 491 Abs.

Crow, J. F. and M. Kimura. 1970. An Introduction to Population Genetics Theory. Harper and Row, New York.

Delius, H., C. Howe and A. W. Kozinski. 1971. Structure of the replicating DNA from bacteriophage T4. Proc. Nat. Acad. Sci. 68: 3049.

Delius, H., N. Mantell and B. Alberts. 1972. Characterization by electron microscopy of the complex formed between T4 bacteriophage gene 32-protein and DNA. J. Mol. Biol. 67: 341.

DeWaard, A., A. V. Paul and I. R. Lehman. 1965. The structural gene for DNA polymerase in bacteriophage T4 and T5. Proc. Nat. Acad. Sci. 54: 1241.

Donachie, W. D. 1968. Relationship between cell size and time of initiation of DNA replication. Nature 219: 1077.

Doty, P., H. Boedtker, J. Fresco, R. Haselkorn and M. Litt. 1959. Secondary structure in ribonucleic acids. Proc. Nat. Acad. Sci. 45: 482.

Dove, W. F., H. Inokuchi and W. F. Stevens. 1971. Replication control in phage lambda. In (A. D. Hershey, ed.) The Bacteriophage Lambda. p. 747. Cold Spring Harbor Laboratory, New York.

Drake, J. W. 1969. Comparative rates of spontaneous mutation. Nature 221: 1132.

Englund, P. T. 1971. The initial step of *in vitro* synthesis of DNA by the T4 DNA polymerase. J. Biol. Chem. 246: 5684.

Epstein, R. H., A. Bolle, C. M. Steinberg, E. Kellenberger, E. Boy de la Tour, R. Chevallez, R. S. Edgar, M. Susman, G. H. Denhardt and A. Lielausis. 1963. Physiological studies of conditional lethal mutants of bacteriophage T4D. Cold Spring Harbor Symp. Quant. Biol. 28: 375.

Fuchs, E. and P. Hanawalt. 1970. Isolation and characteriztion of the DNA replication complex from *Escherichia coli*. J. Mol. Biol. 52: 301.

Goulian, M., Z. J. Lucas and A. Kornberg. 1968. Enzymatic synthesis of DNA. XXV. Purification and properties of DNA polymerase induced by infection with phage T4. J. Biol. Chem. 243: 627.

Gross, J. D. 1972. DNA replication in bacteria. Current Topics in Microbiol. and Immunol. 57: 39.

Helmstetter, C. 1969. Sequence of bacterial reproduction. Ann. Rev. Microbiol. 23: 223.

Helmstetter, C., S. Cooper, O. Pierucci and E. Revelas. 1968. On the bacterial life sequence. Cold Spring Harb. Symp. Quant. Biol. 33: 809.

Herrick, G. and B. Alberts. 1973. A nucleic acid helix-unwinding protein from calf thymus. Fed. Proc. 32: 497 Abs.

Hinkle, D. C. 1973. Bacteriophage T7 DNA replication *in vitro*. Fed. Proc. 32: 492 Abs.

Huberman, J., A. Kornberg and B. Alberts. 1971. The stimulation of T4 DNA polymerase by the protein product of T4 gene 32. J. Mol. Biol. 62: 39.

Inman, R. and M. Schnos. 1971. Structure of branch points in replicating DNA: presence of single-strand connections in lambda DNA brach points. J. Mol. Biol. 56: 319.

Jaenisch, R., A. Mayer and A. Levine. 1971. Replicating SV40 molecules contain closed circular template DNA strands. Nature New Biol. 233: 72.

Keller, W. 1972. RNA-primed DNA synthesis *in vitro*. Proc. Nat. Acad. Sci. 69: 1569.

Klein, A. and F. Bonhoeffer. 1972. DNA replication. Ann. Rev. Biochem. 41: 301.

Kornberg, T. and M. Gefter. 1972. DNA synthesis in cell-free extracts. IV. Purification and properties of DNA polymerase III. J. Biol. Chem. 247: 5369.

Kozinski, A. W. and Z. Felgenhauer. 1967. Molecular recombination in T4 bacteriophage DNA. II. Single-strand breaks and exposure of uncomplemented areas as a prerequisite for recombination. J. Virol. 1: 1193.

Lark, K. G. 1969. Initiation and control of DNA synthesis. Ann. Rev. Biochem. 38: 569.

Lark, K. G. 1972. Evidence for the direct involvement of RNA in the initiation of DNA replication in *E. coli* 15T⁻. J. Mol. Biol. 64: 47.

Lieberman, R. P. and Oishi, M. 1973. Formation of the *recB-recC* DNase by *in vitro* complementation and evidence concerning its subunit nature. Nature New Biol. 243: 75.

Maaløe, O. and N. O. Kjeldgaard. 1966. Control of Macromolecular Synthesis. W. A. Benjamin, Inc., New York.

Marmur, J. and P. Doty. 1962. Determination of the base composition of DNA from its thermal denaturation temperature. J. Mol. Biol. 5: 109.

Marsh, R. C., A. Breschkin and G. Mosig. 1971. Origin and direction of bacteriophage T4 DNA replication. II. A gradient of marker frequencies in partially replicated T4 DNA as assayed by transformation. J. Mol. Biol. 60: 213.

Mathews, C. K. 1972. Biochemistry of DNA-defective amber mutants of bacteriophage T4. III. Nucleotide pools. J. Biol. Chem. 247: 7430.

Miller, R. C. and P. Buckley. 1970. Early intracellular events in the replication of bacteriophage T4 DNA. VI. Newly synthesized proteins in the T4 protein-DNA complex. J. Virol. 5: 502.

Mosig, G., W. Bowden and S. Bock. 1972. *E. coli* DNA polymerase I and other host functions participate in T4 DNA replication and recombination. Nature New Biol. <u>240</u>: 12.

Nüsslein, V., F. Bonhoeffer, A. Klein and B. Otto. 1973. In (R. Wells and R. Inman, eds.) DNA Synthesis *In Vitro*. University Park Press, Baltimore. In press.

Oey, J. L. and R. Knippers. 1972. Properties of the isolated gene 5 protein of bacteriophage fd. J. Mol. Biol. <u>68</u>: 125.

Olivera, B. and F. Bonhoeffer. 1972. Discontinuous DNA replication *in vitro*. I. Two distinct size classes of intermediates. Nature New Biol. <u>240</u>: 233.

Riva, S., A. Cascino and E. P. Geiduschek. 1970. Coupling of late transcription to viral replication in bacteriophage T4 development. J. Mol. Biol. <u>54</u>: 85.

Robberson, D., H. Kasamatsu and J. Vinograd. 1972. Replication of mitochondrial DNA. Circular replicative intermediates in mouse L cells. Proc. Nat. Acad. Sci. <u>69</u>: 737.

Schaller, H., B. Otto, V. Nüsslein, J. Huf, R. Herrman and F. Bonhoeffer. 1972. DNA replication *in vitro*. J. Mol. Biol. <u>63</u>: 183.

Schekman, R., W. Wickner, O. Westergaard, D. Brutlag, K. Geider, L. Bertsch and A. Kornberg. 1972. Initiation of DNA synthesis: synthesis of ϕX174 replicative form requires RNA synthesis resistant to rifampicin. Proc. Nat. Acad. Sci. <u>69</u>: 2691.

Sigal, N., H. Delius, T. Kornberg, M. Gefter and B. Alberts. 1972. A DNA-unwinding protein isolated from *E. coli*: its interaction with DNA and with DNA polymerases. Proc. Nat. Acad. Sci. <u>69</u>: 3537.

Sinha, N. K. and D. P. Snustad. 1971. DNA synthesis in bacteriophage T4-infected *E. coli*: evidence supporting a stoichiometric role for gene 32-product. J. Mol. Biol. <u>62</u>: 267.

Smith, S. M. and N. Symonds. 1973. The unexpected location of a gene conferring abnormal radiation sensitivity on phage T4. Nature <u>241</u>: 395.

Snustad, D. P. 1968. Dominance interactions in *E. coli* cells mixedly infected with bacteriophage T4 wild-type and amber mutants and their possible implications as to type of gene-product function: catalytic vs. stoichiometric. Virology <u>35</u>: 550.

Sompayrac, L. and O. Maaløe. 1973. Autorepressor model for control of DNA replication. Nature New Biol. <u>241</u>: 133.

Stahl, F. W. 1967. Circular genetic maps. J. Cell. Physiol. 70,
Suppl. 1: 1.

Studier, F. W. 1969. Conformational changes of single-stranded
DNA. J. Mol. Biol. 41: 189.

Sugino, A., S. Hirose and R. Okazaki. 1972. RNA-linked nascent
DNA fragments in *Escherichia coli*. Proc. Nat. Acad. Sci. 69: 1863.

Sugino, A. and R. Okazaki. 1972. Mechanism of DNA chain growth.
VII. Direction and rate of growth of T4 nascent short DNA chains.
J. Mol. Biol. 64: 61.

Sugino, A. and R. Okazaki. 1973. RNA-linked DNA fragments *in
vitro*. Proc. Nat. Acad. Sci. 70: 88.

Traub, P. and M. Nomura. 1968. Structure and function of *E. coli*
ribosomes. V. Reconstitution of functionally active 30S ribosomal
particles from RNA and proteins. Proc. Nat. Acad. Sci. 59: 777.

Warner, H. R. and J. E. Barnes. 1966. DNA synthesis in *E. coli*
infected with some DNA polymerase-less mutants of bacteriophage T4.
Virology 28: 100.

Warner, H. R. and M. D. Hobbs. 1967. Incorporation of uracil-C^{14}
into nucleic acids in *Escherichia coli* infected with bacteriophage
T4 and T4 amber mutants. Virology 33: 376.

Werner, R. 1968. Initiation and propagation of growing points in
the DNA of phage T4. Cold Spring Harbor Symp. Quant. Biol. 33: 501.

Westergaard, O., Brutlag, D. and A. Kornberg. 1973. Initiation
of DNA synthesis. IV. Incorporation of the RNA primer into the
phage replicative form. J. Biol. Chem. 248: 1361.

Wickner, R. B., M. Wright, S. Wickner and J. Hurwitz. 1972. Conversion of φX174 and fd single-stranded DNA to replicative forms in
extracts of *Escherichia coli*. Proc. Nat. Acad. Sci. 69: 3233.

Wolfson, J. and D. Dressler. 1972. Regions of single-stranded DNA
in growing points of replicating bacteriophage T7 chromosomes.
Proc. Nat. Acad. Sci. 69: 2682.

Yegian, C. D., M. Mueller, G. Selzer, V. Russo and F. W. Stahl.
1971. Properties of the DNA-delay mutants of bacteriophage T4.
Virology 46: 900.

Yoshikawa, H. and N. Sueoka. 1963. Sequential replication of
Bacillus subtilis chromosome. I. Comparison of marker frequencies
in exponential and stationary growth phases. Proc. Nat. Acad. Sci.
49: 559.

20. REGULATION OF BACTERIAL GENES

Geoffrey Zubay*, Huey-Lang Yang*, Gary Reiness*   and
Michael Cashel[†]

* *Department of Biological Sciences, Columbia University,
New York, New York and [†]Laboratory of Molecular Genetics,
National Institute of Child Health and Human Development,
The National Institutes of Health, Bethesda, Maryland*

It is now apparent that the activities of many bacterial genes
are regulated by several interlocking control apparatuses that
respond to different small molecule effectors. An overview suggests
the existence of a hierarchy of controls (Zubay, 1973). For example, the gene cluster known as the *lac* operon is induced by the
presence of lactose. Lactose is also the substrate of the enzyme
β-galactosidase, which is encoded by the *lac* operon. The induction
of the *lac* operon by lactose is brought about by a highly specific
control process that does not directly affect the activities of
other genes. At a more general level of control, the expression of
the *lac* operon is dependent upon the presence of 3':5'-cyclic AMP
(cAMP). This dependence is characteristic of many genes that encode catabolic enzymes. At an even more general level of control,
we find a mechanism that appears to modulate transcription according
to the gross rate of translation. The small molecule effector for
this control process is probably guanosine tetraphosphate (guanosine bis-diphosphate, ppGpp). The effect this compound has depends
upon the gene - for the *lac* operon ppGpp is stimulatory.

Exploring the detailed biochemical mechanisms of various types
of control processes has led us to investigate gene-directed synthesis of biochemically competent protein or tRNA in cell-free systems
(Zubay, 1973). In such systems one can simulate whole cell conditions and freely manipulate the alleged control elements for a
particular gene while observing the effects on the gene activity.
This makes it possible to demonstrate the function of various control elements and provides a tool for the isolation of control

elements. The studies reported here represent a summary of investigations we are making on several different gene systems.

DESCRIPTION OF CELL-FREE SYSTEM FOR DNA-DIRECTED RNA AND PROTEIN SYNTHESIS

The basic components of the DNA-directed synthetic system are a cell-free extract of E. coli called S-30, the cofactors and substrates necessary for RNA and protein synthesis, and a source of nucleic acid to direct the synthesis (Zubay, 1973). This system is often referred to as a coupled system because transcription and translation take place simultaneously. All the bacterial genes studied here have been isolated in λ or φ80 transducing viruses. Synthesis is usually done for 60 min at 36°. It is now possible to synthesize most bacterial and viral proteins in readily detectable amounts. In previous studies it has been found that the amount of β-galactosidase synthesized in the cell-free system is proportional to the amount of lac operon-containing DNA present (Zubay et al., 1970a). We have continued to use the amounts of active enzyme synthesized as a measure of gene activity because enzyme assays are sensitive, precise and selective. However, one must keep in mind that active protein is an indirect gene product and that controls working at the translation level could affect our conclusions.

STUDIES OF FACTORS AFFECTING THE REGULATION OF THE LAC OPERON

One of the most intensively studied and best understood inducible gene clusters is the lac operon which is involved in the breakdown of lactose to its component monosaccharides, galactose and glucose. The lac operon consists of three structural genes, which code for β-galactosidase, lactose permease, and galactoside transacetylase, and two control elements, a promoter and an operator. The structural genes for these three proteins are adjacent to one another and the controlling elements are located at one end of the gene cluster. In most coupled system studies of the lac operon the level of β-galactosidase synthesis was used as an index of gene activity.

As indicated in the introduction, small molecules of two classes exert a profound effect on the enzyme yield as a result of what appears to be a gene-regulating function. The first class includes inducers of the lac operon, of which isopropylthiogalactopyranoside (IPTG) is the most potent known. In systems isogenic except for the lac operon repressor, IPTG stimulates only that system containing the repressor. If repressor is absent, maximum activity is obtained without IPTG. The interaction of IPTG with the repressor is believed to result in the release of the latter from the operator.

The second class of small molecules exhibiting a regulating effect on enzyme yield are those associated with catabolite repression of which cAMP is a prime example. Cyclic AMP is usually added to the coupled system as its omission results in much lower amounts of β-galactosidase synthesis. The coupled system was used to isolate the protein called CAP (catabolite gene activator protein) which interacts with cAMP to activate the *lac* operon. For this purpose an S-30 is prepared from a CAP mutant that fails to synthesize appreciable β-galactosidase unless a fraction from wild-type cells containing CAP is added. The stimulation of β-galactosidase synthesis by CAP is completely dependent upon the presence of cAMP. Using this assay, CAP can be monitored in crude extracts and extracts purified to varying degrees; this assay has served as an indispensable aid in CAP purification (Zubay *et al.*, 1970b; Zubay, 1969).

In the coupled system one can quantitatively vary the amounts of IPTG inducer, cAMP, CAP and *lac* operon repressor. This has made it possible to do a number of studies on the gene activity as a function of the concentration of various regulatory components. Such studies have helped in determining the mechanism of turning on and off the operon under conditions most closely resembling the *in vivo* state. In order to demonstrate that cyclic AMP and CAP were sufficient for activating the RNA polymerase for *lac* transcription, it was necessary to turn to the use of simpler systems in which transcription could be studied in isolation (Eron and Block, 1971).

STUDIES OF FACTORS AFFECTING THE REGULATION OF THE *ARA* OPERON

The coupled system has also been used to study the *ara* operon. The *ara* operon, like the *lac* operon, is an inducible cluster of structural genes and regulatory elements concerned with a particular catabolic function, *i.e.*, the three step conversion of L-arabinose to D-xylulose 5-phosphate. The *ara* operon is induced when L-arabinose is present in the growth medium. The model for control of the *ara* operon, postulated by Englesberg, Squires and Meronk (1969) contains both a positive and a negative control site. According to this proposal, the C gene encodes a specific regulator protein, the C protein. In the absence of L-arabinose, the C protein acts as a repressor, P_1, binding to the *o* locus. Thus, the *o* locus is a point of negative control like the *o* locus in the *lac* operon. P_1 is displaced from *o* by L-arabinose, which stimulates the conversion of P_1 to an alternate conformation P_2. P_2 has a high affinity for the *I* locus on the DNA. The binding of P_2 to *I* is required for a high level of gene expression for the *ara* operon; the *I* locus is called a site for positive gene control. The *ara* operon, like the *lac* operon, requires cAMP and CAP for gene expression. The promoter element is presumed to reside somewhere in the *I* region as is the site for binding of CAP.

A DNA-directed cell-free system that synthesizes the L-ribulo-
kinase coded by the *ara* operon has been developed (Zubay *et al.*,
1971; Greenblatt and Schleif, 1971). L-arabinose and cAMP are required for the expression of this operon. The C protein is also
required and can be supplied either by *de novo* synthesis in the cell-
free system or added back from extracts of whole cells. Since,
according to the model described above, the C protein is required
for activating the operon, it was anticipated that active S-30 extracts would have to be made from strains carrying the C gene.
Therefore it came as a great surprise when it was found that equally effective S-30's could be prepared from strains with or without
the C gene. It was eventually found that C protein does not survive
S-30 preparation and that ribulokinase is made in a DNA-directed
cell-free system only after the C protein itself has been synthesized (Yang and Zubay, 1973a). Therefore the presence of the C gene
on the λ*ara* DNA used should be obligatory (the C gene is normally
located immediately adjacent to the control elements of the *ara*
operon) for ribulokinase synthesis to occur. This was confirmed by
showing that when λ*ara* DNA lacking the C gene is used, no ribulokinase is made. Active C protein can be supplied from protein extracts of whole cells if great care is taken in their preparation;
we have found that prior to use such extracts must be kept cold and
must contain arabinose and p-toluene sulfonyl fluoride, a serine
proteinase inhibitor. Attempts are being made to purify the C
protein using the stimulatory effect on ribulokinase synthesis to
assay the protein at different stages during purification.

The loss of the C protein activity in the preparation of S-30
extracts has led us to wonder if other gene regulating proteins
might be missing or inactive in the S-30's. This has resulted in
a new approach to finding regulatory proteins, which is described
below.

STUDIES OF FACTORS AFFECTING THE REGULATION
OF THE *TRP* AND *ARG* OPERONS

Two repressible operons have been studied in the coupled system: the *trp* and *arg* operons. These operons encode enzymes essential for the synthesis of tryptophan and arginine; they have control elements adjacent to structural genes in much the same way as
the inducible operon systems. Whereas all five structural genes
associated with tryptophan biosynthesis exist in one cluster, the
nine structural genes associated with arginine biosynthesis are
broken up into 6 separate regions each with its own promoter-operator control elements. Also associated with each amino-acid system
at an unlinked location is a specific regulator gene R, which is
believed to encode a protein repressor molecule. *In vivo*, it is

known that each of these operons are repressed at high levels of
amino acid and derepressed at low levels of amino acid. The proposed mechanism for repressing the operon involves complex formation
between the operator site on the DNA and the repressor in combination with either the amino acid or a derivative thereof.

Studies of the *trp* operon in the coupled system have been made
with both λ*trp* DNA (Pouwels and Van Rotterdam, 1972) and λ*trp-lac*
DNA (Zubay *et al.*, 1972). The λ*trp-lac* DNA carries a fusion of the
trp and *lac* operons so that the synthesis of β-galactosidase is
under control of the normal *trp* operon control elements. The use
of λ*trp-lac* DNA has been very convenient because of the β-galactosidase enzyme assay. When using λ*trp-lac* DNA, synthesis in extracts
of *trp* R⁻ cells is progressively reduced by increased additions of
extract from *trp* R⁺ cells. With DNA containing the normal *lac*
operon such as λ*dlac* DNA no inhibition of β-galactosidase synthesis
is seen when *trp* R⁺ product is added. This highly sensitive and
specific assay has facilitated quantitation and partial purification
of the *trp* repressor. The same basic approach is being used to
assay for and purify the *arg* repressor (Urm *et al.*, 1973). The
partially purified *trp* repressor has been studied further in a transcriptional system containing, in addition to the partially purified
repressor, λ*trp* DNA, RNA polymerase and the salts and substrates required for transcription (Rose *et al.*, 1973). In such a system it
has been possible to show that the *trp* repressor specifically inhibits up to 90 percent of the transcription from the *trp* operon
with an absolute requirement for tryptophan. In the purified transcriptional system there is little chance of making appreciable
quantities of any tryptophan derivative. Therefore these observations provide strong support for the notion that tryptophan itself
functions as the corepressor of the *trp* operon. The coupled system
could not be used to make this observation since both amino acid and
tryptophanyl-tRNA are invariably present. On the other hand the
purified transcriptional system could not be used as an assay for
trp repressor particularly on crude extracts because the *trp* R⁺
effects are obscured by the nonspecific effects of other proteins.
This study demonstrates the relative merits of the coupled system
and the simpler transcription system at different stages in an investigation.

STUDIES OF RELATIVELY UNSTABLE PROTEIN FACTORS
INVOLVED IN REGULATION

Whereas S-30 extracts seem to contain all the proteins necessary for transcription and translation there is evidence that some
regulatory proteins, such as the *ara* C protein (discussed above) are
missing as a result of inactivation. Such deficiencies in the S-30

could be exploited in cases where mutants are lacking. Consider the
situation in which an S-30 lacks a particular regulatory protein
which can be supplied from protein extracts prepared otherwise as in
the case of the *ara* C protein. In such a situation an *in vitro*
complementation assay could be developed just as in the case where
normal and mutant extracts are available. Thus far two new protein
factors have been found in this way: a possible termination factor
for bacterial operons and a possible stimulation factor for anabolic
operons. The evidence for such factors is described below.

The evidence for a bacterial termination factor came to light
in a comparison of the cAMP effects on the stimulation of β-galactosidase synthesis when using λ*dlac* DNA and λ*plac* DNA (Yang and
Zubay, 1973b). When λ*dlac* DNA is used in the absence of cAMP only
5 percent of normal β-galactosidase synthesis occurs. In contrast
when λ*plac* DNA is used in the absence of cAMP only a 50 percent
reduction of β-galactosidase synthesis occurs. These differences
cannot be due to the *lac* control elements since these are known to
be the same in both DNAs. Both DNAs also contain at least part of
the *i* gene, which is situated immediately adjacent to the *lac* control elements; this gene is known to end with a normal termination
signal. To account for the high level of β-galactosidase synthesis
with λ*plac* DNA in the absence of cAMP, we have hypothesized that
the *lac* operon in this DNA is located near an initiation site on the
virus genome, which 'reads through' the *lac* operon due to a deficiency of a normal bacterial termination factor. To test this possibility a nonpreincubated protein extract was added back to the
S-30 and λ*plac* DNA was used to direct β-galactosidase synthesis.
Under these conditions all of the β-galactosidase synthesis in the
absence of cAMP was eliminated without any major change in the cAMP-
stimulated β-galactosidase synthesis. Apparently the nonpreincubated extract contains the factor necessary to prevent 'read-through'.
This inhibitory effect is being used as an assay to guide the purification of a protein from the crude extract; the protein has a
molecular weight greater than 100,000 as judged by its near exclusion from G-100 Sephadex. The relationship between this bacterial
termination factor and the ρ termination factor of λ phage discovered by Roberts (1969) has not been determined.

Another protein factor that appears to be deficient in S-30's
shows a stimulatory effect on the *trp* operon. This factor stimulates
(a maximum of 4-fold stimulation has been obtained) β-galactosidase
synthesis when λ*trp-lac* is used but not when either λ*dlac* DNA or
λ*plac* DNA are used (Yang and Zubay, 1973b). Only the first DNA is
responsive to normal *trp* operon control elements. This stimulation
factor is being purified using the coupled system as a monitor.
Our working hypothesis is that this protein is part of a positive
control system for stimulating the *trp* and possibly other anabolic
operons.

STUDIES OF A POSSIBLE MASTER CONTROL FOR RNA SYNTHESIS
INVOLVING pppGpp AND ppGpp

In vivo and *in vitro* studies have shown that the guanine nucleotides, pppGpp and ppGpp, are synthesized on the ribosome at a rate
that is an inverse function to the rate of protein synthesis and
RNA accumulation (Lazzarini *et al.*, 1971). A reasonable working
hypothesis would be that these compounds modulate transcription
according to the overall rate of translation. In the cell-free
system under conditions of coupled transcription and translation,
pppGpp is rapidly hydrolyzed to ppGpp while ppGpp itself is quite
stable (Yang *et al.*, 1973). Adding either ppGpp or pppGpp (which
is rapidly converted to ppGpp) results in a stimulation of about
2.5 fold of the activities of the *ara*, *lac* and *trp* operons and an
inhibition of about 10 fold of the *arg* operon. When the hydrolysis-
resistant analog of pppGpp (pCH$_2$ppGpp) is used in place of pppGpp
the same inhibitory potency is observed for the *arg* operon. This
suggests that inhibition can occur with both ppGpp and pppGpp. In
contrast to this apparent lack of specificity, pCH$_2$ppGpp gives no
stimulation of the *ara*, *lac* or *trp* operons; thus the stimulatory
effect is specific for ppGpp. Further studies show that ppG, pGp
and pppGp lack the stimulatory activity of ppGpp, again indicating
a high degree of specificity.

Parallel studies of the DNA-directed synthesis of tRNA^{Tyr} show
no effect at moderate levels of ppGpp or pppGpp and only slight
inhibition of tRNA synthesis by very high levels of ppGpp which are
on the borderline of concentrations of any guanine nucleotides that
yield nonspecific inhibition. By this measure, ppGpp and pppGpp do
not function as modulators of tRNA synthesis.

It is possible experimentally to isolate the translational
component of the coupled system by substituting mRNA in place of
DNA in the cell-free system. With β-galactosidase messenger as well
as MS2 viral RNA, ppGpp and pppGpp show only a slight inhibitory
effect on messenger-directed protein synthesis. These observations
together with the fact that in the same system these nucleotides do
affect coupled transcription and translation, lead us to surmise
that the activities of pppGpp and ppGpp are exerted at the level of
RNA polymerase activity. We are led to propose that the guanosine
nucleotides affect transcription by interacting with the RNA polymerase, an idea that is supported by Cashel's observations (1970)
that the ppGpp binds to RNA polymerase and that at saturating levels
this binding results in the inhibition of about 60% of the RNA synthesis that begin with a guanine residue. From all this we conclude
that ppGpp or pppGpp influence transcription in a positive, negative
or negligible way according to the manner in which the (p)ppGpp-
polymerase complex interacts with the promoter. In this way the
guanine nucleotides produced in response to a retardation of protein

synthesis could modulate the transcription from all genes. Conclusive proof of this mechanism awaits the isolation of mutant polymerases that do not respond to the guanine nucleotides *in vitro* or *in vivo*.

ACKNOWLEDGMENT

The work described herein involved an extensive collaboration with several laboratories that supplied bacterial and viral strains. In this regard I would like to acknowledge J. Beckwith, E. Englesberg, W. Maas, J. Miller, D. Morse and J. Schrenk. Financial support was obtained from the National Institutes of Health (P.H.S. 5201 GM 16648-05), the American Cancer Society (ACS NP-12B) and the National Science Foundation (NSF GB 18733).

REFERENCES

Cashel, M. 1970. Inhibition of RNA polymerase by ppGpp, a nucleotide accumulated during stringent response to amino acid starvation in *E. coli*. Cold Spring Harbor Symp. Quant. Biol. 35: 407.

Englesberg, E., C. Squires and F. Meronk. 1969. The L-arabinose operon in *Escherichia coli* B/r: a genetic demonstration of two functional states of the product of a regulator gene. Proc. Nat. Acad. Sci. 62: 1100.

Eron, L. and R. Block. 1971. Mechanism of initiation and repression of *in vitro* transcription of the *lac* operon of *Escherichia coli*. Proc. Nat. Acad. Sci. 68: 1828.

Greenblatt, J. and R. Schleif. 1971. Regulation of the arabinose operon in a cell-free system. Nature New Biol. 233: 166.

Lazzarini, R. H., M. Cashel and J. Gallant. 1971. On the regulation of guanosine tetraphosphate levels in stringent and relaxed strains of *E. coli*. J. Biol. Chem. 246: 4381.

Pouwels, P. H. and J. Van Rotterdam. 1972. *In vitro* synthesis of enzymes of the tryptophan operon of *Escherichia coli*. Proc. Nat. Acad. Sci. 69: 1786.

Roberts, J. W. 1969. Termination factor for RNA synthesis. Nature 224: 1168.

Rose, J. K., C. L. Squires, C. Yanofsky, H.-L. Yang and G. Zubay. 1973. *In vitro* transcription of the tryptophan operon by purified RNA polymerase: regulation in the presence of partially purified repressor and tryptophan. Nature New Biol. in press.

Urm, E., N. Kelker, H.-L. Yang, G. Zubay and W. Maas. 1973. *In vitro* repression of N-α-acetyl-L-ornithinase synthesis in *Escherichia coli*. Mol. Gen. Genet. <u>121</u>: 1.

Yang, H.-L. and G. Zubay. 1973a. Synthesis of the arabinose operon regulator protein in a cell-free system. Mol. Gen. Genet. <u>122</u>: 131.

Yang, H.-L. and G. Zubay. 1973b. Unstable proteins involved in regulation of transcription. Proc. Nat. Acad. Sci. in press.

Yang, H.-L., G. Zubay, E. Urm, G. Reiness and M. Cashel. 1973. The effects of guanosine tetraphosphate (ppGpp), guanosine pentaphosphate (pppGpp) and β-γ methylenyl-guanosine pentaphosphate (pCH$_2$ppGpp) on *Escherichia coli* gene expression *in vitro*. Proc. Nat. Acad. Sci. in press.

Zubay, G. 1969. The mechanism of activation of catabolite-sensitive genes: a positive system. In (T. W. Rall, M. Rodbell and P. Condliffe, eds.) THE ROLE OF ADENYL CYCLASE AND CYCLIC 3'5'-AMP IN BIOLOGICAL SYSTEMS. p. 231. National Institutes of Health, Bethesda.

Zubay, G. 1973. *In vitro* synthesis of protein in microbial systems. Ann. Rev. Genetics in press.

Zubay, G., D. A. Chambers and L. C. Cheong. 1970a. Cell-free studies on the regulation of the *lac* operon. In (D. Zipser and J.R. Beckwith, eds.) THE *LAC* OPERON. p. 375. Cold Spring Harbor Laboratory, New York.

Zubay, G., D. Schwartz and J. Beckwith. 1970b. Mechanism of activation of carabolite-sensitive genes: a positive control system. Proc. Nat. Acad. Sci. <u>66</u>: 104.

Zubay, G., L. Gielow and E. Englesberg. 1971. Cell-free studies on the regulation of the arabinose operon. Nature New Biol. <u>233</u>: 164.

Zubay, G., D. E. Morse, W. J. Schrenk and J. H. M. Miller. 1972. Detection and isolation of the repressor protein for the tryptophan operon of *Escherichia coli*. Proc. Nat. Acad. Sci. <u>69</u>: 1100.

21. HOST-DEPENDENT GENE EXPRESSION OF BACTERIOPHAGES T3 AND T7

Rudolf Hausmann

Institut f. Biologie III der Universität, Freiburg i. Br., W. Germany

A viral genome codes for only part of the genetic information necessary for its self-replication. The host contributes the machinery for energy production, the building blocks of viral nucleic acids and proteins, and a transcription-translation apparatus. Despite the universality of the genetic code and of basic metabolic pathways, however, a wild-type viral genome that succeeds in invading a given, normally metabolizing host cell may possibly not yield progeny: for normal virus growth, the viral genome apparently has to be in tune with the genome of the host in regard to factors that are highly specific for a given virus. In addition to examples of such situations in animal virology (Dulbecco, 1969; Bang, 1972), several phage-bacteria systems are known in which virus infection is abortive, or results in a low yield of progeny virus. In phage genetics, the most extensively investigated mechanism of abortive infection by wild-type viruses is that of DNA restriction: the injected viral DNA is cut to pieces by the action of nucleotide sequence-specific restriction enzymes of the host (see review: Meselson *et al.*, 1972). The physical destruction of the invading phage genome is an efficient, straightforward way of interfering with the normal course of viral development. However, several other examples of abortive infection by wild-type phages are known, in which interference with the physical integrity of the invading genome does not seem to be the cause for failure of phage growth (Hausmann *et al.*, 1968; Morrison and Malamy, 1971; Georgopoulos, 1971; Moyer *et al.*, 1972). In such cases, at what stages of viral development and by which mechanisms does the block occur?

As a model system for investigating this question, I have chosen a series of enterobacterial hosts that are nonpermissive for phage T7. This system has the following advantages: (a) The

genetics and physiology of T7 - a relatively small, virulent,
double-stranded DNA phage - have been well investigated (see reviews: Studier, 1972; Summers, 1972; Hausmann, 1973). (b) Phage
T3, which is closely related to T7, differs in its ability to grow
on these hosts. Since T3 and T7 can be crossed, genetic analysis
of viral determinants of abortive infection is possible even when
no T7 mutants with altered growth properties can be found. (c) Previous work on abortive infection of some enterobacterial strains
by T7 (Hausmann *et al.*, 1969; Hausmann and Härle, 1971; Morrison
and Malamy, 1971) indicated that a variety of different mechanisms
might be found. Studies of such mechanisms may contribute to shape
our views on the molecular strategy of infection used by these
phages to take over the metabolic apparatus of the host.

IDENTIFICATION OF NONPERMISSIVE HOSTS

About 150 *Escherichia coli* strains - isolated from patients
examined at the Public Health Institute of Cologne - were streaked
out on nutrient agar plates, and spot-tested with concentrated
suspensions (10^{12} particles/ml) of the wild types of T3 and T7.
The cells of 12 strains were shown to be killed by both phages.
Of these, five strains were eliminated from this study because they
adsorbed poorly at least one of the phages; two other strains
supported normal growth of both, T3 and T7, and were also eliminated. The other five strains: E8, Igk-G, Igk-L, Igk-M and Igk-N
(henceforth called E, G, L, M and N, respectively) were efficiently
killed by T3 and T7, but produced very small, or no plaques when
T7 was plated in dilute suspensions (10^4 particles/ml). [Strain E
has been used in previous work (Hausmann and Härle, 1971).] Ten
common laboratory strains of *E. coli* were also tested as in the
series above. Of these, *E. coli* F (the usual laboratory host for
T5; obtained from Y. T. Lanni) turned out to be nonpermissive for
T7, but it plated T3 normally. Three further nonpermissive hosts
for T7 were included in this study: *Shigella sonnei* D_2 371-48
(henceforth called D), described earlier (Hausmann *et al.*, 1968);
E. coli B(P1), obtained from W. Arber; and *E. coli* 560F$^+$, from R.
Knippers. Strain B(P1) was included because the prophage P1 is
known to restrict T3 and T7 (Eskridge, Weinfeld, and Paigen, 1967),
but the restriction mechanism had not been investigated. Strain
560F$^+$, which is nonpermissive for T7 by virtue of the sex factor F,
was included for comparative purposes, since the physiology of F-
determined abortive infection has been investigated in some detail
(see review: Summers, 1972). As a permissive host (norm) *E. coli*
B was used. This host, as well as the phages, have been referred
to previously (Hausmann *et al.*, 1968).

Since various sex factor-like episomes are known to interfere
with T7 growth (Watanabe *et al.*, 1966; Morrison and Malamy, 1971;

Hausmann and Härle, 1971), the nonpermissive hosts used here were
spot-tested with the male-specific phages μ_2 and Qβ. Except for
560F[+], none was sensitive to these phages. Also, none of the hosts
produced a colicin active on B.

FATE OF PARENTAL T7 DNA

Since the destruction of the invading phage genome by a DNA
restriction mechanism would prevent detection of more subtle mis-
fits between viral DNA and its host environment, an attempt was
made to eliminate from this study the nonpermissive hosts in which
DNA restriction seemed obviously involved in abortive infection.
Cells of the various host strains were exposed to ^{32}P-labeled T7
particles, and infection was allowed to proceed at 37°C for 9 min
(which corresponds to about 2/3 of the normal latent period).
Samples of infected cultures were then lysed and subjected to sedimentation analysis in neutral sucrose gradients (Fig. 1). Only in
hosts L, N, and D was extensive scission of parental T7 DNA mole-

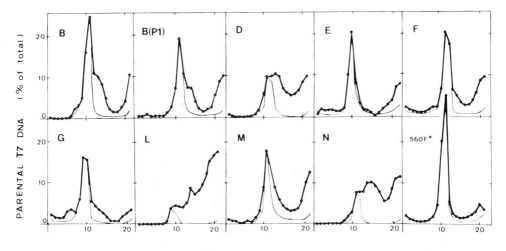

Figure 1. Fate of parental T7 DNA. ^{32}P-labeled T7 (10 particles/
cell) were adsorbed to concentrated host bacteria (6 X 10^9 cells/ml)
for 3 min. After a 20-fold dilution into cold medium (5°C), unad-
sorbed particles were removed by centrifugation. Infected cells
were resuspended in warm nutrient medium (2 X 10^8 cells/ml) and incubated for 9 min at 37°C. Samples were then lysed with lysozyme-
EDTA-sodium dodecyl sulfate. ^{3}H-labeled T7 DNA was added as a marker (thin lines; peaks normalized to ^{32}P counts in corresponding
fractions). Centrifugation was in a Spinco SW39 rotor for 150 min
at 39,000 rpm. Bottom fractions are to the left. Details on media,
solutions, lysis conditions and preparation of labeled phage are
in Hausmann (1968).

cules observed. In D, fragmentation of invading T7 DNA could be
prevented by addition of chloramphenicol (300 µg/ml, final concentration) as late as 3 min after infection (37°C). This was in
accordance with previous work (Hausmann *et al.*, 1968), where breakdown of T7 DNA was attributed to the expression of a nonessential,
conditional lethal phage function. Fragmentation of parental T7
DNA was not inhibited by addition of chloramphenicol to L or N
cells prior to, or during phage infection. It was thought, therefore, that abortive infection in these two cases was probably due
to the action of a DNA restriction enzyme present in the host before infection. Thus, hosts L and N were not further analyzed in
the course of this study. In the other six nonpermissive hosts,
accumulation of parental T7 DNA fragments that sedimented more
slowly than full-length genomes was not more pronounced than in the
normal host. Since a large proportion of the parental DNA co-
sedimented with marker DNA from mature phage (Fig. 1), DNA restriction was considered an unlikely mechanism for abortive infection
in these cases.

LYSIS PATTERNS AND BURST SIZES

For a quantitative evaluation of the degrees of nonpermissive-
ness of the different host strains, one-step growth curves were
obtained for T3 and T7 infecting these hosts. Phage production
was checked under conditions of premature lysis, since the possibility existed that some strains that did not lyse after infection did
produce phage but could not liberate them. Other samples of the
infected cultures were used for measurements at A_{260} nm to check
their ability to lyse spontaneously. The eight hosts tested could
thus be divided into several phenotypes, according to lysis pattern
and ability of phage production (Fig. 2). Some nonpermissive hosts,
like F, G, and $560F^+$, showed no optical density increase, or a reduced one, after T7 infection – in contrast to the normal situation.
For host $560F^+$, the rate of net protein synthesis was measured after
T7 infection: within about one minute this rate was reduced to less
than 10% of the pre-infection rate. Further, T7-infected $560F^+$
cultures, at higher multiplicities (20-50), showed a progressive
decrease in optical density that started immediately after phage
addition (lysis from without). This sensitivity to higher multiplicities, in a range that did not affect the normal host, and the
speed of change in the rate of protein synthesis, suggest that inability of the host to repair membrane damage during infection
could be a factor of abortive infection. It remains to be investigated to what extent this is related to the translational control
mechanisms (Morrison and Malamy, 1971; Scheps *et al.*, 1972) proposed to be specifically inhibited during F^+-mediated T7 abortion.
Upon T7 infection of B(P1) cells, the optical density continued to
increase for several hours; microscopic examination revealed filamentous growth of these cells.

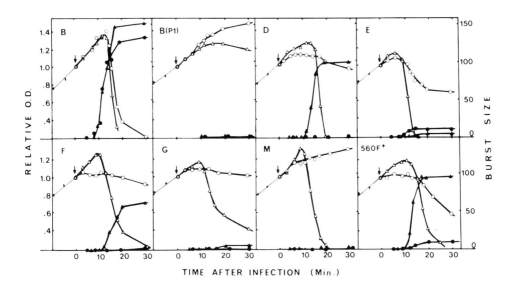

Figure 2. Patterns of lysis (open symbols) and burst sizes (filled symbols) after infection of various hosts by T3 (triangles) or T7 (circles). Phage at a multiplicity of 10 were added (arrows) to exponentially growing nutrient broth cultures (2 X 10^8 cells/ml) at 37°C. At intervals, samples were withdrawn for (a) monitoring lysis by measurements of A_{600}, or (b) assaying phage particles, after disruption of the cells with low intensity ultrasound (a treatment that does not affect phage viability).

PHAGE-DIRECTED PROTEIN SYNTHESIS

To monitor the kinetics of synthesis of specific phage-coded proteins by nonpermissive hosts, S-adenosylmethionine-cleaving enzyme (AdoMet-ase; possibly the product of gene 0.3 of T3, not produced by T7) and phage RNA polymerase (gene 1 product) were chosen as "early" proteins; as representatives of "late" proteins (*i.e.* proteins whose structural genes are transcribed normally by the phage RNA polymerase), endonuclease (gene 3 product), lysozyme (gene 3,5 product), and serum blocking protein (SBP, a tail protein; gene 17 product) were tested.

In T3 infections, except for infectin of B(P1), the times of appearance of the tested phage enzymes were normal; however, the levels of enzyme activity (per mg protein in cell extracts) were often 30-60% below normal. These low activities, although probably reflecting a less than ideal adjustment of the phage genome to the

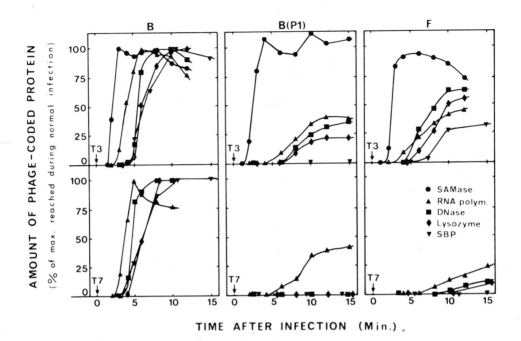

TIME AFTER INFECTION (Min.).

Figure 3. Time course of synthesis of some T3- or T7-coded proteins
in the hosts B, B(P1) and F. Exponentially growing cells were infected with phage (10 particles/cell) and incubated at 37°C. At
intervals, samples were withdrawn for preparation of cell-free
extracts; these were used as a source of enzyme. Assays were done
according to Hausmann and Härle (1971).

corresponding host environment, cannot directly be related to abortive infection by T3, since the progeny-yielding host F, for instance, also showed these low levels of T3 enzymes (Fig. 3). Upon
T3 infection of B(P1), the pattern of AdoMet-ase synthesis was
normal, but synthesis of phage RNA polymerase, DNase, and lysozyme,
was delayed and proceeded at a low rate. T3 SBP-synthesis in B(P1),
E, and M, reached less than 5% of that in B; and it varied between
25 and 60% of norm in the other hosts.

Upon infection with T7 the patterns of synthesis of RNA polymerase, DNase, and lysozyme were normal or nearly normal in the
hosts D, E, and G. In M, the level of lysozyme was low (10-20%
of norm) but the time of its appearance was normal. In F, and
560F+ cells, the rate of synthesis of all tested T7-directed enzymes was less than 10% of norm; in B(P1) T7 RNA polymerase
reached levels of about 50% of norm, but no other enzyme activities
could be detected (Fig. 3). Cells of F, B(P1) and M, synthesized
less than about 5% of T7 SBP, compared to B; in the other hosts
values varied between 10 and 30%.

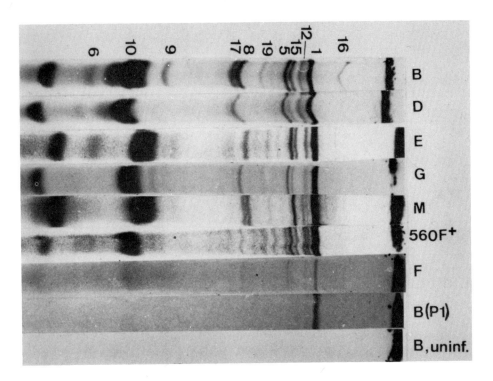

Figure 4. Patterns of T7-coded proteins synthesized in various
hosts. Cells in minimal medium were UV-irradiated to inhibit host
protein synthesis; ^{14}C-labeled amino acids (20 µCi/ml) and phage
(5 particles/cell) were added. After 30 min incubation at 37°C,
samples were treated with 5% trichloroacetic acid. The precipitated proteins were dissolved in 1% sodium dodecyl sulfate and analyzed through electrophoresis in 10% polyacrylamide gels (with sodium
dodecyl sulfate), followed by autoradiography. The origin is at
the top. The technique was essentially as described by Studier
and Maizel (1969). Numbers at the left refer to the structural
genes of the banded proteins (Studier and Maizel, 1969; Studier,
1972).

    Another approach for studying protein synthesis in the non-
permissive hosts was through the gel electrophoresis-autoradiography
method which was successfully applied by Studier and Maizel (1969)
and by Studier (1972) to the analysis of patterns of T7-directed
protein synthesis in the normal host. As shown in Fig. 4, only
RNA polymerase was synthesized after T7 infection of B(P1) while
in the autoradiogram of F several weak bands of T7 proteins were
detectable. This is in agreement with findings of Fig. 3. In the
other hosts, individual bands of T7 proteins could vary in their

relative intensities, when compared to the B pattern. However, no
particular interpretation is possible at this stage. The relatively high level of radioactivity in T7 proteins synthesized by 560F$^+$
seems to be in contradiction with the reduced rate of protein synthesis in these cells, observed in the experiment of Fig. 3. The
explanation seems to lie in the marked sensitivity to higher multiplicities of these cells. (A multiplicity of only about 5 was used
for the gel-electrophoresis autoradiography experiment.)

BREAKDOWN OF HOST DNA

To study the DNA metabolism of phage-infected nonpermissive
hosts, the ability of the invading phage to break down the host
DNA was first checked: [^{3}H]thymidine-labeled cells growing in non-
radioactive medium were infected with amber mutants of T3 or T7,
defective in gene 5 (DNA polymerase). (These mutants were chosen
in order to avoid masking of host DNA breakdown by eventually synthesized phage DNA. Gene 5 is essential for phage DNA synthesis
but not for breaking down the host DNA.) At intervals, samples
were checked for acid-precipitable counts. It was shown that, in
most cases, breakdown of host DNA upon infection followed the normal pattern (Fig. 5). Noteworthy is that T7 was unable to promote
intracellular DNA breakdown in the hosts 560F$^+$ (in agreement with
Morrison and Malamy, 1971), and B(P1). In F, T7-directed host DNA
breakdown started prematurely but proceeded at less than 1/5 of
the normal rate. T3 did not promote host DNA breakdown in G, and
promoted breakdown of B(P1) DNA at about half the normal rate.

PHAGE-DIRECTED THYMIDINE INCORPORATION

As a second aspect of DNA metabolism of infected nonpermissive
hosts, their capacity to synthesize phage-directed DNA was examined.
A quantitative appraisal was made by measuring phage-directed [^{3}H]-
thymidine incorporation into acid-precipitable material in host
cells whose own DNA synthesis had been blocked through UV irradia-
tion shortly before infection. Hosts E (Hausmann and Härle, 1971),
B(P1), and G, were the only ones unable to support T3-directed DNA
synthesis; all the others, including M, which is nonpermissive for
T3, showed a normal pattern. However, upon infection with T7, only
E showed normal thymidine incorporation; hosts B(P1), F, and 560F$^+$
did not incorporate thymidine. In the hosts D, G, and M, incorporation started at the normal time, about 4 min after infection, but
came to a halt at about 8 min; the incorporated counts were then
resolubilized (Fig. 6). [This pattern had already been observed
for D (Hausmann *et al.*, 1968), which was here reexamined for comparison.] The similarity of the patterns in D, G, and M, suggested
that similar mechanisms of T7 abortion might be at work in these
hosts. To test this, T7 *ss1−*, *i.e.* a T7 mutant able to grow normal-

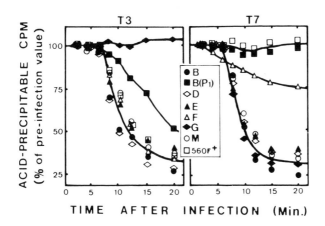

Figure 5. Breakdown of bacterial DNA in various hosts after infection by T3*am*H2 or T7*am*N71. Cells were grown in the presence of
[^{3}H]thymidine for several generations, transferred to nonradioactive
medium and further incubated at 37°C. Phage (10 particles/cell)
were added and samples were withdrawn at intervals and assayed for
acid-precipitable radioactivity. Experimental details are in
Hausmann *et al.* (1968).

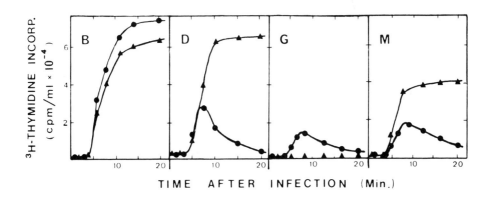

Figure 6. Phage DNA synthesis after infection of hosts B, D, G,
and M by T3 (triangles) or by T7 (circles). Exponentially growing
cultures (2 X 10^8 cells/ml) were UV-irradiated to inhibit synthesis
of bacterial DNA. [^{3}H]thymidine (10 μCi/ml) and phage (10 parti-
cles/cell) were then added. After incubation for various times at
37°C, samples were taken and assayed for acid precipitable radioactivity. Experimental details are in Hausmann *et al.* (1968).

ly on D (Hausmann *et al.*, 1968), was used for infection of G and
M. In these two hosts, T7 *ss*1⁻ could not grow: this mutant was
undistinguishable from wild type with regard to DNA synthesis.
Thus, the mechanism of T7 abortion in D must be different from that
in G and M. (As noted above, G and M differ markedly with regard
to T3-directed DNA synthesis.)

SEDIMENTATION ANALYSIS OF PHAGE-DIRECTED DNA

As previously shown (Hausmann and Härle, 1971), during T7 infection of E the newly synthesized phage DNA accumulated as a material sedimenting faster than DNA from phage particles. And it is
known (Hausmann, 1968), that during T7 infection of D the newly
synthesized phage DNA is cut to pieces smaller than mature phage
DNA. Thus, it was of interest to investigate sedimentation of newly synthesized T7 DNA in G and M cells, and that of T3 DNA in M
cells (*i.e.*, the not yet examined situations where phage DNA synthesis occurred during abortive infection). Host cultures were UV-
irradiated, and [³H]thymidine and phage were added; at 9 min after
infection, samples were taken and prepared for sedimentation analysis in neutral sucrose gradients. Sedimentation of T3 DNA synthesized in M apparently was not significantly different from that of
T3 DNA synthesized in the normal host, B. T7 DNA synthesized in
G or M, however, was broken down to pieces smaller than mature phage
DNA. Compared to D, fragmentation was more extensive in G, but much
less pronounced in M (Fig. 7).

PHAGE MUTANTS WITH EXTENDED RANGE OF PERMISSIVE HOSTS

The fact that wild-type particles of T3 and T7 do not grow on
many of the hosts they invade provides simple selective systems for
the isolation of putative mutants able to grow on these hosts. T7
mutants able to grow on D were indeed found during previous work
(Hausmann *et al.*, 1968). However, it was not possible to find
either spontaneous or hydroxylamine-induced T3 or T7 mutants able
to grow normally on a nonpermissive host other than D.

T7 mutants able to grow on D (*ss*⁻ mutants) were shown to be
defective in the function of the *ss*⁺ gene, which is nonessential
for growth on B and which is lethal on D (Hausmann *et al.*, 1968).
In the course of the present work more *ss*⁻ mutants were isolated
by their ability to produce plaques on D. Some of these mutants
were "leaky", *i.e.*, their plaques were smaller than those of true
ss⁻ mutants. Two of such leaky *ss*⁻ mutants, *ss*4 and *ss*6, were
crossed with each other and with the mutant *ss*1⁻. The progeny was
plated on a mixed indicator lawn of B and D, as described (Hausmann *et al.*, 1968). On this mixed indicator, *ss*⁺, *ss*⁻, and leaky

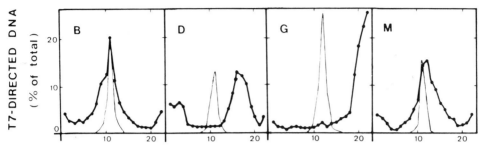

Figure 7. Sedimentation patterns in neutral 5-20% sucrose gradients
of T7-directed DNA, synthesized in hosts B, D, G and M. At 9 min
after infection, in the experiment in Fig. 6, a sample was taken
from each culture and lysed with lysozyme-EDTA-sodium dodecyl sulfate. ^{32}P-labeled T7 DNA was added as a marker (thin lines; peaks
normalized to fraction with highest ^{3}H-counts). Centrifugation
was in a Spinco SW39 rotor for 150 min at 39,000 rpm. The fractions
were assayed for acid-precipitable radioactivity (see legend to
Fig. 1).

δδ plaques could be distinguished. The percentage of δδ$^+$ recombinants in the cross δδ4 X δδ1$^-$ was less than 0.2%; the cross δδ6
X δδ1$^-$ gave about 3% δδ$^+$ recombinants. In the cross δδ4 X δδ6,
two recombinant types, with the phenotypes of δδ$^+$ and δδ$^-$, were
found in about equal proportions; the recombination percentage was
5%. Thus, by comparison with previous work (Hausmann *et al.*, 1968)
the two leaky δδ mutations seem to be located close to each end of
the δδ gene. The recombinants with the phenotype of δδ$^-$, from the
cross δδ4 X δδ6, were shown to be double mutants, since in back-
crosses to T7 wild type (δδ$^+$) they gave about 5% recombinants with
the phenotype of leaky δδ. These recombinants were either of δδ4
or δδ6 genotype, as could be shown by appropriate crosses.

The leaky δδ mutants, δδ4 and δδ6, as well as their reciprocal
recombinants δδ4$^+$·δδ6$^+$ (wild type) and δδ4·δδ6 (double mutant) were
then investigated with regard to phage DNA synthesis in the host
D. Resolubilization of newly incorporated [^{3}H]thymidine was less
pronounced during infection with leaky δδ mutants, as compared to
wild type infection. Sedimentation analysis of samples taken at
various intervals after infection showed that the progressive
scission of newly synthesized DNA also was much less accentuated
during infection with the leaky δδ types, as compared to wild
type (Fig. 8). In the double mutant δδ4·δδ6, the δδ-function
seemed totally defective, since T7 DNA synthesis proceeded normally,

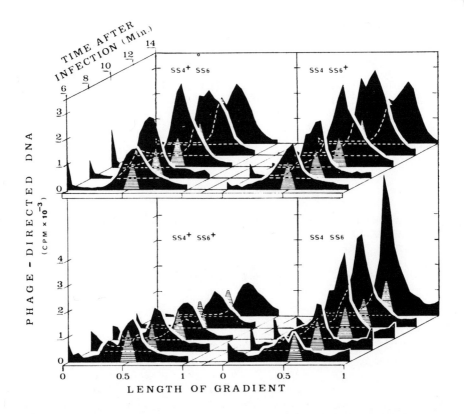

Figure 8. Sedimentation in neutral 5-20% sucrose gradients of
phage DNA synthesized in host D by T7𝛿𝛿4, T7𝛿𝛿6 and the two reciprocal recombinants from a cross 𝛿𝛿4 X 𝛿𝛿6. [³H]thymidine (10 μCi/
ml) and phage (10 particles/cell) were added to cultures of UV-
irradiated D cells. At intervals, samples were lysed with lysozyme-
EDTA-sodium dodecyl sulfate. ³²P-labeled T7 DNA was added as a
marker (striped triangles). Centrifugation was in a Spinco SW39
rotor for 150 min at 39,000 rpm. The profiles represent phage-
directed cumulative incorporation of [³H]thymidine into acid-precipitable material (see legend to Fig. 1).

as in the 𝛿𝛿1⁻ mutant characterized in previous work (Hausmann *et
al.*, 1968).

     Clues to the nature of the 𝛿𝛿-function are still missing, al-
though a genetic determinant of the host, which is required for
lethal expression of the 𝛿𝛿⁺ function, has now been mapped between
thr and *leu* on the D chromosome by P1 transduction (Gatzojas and
Hausmann, in preparation). However, it is not clear whether a

functional gene product of D interacts with the ss^+ product to bring about T7 abortion, or whether a functional product of B, absent from D, is required to protect the phage DNA from ss^+-induced self-digestion.

SUMMARY AND CONCLUSIONS

Among 12 newly isolated *E. coli* strains sensitive to the related phages T3 and T7, only two produced normal phage bursts: permissiveness seems not to be the rule for sensitive hosts. Besides DNA restriction, there was a variety of phenotypically distinguishable mechanisms of abortion. In a series of seven nonpermissive hosts for T7, where DNA restriction was not involved, the physiology of abortive infection was different for each host. In 3 cases (hosts D, F, and $560F^+$), T3 grew normally. There was no T3 DNA synthesis after infection of hosts B(P1), E, and G, but in M synthesis of T3 DNA was normal. T7 DNA synthesis did not occur in B(P1) – whose cells grew filamentously after infection – F, and $560F^+$. During T7 infection of E, phage DNA accumulated as fast-sedimenting material; during T7 infection of D, G, and M, the newly synthesized phage DNA was broken down to small pieces. Further host-specific differences in the physiology of abortive infection by T3 or T7 lie in the ability of the phage to breakdown the host DNA to acid-soluble material, in the patterns of phage protein synthesis, and in cell lysis. Elucidation of the molecular mechanisms of abortion has to await further genetic and biochemical analysis, but the multiplicity of patterns of nonpermissive infection suggests that virulent phages like T3 and T7 depend on the host for a variety of highly specific functions. Detailed information on these functions may provide new insights into host-virus relationships.

ACKNOWLEDGMENTS

I wish to thank Miss Carolyn Tomkiewicz and Miss Ulrike Schulz for their dedicated technical assistances. I am grateful to Dr. E. Härle for many helpful discussions and valuable assistance in gel electrophoresis and autoradiography. This investigation was supported by grants Nos. Ha-709/1 and Ha-709/2 from the Deutsche Forschungsgemeinschaft.

REFERENCES

Bang, F. B. 1972. Specificity of viruses for tissues and hosts. Symp. Soc. Gen. Microbiol. 22: 415.

Dulbecco, R. 1969. Cell transformation by viruses. Science 166: 962.

Georgopoulos, C. P. 1971. A bacterial mutation affecting N function. In (A.D. Hershey, ed.) The Bacteriophage Lambda p. 639. Cold Spring Harbor Laboratory, New York.

Eskridge, R. W., H. Weinfeld and K. Paigen. 1967. Susceptibility of different coliphage genomes to host-controlled variation. J. Bacteriol. 93: 835.

Hausmann, R. 1968. Sedimentation analysis of phage T7-directed DNA synthesized in the presence of a dominant conditional lethal phage gene. Biochem. Biophys. Res. Commun. 31: 609.

Hausmann, R. 1973. The genetics of T-odd phages. Ann. Rev. Microbiol. 27: in press.

Hausmann, R., B. Gomez and B. Moody. 1968. Physiological and genetic aspects of abortive infection of a Shigella sonnei strain by coliphage T7. J. Virol. 2: 335.

Hausmann, R. and E. Härle. 1971. Expression of the genomes of the related bacteriophages T3 and T7. Wien. med. Akad. 1: 467.

Meselson, M., R. Uyan and J. Heywood. 1972. Restriction and modification of DNA. Ann. Rev. Biochem. 41: 447.

Morrison, T. G. and M. H. Malamy. 1971. T7 translational control mechanisms and their inhibition by F factors. Nature New Biol. 231: 37.

Moyer, R. W., A. S. Fu and C. Szabo. 1972. Regulation of bacteriophage T5 development by ColI factors. J. Virol. 9: 804.

Scheps, R., H. Zeller and M. Revel. 1972. Deficiency in initiation factors or protein synthesis induced by phage T7 in E. coli F⁺ strains. FEBS Lett. 27: 1.

Studier, F. W. 1972. Bacteriophage T7. Science 176: 367.

Studier, F. W. and J. V. Maizel, Jr. 1969. T7-directed protein synthesis. Virology 39: 575.

Summers, W. C. 1972. Regulation of RNA metabolism of T7 and related phages. Ann. Rev. Genet. 6: 191.

Watanabe, T., T. Takano, T. Arai, H. Nishida and S. Sato. 1966. Episome-mediated transfer of drug resistance in Enterobacteriaceae. J. Bacteriol. 92: 477.

22. SYNTHESIS OF RNA PRIMER FOR LAMBDA DNA REPLICATION IS

CONTROLLED BY PHAGE AND HOST

Sidney Hayes and Waclaw Szybalski

McArdle Laboratory for Cancer Research, University of Wisconsin, Madison Wisconsin

As discussed in this Symposium by Dr. Alberts, there appear to be two kinds of initiation of DNA synthesis: (1) primary initiation from a specific site (origin or *ori* site) on double-stranded DNA leading to the formation of a replication fork, and (2) frequent discontinuous initiations restricted mainly to the "lagging" strand of DNA within the moving fork and leading to the formation of so-called Okazaki fragments. The first step in both kinds of initiation probably involves the synthesis of an RNA primer, since DNA polymerases require the 3'-OH terminus of a pre-existing primer, and RNA polymerase can initiate RNA synthesis from a DNA template without a primer.

We would like to present data showing that, for bacteriophage lambda, a unique 4S RNA is synthesized at the *ori* site, from which bidirectional λ DNA synthesis starts, and that this RNA, which we call *oop*, probably primes the initiation of λ DNA synthesis at the *ori* site and participates in formation of the replication fork (Hayes and Szybalski, 1973). A more complete account of these studies will be published elsewhere.

LOCALIZATION AND CHARACTERIZATION OF *OOP* RNA

The *oop* RNA is coded by the *l* strand of λ DNA within a region of about 500 nucleotide pairs in length, defined by the right endpoints of two substitutions, *imm*21 and *hy*42, and containing the *ori* site (Fig. 1). This 4S RNA most probably corresponds to the one observed by Champoux (1970) and to the 81 nucleotide-long "minor leftward RNA" synthesized *in vitro* (Blattner and Dahlberg,

277

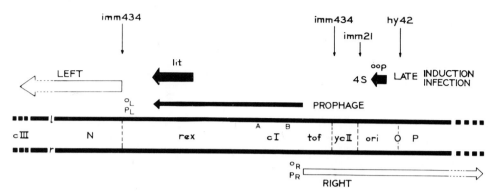

Figure 1. Physical and genetic map of the immunity and neighboring regions of coliphage λ. The endpoints of the substitutions, which delete DNA in the immunity region, are indicated by vertical arrows and are drawn to scale (Fiandt and Szybalski, 1973). For the designation of the genes see Szybalski *et al.* (1970). The open arrows indicate the major leftward and rightward transcripts. The black arrows indicate the immunity transcription in the prophage (*cl-rex*) or after induction (*oop* and *lit*). The late immunity transcription (*lit*) RNA is always produced coordinately with the *oop* RNA (Hayes, 1972). The heavy lines represent the *l* and *r* DNA strands.

1972) and *in vivo* (Lozeron, Dahlberg and Szybalski, in preparation) and sequenced by Dahlberg and Blattner (1973). The *oop* RNA is synthesized from the noninduced prophage, but at a barely detectable level, *i.e.*, 0.001 to 0.002% of the total pulse-labeled RNA. The *oop* transcription, however, increases 30 to 100-fold between 5 and 10 minutes after thermal induction (Table 1).

EFFECT OF MUTATIONS AND INHIBITORS ON *OOP* RNA SYNTHESIS

As shown in Table 1, *oop* RNA synthesis increased about 50-fold after thermal induction of the λcl857 lysogen, in parallel with the increase in λ DNA copies. Is there a relationship between *oop* synthesis and λ DNA replication? Table 2 shows that several host (*dna*B and *dna*G) and phage (*ori*⁻, *O*⁻ and *P*⁻) mutations inhibit both λ DNA replication and *oop* RNA synthesis. The *dna*E mutation, however, abolishes λ DNA replication, but does not prevent *oop* synthesis. Similarly, *oop* transcription is not depressed when λ DNA replication is inhibited by nalidixic acid (Table 1).

Table 1 also shows that *oop* RNA synthesis is sensitive to rifampicin, which inhibits RNA synthesis initiation. When this inhibitor was added 1.5 minutes before the [³H]uridine pulse, *oop* synthesis was reduced about 60-fold, whereas the total pulse-labeled RNA declined 17-fold. Preferential inhibition of *oop* RNA synthesis would be expected under these conditions, since *oop* RNA is very short.

Table 1. Effect of prophage induction on λ DNA and *oop* RNA syntheses in the absence or presence of inhibitors of DNA replication and transcription.

Time(min)[a]	Temp.(°C)	λ DNA Replication[b]	*oop* RNA Synthesis[c]	Total RNA Synthesis[d]
0	30	1	1	75
5	42.5	1-2	3	102
15	42.5	6	27	88
21	42.5	10	47	89
25	42.5	17	46	84
25(Nal)[e]	42.5	4	99	29
25(Rif)[f]	42.5	17	12	5

[a] To measure RNA synthesis, the lysogens were pulsed with [^{3}H]-uridine for 1 minute either at 30°C (0 time) or at the indicated times after transferring the W3350(λcI857) culture to 42.5°C (Bøvre, Lozeron and Szybalski, 1971).

[b] λ DNA assay was described by Stevens *et al.* (1971). The results are the averages for the *att-N* and *x-0-P* tester [^{3}H]RNA's and indicate the number of λ DNA copies per lysogen.

[c] Percent of total (λ plus host) pulse-labeled RNA (X10^3) which hybridized with the *l* strand of λ DNA between the *imm*21 and *hy*42 endpoints (see Fig. 1). About 0.5 ml of [^{3}H]RNA extract (see footnote d) was used for each multi-step hybridization to determine *oop* RNA.

[d] Total trichloroacetic acid-precipitable RNA (cpm X 10^{-3}/5µl of [^{3}H]RNA extract).

[e] Nalidixic acid (250 µg/ml) was added immediately before transfer to 42.5°C.

[f] Rifampicin (200 µg/ml) was added at 1.5 minutes before the [^{3}H]uridine pulse.

EFFECT OF REPRESSOR ON *OOP* RNA

Since *oop* RNA synthesis is very low in the repressed prophage, we decided to investigate the effect of the λ repressor on fully expressed *oop* synthesis. This was possible because the denaturation of the cI857-coded repressor is reversible. Thus, repression can be lifted by heating the λcI857 lysogen and then quickly restored

Table 2. Effect of phage and host mutations on λ DNA replication and *oop* RNA synthesis

Phage mutant	λ DNA	*oop*	Host mutant	λ DNA	*oop*
+	13	50	*dna*A	17	72
O-	1	1	*dna*F	15	75
P-	1	1	*dna*B	1	3
ori-	1	3	*dna*G	1.5	1
+(noninduced)	1	1-2	*dna*E	1	70

For details see the legend to Table 1. The *oop* RNA was measured in lysogens pulsed with [³H]uridine from 20.5 to 21.5 minutes after transfer from 30°C to 42.5°C, with the exception of the noninduced λ⁺ lysogens, which were always kept at 30°C (last line). The increase in λ DNA above that of the noninduced control was assayed at 20 minutes after thermal induction.

Table 3. The effect of repressor on *oop* and *att-N* transcription

Induction and repression of the λc1857 lysogen		ℓ-strand transcripts (% of total [³H]RNA X 10³)	
		oop	*att-N*
Induced	0-3.5 min at 43°C	1	10,468
Induced	0-21.5 min at 43°C	45	1,540
Induced and repressed	0-15 min at 43°C 15-21.5 min at 30°C	40	40

For details see the legend to Table 1. The lysogen was labeled with [³H]uridine at 2.5 to 3.5 minutes (first line) or at 20.5 to 21.5 minutes after thermal induction. The *att-N* transcription corresponds to the difference between the hybridization values for the ℓ strands of λ and λ*bio*3h-1.

by rapidly cooling the culture to 30°C. Table 3 shows that restoration of repressor, which blocks the major o_L-controlled leftward *att-N* transcription, had no effect on *oop* RNA synthesis.

CONCLUSIONS AND SUMMARY

The data presented can be conveniently summarized by the model shown in Fig. 2. Synthesis of *oop* RNA starts at the *ori* site, where λ DNA replication begins (Dove *et al.*, 1971; Stevens *et al.*, 1971). We propose that *oop* RNA is a primer for the initiation of leftward λ DNA synthesis.

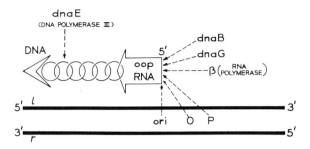

Figure 2. A model for the role of *oop* RNA in the initiation of
leftward DNA synthesis. The *oop* RNA synthesis starts at the *ori*
site and requires the products of genes *O* and *P* and of host genes
*dna*B and *dna*G in addition to the host RNA polymerase for its full
expression. The 3'OH terminus of the *oop* RNA primer is extended
by the host DNA polymerase III, the product of gene *dna*E.

        After induction, the synthesis of *oop* RNA was shown to increase
30 to 100 fold over the extremely low level of synthesis from the
noninduced prophage. The requirements for this greatly enhanced
oop transcription include, in addition to the *E. coli* RNA polymerase
(or at least its β-subunit, since the accelerated *oop* synthesis
remains rifampicin sensitive), the product of λ genes *O* and *P*, a
cis-dominant *ori* site, and two products of host genes *dna*B and *dna*G.
These genes are all known to be required for λ DNA replication
(Dove *et al.*, 1971; Stevens *et al.*, 1971; Wechsler and Gross,
1971). These five gene products might interact with the DNA template at the *ori* site or act as cofactors for the RNA polymerase,
thus stimulating the synthesis of the *oop* RNA primer. They do not
seem to participate directly in λ DNA synthesis, which is accomplished by DNA polymerase III, the product of host gene *dna*E (Gefter *et
al.*, 1971), as shown in Fig. 2.

        A more rigorous proof of the role of *oop* RNA in priming λ DNA
replication would be to demonstrate a covalent linkage between λ
DNA and *oop* RNA (see the top of the *oop* arrow in Fig. 2). In experiments to be reported elsewhere, Cs_2SO_4 equilibrium gradient
centrifugation and various hybridization procedures were used to
detect a product of density intermediate between DNA and RNA that
corresponds to DNA covalently bound to *oop* RNA.

        Early λ DNA replication is bidirectional (Schnös and Inman,
1970; Stevens *et al.*, 1971), whereas late λ DNA replication appears
to be predominantly leftward (LePecq and Baldwin, 1968). The *oop*
RNA is a good candidate for a primer for initiation of the leftward
λ DNA replication. Is there also a primer for continuous rightward
DNA replication? It has been demonstrated by Dove *et al.* (1969,

1971) that rightward transcription near the *ori* region is required for the initiation of λ DNA replication. It is possible that a processed *ori*-proximal RNA product of the P_R-*ori*-O-P major rightward λ transcript could be utilized as a primer for the early rightward λ DNA replication. It might be significant that rather intensive synthesis of both the rightward *ori* transcripts and *oop* RNA are required for initiating λ DNA replication. Conceivably, critical concentrations of the RNA primers might be necessary for their efficient utilization in the priming process.

ACKNOWLEDGMENT

These studies were supported by grants from the National Cancer Institute (CA-07175) and the National Science Foundation (GB-2096). We are indebted to Drs. W. F. Dove and J. A. Wechsler for the phage and bacterial strains and to Mrs. Barbara K. Roe for the very able technical assistance.

REFERENCES

Blattner, F. R. and J. E. Dahlberg. 1972. RNA synthesis startpoints in bacteriophage λ: Are the promoter and operator transcribed? Nature New Biol. 237: 227.

Bøvre, K., H. A. Lozeron and W. Szybalski. 1971. Techniques of RNA-DNA hybridization in solution for the study of viral transcription. Methods in Virology 5: 271.

Champoux, J. J. 1970. The sequence and orientation of transcription in bacteriophage λ. Cold Spring Harbor Symp. Quant. Biol. 35: 319.

Dahlberg, J. E. and F. R. Blattner. 1973. Sequence of self-terminating RNA made near the origin of DNA replication of phage lambda. Fed. Proc. 32: 664Abs.

Dove, W. F., E. Hargrove, M. Ohashi, F. Haugli and A. Guha. 1969. Replication activation in lambda. Japan J. Genet. 44, suppl. 1: 11.

Dove, W. F., H. Inokuchi and W. F. Stevens. 1971. Replication control in phage lambda. In (A. D. Hershey, ed.) The Bacteriophage Lambda. p. 747. Cold Spring Harbor Laboratory, Cold Spring Harbor.

Fiandt, M. and W. Szybalski. 1973. Electron microscopy of the immunity region in coliphage lambda. Abstracts of the Ann. Meet. of the Amer. Soc. for Microbiol., p. 218.

Gefter, M. L., Y. Hirota, T. Kornberg, J. A. Wechsler and C. Barnoux. 1971. Analysis of DNA polymerases II and III in mutants of *Escherichia coli* thermosensitive for DNA synthesis. Proc. Nat. Acad. Sci. 68: 3150.

Hayes, S. J. 1972. Regulation of lambda repressor transcription. Fed. Proc. 31: 444Abs.

Hayes, S. and W. Szybalski. 1973. Possible primer for DNA replication in coliphage lambda. Fed. Proc. 32: 529Abs.

LePecq, J. B. and R. L. Baldwin. 1968. The starting point and direction of λ DNA replication. Cold Spring Harbor Symp. Quant. Biol. 33: 609.

Schnös, M. and R. B. Inman. 1970. Position of branch points in replicating λ DNA. J. Mol. Biol. 51: 61.

Stevens, W. F., S. Adhya and W. Szybalski. 1971. Origin and bidirectional orientation of DNA replication in coliphage lambda. In (A. D. Hershey, ed.) The Bacteriophage Lambda. p. 575. Cold Spring Harbor Laboratory, Cold Spring Harbor.

Szybalski, W., K. Bøvre, M. Fiandt, S. Hayes, Z. Hradecna, S. Kumar, H. A. Lozeron, H. J. J. Nijkamp and W. F. Stevens. 1970. Transcriptional units and their controls in *Escherichia coli* phage λ: Operons and scriptons. Cold Spring Harbor Symp. Quant. Biol. 35: 341.

Wechsler, J. A. and J. D. Gross. 1971. *Escherichia coli* mutants temperature-sensitive for DNA synthesis. Molec. Gen. Genetics 113: 273.

23. INTERACTION IN DNA REPLICATION OF THE GENE 32 AND *r*II PRODUCTS

OF PHAGE T4 WITH THE *dna* C PRODUCT OF THE HOST

Gisela Mosig and Alan Breschkin

Vanderbilt University, Nashville, Tennessee

To gain a better understanding of DNA replication in general, we are interested in the interactions between host and phage functions in phage growth. It has been tacitly assumed that DNA replication of bacteriophage T4 is independent of host functions, since T4 codes for several functions that are essential for DNA replication (Epstein *et al.*, 1963) and since T4 produces progeny in all mutant hosts that are defective in their own DNA replication (for review, see Gross, 1972 and Alberts, this Symposium). However, we must keep in mind that the tested mutant hosts do not lack the respective proteins, but rather produce altered proteins. Any such protein, though temperature sensitive in replication of bacterial DNA, may still be capable of interacting with components of the T4 replicating apparatus.

Recently, we have shown that several *E. coli* functions (coded for by the *dna* B, *dna* E, *dna* C, *dna* G and *pol* A genes) can participate in T4 DNA replication and/or recombination (Mosig *et al.*, 1972). Our present results indicate that *in vivo* the *dna* C product of *E. coli* (which is required for initiation of *E. coli* DNA replication; for review, see Gross, 1972) interacts with the gene 32 product of T4. Furthermore, the *r*II proteins of T4 must be involved in this interaction.

The T4 gene 32 protein is apparently essential in genetic recombination (Tomizawa, 1967; Kozinski and Felgenhauer, 1967) and in DNA replication (Epstein *et al.*, 1963). Alberts and his collaborators have elegantly characterized properties and functions of this protein; this work is summarized in this symposium (Alberts). Presumably, gene 32 protein is required both for initiation and

285

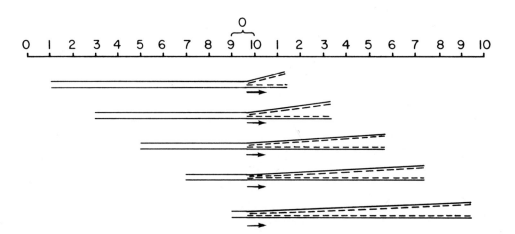

Figure 1. The postulated pattern of replication of normal T4 chromosomes in the absence of recombination within the terminal redundancies. The upper line represents twice the length of the complete
genome, the other lines show the replication of five random chromosomes from the origin region, 0, in the direction of the arrows.

chain elongation in DNA replication, in addition to its function
in recombination.

     Our present studies follow from our previous observations that
incomplete T4 chromosomes containing gene 43 (DNA polymerase), replicated on the average half of their parental DNA in wild type hosts,
although many of them must lack gene 32 (Mosig and Werner, 1969;
Marsh *et al.*, 1971). On the other hand, in *dna* C mutant hosts, incomplete T4 chromosomes lacking gene 32 replicated little or none
of their DNA (Mosig *et al.*, 1972). This suggested that either the
dna C function can substitute for a missing gene 32 protein, or that
the *dna* C product has to interact with the gene 32 protein (*e.g.* in
initiation). We have also concluded from the above mentioned studies
that the first round of T4 DNA replication starts at an origin region near gene 43 and proceeds predominantly in the clockwise direction to the end of the molecule.   In our model, recombination (presumably within the terminal redundancies) is required for complete
replication of all T4 chromosomes. If gene 32 protein is essential
for recombination, in its absence about one half of the parental
DNA should remain unreplicated (Fig. 1). This consideration com-
plicated possible interpretations of our results. To clarify further the relationship of the bacterial *dna* C and the T4 gene 32 proteins, we have investigated the possibility that some gene 32
mutants might be differentially defective in DNA replication or
recombination.

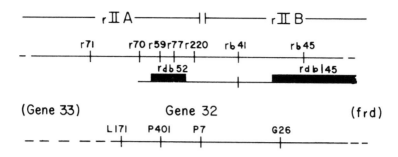

Figure 2. Approximate map position within the genes *rIIA*, *rIIB* and 32 of the mutations used in our studies.

Different gene 32 *ts* mutants differ in their response (cessation of [^{3}H]thymidine incorporation) to a temperature shift from the permissive to the restrictive temperature (Riva *et al.*, 1970), although none of the mutants produces viable progeny at 42°C. We reasoned that these different responses might reflect differential functional damages in the respective proteins and compared growth and DNA replication of the "tightest" mutant P 7 and the most "leaky" mutant L 171 (for their map position see Fig. 2) in wild type and *dna* C hosts. We measured the decrease in density of $^{13}C^{15}N^{32}P$-labeled parental phage DNA and the production of light phage DNA following single infection of light bacteria in the presence of [^{3}H]thymidine. In neutral Cs_2SO_4 gradients of sheared lysates, replicated and unreplicated T4 DNA's are well separated from each other and from bacterial DNA (Mosig *et al.*, 1972) and the proportion of the total parental DNA that was replicated can be readily determined. Neither P 7 nor L 171 replicated more than one half of their parental DNA (Table 1; gradients are not shown in this paper). We also followed the distribution of unsheared DNA from these lysates in neutral Cs_2SO_4 gradients. Under these conditions, partially replicated parental DNA would band at hybrid or slightly denser than hybrid position. Parental ^{32}P-label would move to lighter than hybrid density only if light progeny DNA was produced and remained attached to the parental DNA molecules (Werner, 1968), or if parental DNA strands recombined with the light progeny DNA (Kozinski and Felgenhauer, 1967).

Most of the unsheared ^{32}P-containing P 7 or L 171 DNA banded at denser than hybrid and little or none at lighter than hybrid positions (for a representative example see Fig. A). These results suggest that most chromosomes were only partially replicated and that both P 7 and L 171 are defective in recombination. However, P 7 and L 171 differed in two respects: 1) While L 171 produced small but measurable amounts of light phage DNA (Fig. 3A), P 7 produced none. 2) The proportion of L 171 DNA that replicated

Table 1. Normalized proportion (as %) of parental T4 DNA that was replicated at 42°C

Phage	Bacteria	
	wild type (B or DG 75)	*dna* C PC 2
wild type	100	90
*r*71	90	90
32 deleted*	48 – 50	<3
P 7	48 – 50	20 – 22
L 171	47 – 50	47 – 50
L 171 *r*71	63	48 – 50

Experimental conditions and host strains were as described by Mosig *et al.* (1972). The proportion of wild type DNA that replicated in wild type hosts (70%) was arbitrarily taken as 100 percent and all other data were normalized for these values.

*These values (from Mosig *et al.*, 1972) are based on the probability that incomplete chromosomes containing gene 43, lack gene 32.

was similar in *dna* C as in wild type bacteria, while the residual replication of P 7 DNA was severely reduced in *dna* C hosts (Table 1). These results, together with our previous results (Mosig *et al.*, 1972) are best explained by the following hypothesis: the *dna* C product has to interact with another bacterial protein or with gene 32 protein during initiation of T4 DNA replication. In the absence of gene 32 protein but in the presence of *dna* C⁺ protein, the presumptive bacterial protein may suffice for the first initiation of T4 replication. However, the defective L 171 or P 7 proteins compete with the bacterial protein for the interaction with the *dna* C product, and the L 171 *dna* C⁻ complex shows more residual functional activity than the P 7 *dna* C⁻ complex.

Further support for this hypothesis comes from the pattern of partial suppression of L 171 by certain *r*II mutations (Mosig, Breschkin and Berquist, in preparation). Some L 171 *r*II double mutants (*r*71, *r*70, *r*77, *r*b41) produced average burst sizes of about 8 in *E. coli* B at 42°C (as compared with <0.3 for the single L 171 mutant). None of the other *r*II mutants tested (Fig. 2) had suppressing activity and none of the other gene 32 mutations suppressed the *r*II plaque morphology at intermediate temperatures. (The inability to grow on K(λ) was not suppressed.) These observations taken together suggest that this suppression reflects the direct interaction of the two proteins, rather than a general physiological effect. By contrast, no *r*II suppression occurred in *dna* C hosts; at 42°C, single L 171 or L 171 *r*II mutants gave burst sizes below 0.1.

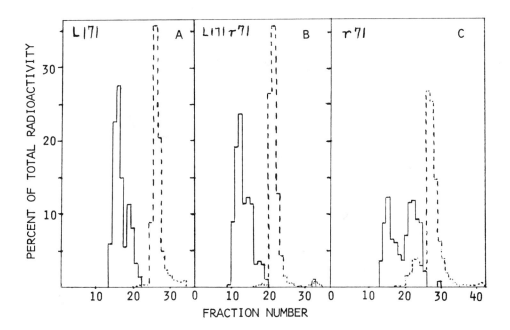

Figure 3. Density distribution in neutral Cs_2SO_4 gradients of unsheared DNA, isolated from E. coli DG 75, 26 min after single infection at 42°C with $^{13}C^{15}N^{32}P$-labeled L 171⁻(A), L 171 r71⁻(B) and
r71⁻(C) particles. Growth conditions and lysis were as described
(Mosig et al., 1972). For example, the four peaks in B represent,
from left to right, heavy T4 DNA, hybrid T4 DNA, light T4 DNA and
bacterial DNA.

     The DNA replication pattern of the L 171 r71 double mutant
completely corroborated these findings. In wild type hosts, the
double mutant replicated more than 60% of its total DNA (Table 1)
and in Cs_2SO_4 gradients of unsheared DNA more than 10% of the parental DNA banded at lighter than hybrid density (Fig. 3B). We
conclude that some but not all rII⁻ mutations partially restore the
recombination function of L 171. Consequently, those parental DNA
molecules that successfully recombine can replicate all of their
DNA and produce viable progeny. Consistent with this hypothesis,
we found in preliminary single burst experiments, that 10-15% of
the infected bacteria produce 10-60 progeny particles each. In
dna C mutant hosts, neither L 171 nor L 171 r71 replicated more
than half of their DNA and no unsheared DNA banded at lighter than
hybrid density. Thus we must conclude that the partial suppression by rII mutations of L 171 requires a functional dna C⁺ product.
It is interesting to note that both the origin region of T4 DNA
replication (Marsh et al., 1971) and the rII proteins (Weintraub

and Frankel, 1972) are associated with the bacterial cell envelope.
Our present experiments do not yet determine whether the suppressing *r*II mutations permit complete replication of some L 171 chromosomes because they restore recombination within the terminal redundancies or because they permit bidirectional initiation of DNA
replication.

ACKNOWLEDGMENTS

    We thank Mrs. Susan Bock for excellent technical assistance.
Supported by NIH grant GM 13221.

REFERENCES

Epstein, R. H., A. Bolle, C. M. Steinberg, E. Kellenberger, E.
BoyDeLaTour, R. Chevalley, R. S. Edgar, M. Susman, G. H. Denhardt
and A. Lielaulis. 1963. Physiological studies of conditional
lethal mutants of bacteriophage T4d. Cold Spring Harbor Symp. Quant.
Biol. 28: 375.

Gross, J. D. 1972. DNA replication in bacteria. Current Topics
in Microbiol. and Immunol. 57: 39.

Kozinski, A. and Z. Felgenhauer. 1967. Molecular recombination in
T4 bacteriophage deoxyribonucleic acid II. Single-strand breaks
and exposure of uncomplemented areas as a prerequisite for recombination. J. Virol. 1: 1193.

Marsh, R. C., A. M. Breschkin and G. Mosig. 1971. Origin and direction of bacteriophage T4 DNA replication. II. A gradient of
marker frequencies in partially replicated T4 DNA as assayed by
transformation. J. Mol. Biol. 60: 213.

Mosig, G. and R. Werner. 1969. On the replication of incomplete
chromosomes of phage T4. Proc. Nat. Acad. Sci. 64: 747.

Mosig, G., D. W. Bowden and S. Bock. 1972. *E. coli* DNA polymerase
I and other host functions participate in T4 DNA replication and
recombination. Nature New Biol. 240: 12.

Riva, S., A. Cascino and E. P. Geiduschek. 1970. Coupling of late
transcription to viral replication in bacteriophage T4 development.
J. Mol. Biol. 54: 85.

Tomizawa, J.-I. 1967. Molecular mechanisms of genetic recombination
in bacteriophage: Joint molecules and their conversion to recombinant molecules. J. Cell Physiol. 70: 201.

Weintraub, S. B. and F. R. Frankel. 1972. Identification of the T4*r*IIB gene product as a membrane protein. J. Mol. Biol. $\underline{70}$: 589.

Werner, R. 1968. Initiation and propagation of growing points in the DNA of phage T4. Cold Spring Harbor Symp. Quant. Biol. $\underline{33}$: 50.

24. SOME CONSIDERATIONS REGARDING THE STRUCTURE AND FUNCTION OF

PROMOTER-OPERATOR REGIONS

Frederick R. Blattner

McArdle Laboratory for Cancer Research, The University of Wisconsin, Madison, Wisconsin

A well known property of efficient chemical catalysts is that they usually possess large surface areas. This generally is to provide a high concentration of accessible catalytic sites. However, some solid catalysts also employ catalytically inert portions of their surface for lateral diffusion of adsorbed molecules. In such cases efficient catalysis can occur despite a relatively low concentration of active sites (Haensel and Burwell, 1971). In many biologically important cases, enzymes are present at low concentration and it becomes advantageous to embed the catalyst in a membrane. Substrates can then adsorb first to the membrane and find the enzyme by a two-dimensional diffusion process. This strategy for speeding up a reaction by reducing the dimensionality of the space in which a rate limiting diffusion process takes place was proposed and analyzed in detail by Adam and our chairman for today, Dr. Max Delbrück (Adam and Delbrück, 1967).

IN VITRO STUDIES OF THE LEFT OPERON OF λ

We have recently suggested that a similar strategy may be employed by RNA polymerase in finding RNA startpoints on DNA molecules which are also at very low concentrations in cells. The basis for this suggestion came from experiments by Jim Dahlberg, Waclaw Szybalski, Julie Boettiger, Mike Fiandt, and myself in which we used an *in vitro* transcription system to map RNA startpoints in bacteriophage λ. In these experiments we employed a combination of techniques including RNA sequencing, DNA·RNA hybridization, electron micrography and recombinational deletion mapping to produce a high resolution map of the promoter-operator region of the major leftward

293

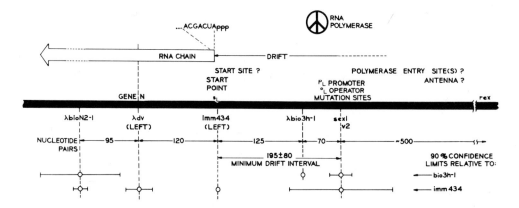

Figure 1. A map of the leftward promoter-operator region of phage
λ.

operon of this phage (Blattner and Dahlberg, 1972; Blattner *et al.*,
1972). This map, illustrated in Fig. 1, shows that the promoter-
operator region is quite large in relation to the dimensions of RNA
polymerase. A minimum estimate for its size is the distance from
the RNA startpoint to the site of the *sex*l promoter mutation.

A series of deletion and substitution mutants of λ with endpoints in this area were examined, and two were found which cut
between *sex*l and the RNA startsite denoted s_L. The distance was
thus divided into three parts which were measured independently.
The first, from s_L to *imm*434 was measured by determining the sequence
from s_L to the λdv endpoint and subtracting this number of nucleotides from the electron micrographically determined length of the
dv-*imm*434 interval (Fig. 1). The second, from *imm*434 to 3h-l, was
measured electron micrographically, and the third, from 3h-l *sex*l,
was estimated by recombination measurements calibrated by physical
mapping. The total distance was 195 ± 80 nucleotide pairs or three
to ten 100 Å diameters of the RNA polymerase protein. This of
course is a minimum estimate for the size of the promoter. A maximum estimate could be the distance from the startpoint to the
terminus of the next operon upstream which Hayes and Szybalski
estimate to be 580 nucleotide pairs (Hayes and Szybalski, 1973).

An important conclusion of this work is that nucleotide sequences involved in control of transcription (both *in vivo* and *in
vitro*) are not themselves transcribed into RNA (Lozeron *et al.*,
1972). This is based not only on mapping data but on nucleotide
sequence analysis of the initial portions of *in vitro* transcripts
from various promoter and operator mutant templates. The templates
we examined included the promoter *sex*l, operator mutants v2 and

υlυ3, and the heteroimmune substitution mutant λ*imm*434. None of these showed pertinent changes in initial sequence as a result of the presence of the mutations.

To interpret these results a number of possibilities should be considered (Blattner *et al.*, 1972) including condensation or folding of the DNA to bring sequences at the extremes of the promoter-operator region closer together. Two considerations tend to mitigate against this possibility. First, there are theoretical difficulties in folding native DNA on such a short radius relative to the persistence length of DNA without unwinding the helix (Tribel *et al.*, 1971). The experiments of Sucier and Wang (1972) show that polymerase doesn't denature DNA very much. Second, the pieces of DNA that are resistant to DNase digestion because of protection by RNA polymerase measure only about one polymerase diameter in length (Blattner, 1968).

An alternative hypothesis embodying RNA polymerase movement without production of RNA chains is presented in Fig. 2. In this model, the promoter-operator is divided into three parts, the entry, drift, and start regions. The first effective interaction between polymerase and DNA takes place at the entry region which in principle could be a small polymerase-sized site. More probably it consists of a larger stretch of DNA which we call an "antenna". As Chamberlin calculated earlier in the Symposium, it would take 8000 seconds for an enzyme molecule to find directly a site measuring 30 nucleotides within a DNA molecule of λ size whereas an "antenna" of 130 nucleotides containing 100 overlapping 30 nucleotide targets or one of 3000 nucleotides containing 100 tandemly arranged non-overlapping targets could reduce this time to 80 seconds. The entry region of course could be even larger perhaps comprising a substantial percentage of the phage chromosome.

The leftward operon of λ is under control of two repressors, the cI-coded repressor which binds to an operator site O_L and the *to*$_6$ gene product which is also presumably a repressor. The latest measurements by Maniatis and Ptashne (1973) place the size of the cI repressor binding site(s) at 110 nucleotide pairs. In Fig. 2 we have placed this site and (hypothetically) a similar sized target for the *to*$_6$ repressor in the drift region in between entry region and RNA startpoint. Control would thus be achieved by controlling the access of polymerase to the startsite. Quite possibly promoter mutants such as *s*ex1 work in a similar manner by introducing sequences that are more or less difficult for the enzyme to drift through.

The third element of the promoter-operator region which we call the startsite is a recognition sequence which triggers initiation of RNA synthesis at the specific nucleotide on the template

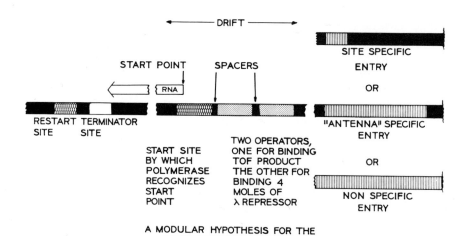

Figure 2.   Hypothetical structure of a promoter-operator region.

corresponding to the RNA startpoint. Once the enzyme has reached
this site it becomes stably bound and capable of rapid starting.
Presumably the class A binding sites on T7 DNA described by Hinkle
and Chamberlin (1972) correspond to startsites.

     Heyden *et al.* (1972) recently have carried the DNA protection
by RNA polymerase technique to new levels of refinement. They obtained a unique 30 nucleotide protected fragment from DNA of phage
fd which presumably includes a startsite. This fragment contains
the RNA startpoint of one of the phage promoters as well as the
first 6 nucleotides of the RNA. Although the duplex DNA fragment
as isolated is bound tightly to RNA polymerase, it does not easily
rebind to the enzyme once it has been released. We assume this is
because DNase digestion removes the entry site or antenna that
would normally be at some distance from the startsite (H. Schaller,
personal communication).

     An important unresolved question concerns the extent to which
the various sites in the promoter-operator region overlap. In Fig.
2 we depict an extreme view, which we call a modular hypothesis,
in which each site is physically separate and optional spacers have
been included in between them. This arrangement has practical and
evolutionary advantages in that lines of control can be kept independent, and recognition sequences for different control elements
are free to evolve independently. This scheme also permits evolution of control circuits by insertion or deletion of modules. It
is equally possible however, that some or all of the sites overlap
or interpenetrate, and this could also have advantages. It will
probably be necessary to determine the complete nucleotide sequence

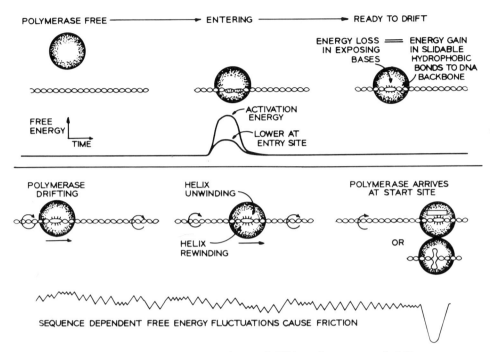

Figure 3. Hypothetical mechanism of RNA polymerase drift.

of a promoter-operator region both for wild types as well as for
some mutants before meaningful progress can be made.

As we have mentioned, our proposal for the structure of the
promoter-operator region assumes that RNA polymerase is capable
of moving along DNA without production of RNA chains. Some suggestions for the mechanism of this movement are presented in Fig. 3.
Initially RNA polymerase and DNA are separated in solution and the
free energy of the system is at some reference value. The initial
attachment to DNA we suppose involves an activation energy which is
rather high at most points of the DNA, but which is lower at the
antenna or entry site. Thus, although the binding energy is not a
strong function of where on the DNA an already bound enzyme might
be located, entry occurs primarily at entry sites because there is
less of an activation barrier there.

Once the polymerase has entered, it is free to move laterally
into regions that would have been difficult to enter directly. To
conform with the measurements of Saucier and Wang (1972), the equivalent of 4-5 bases or 1/2 turn of the helix is assumed to be unwound per enzyme molecule as it drifts. As the polymerase moves
the unwound portion moves with it by separation of the helix in

front and closure behind. In this way the unbounded base pairs
would be available for inspection as the enzyme moved along so that
the startsite can eventually be recognized.

Bonds to the phosphate-sugar backbone are probably needed to
align the DNA on the surface of the enzyme and the energy of these
bonds per nucleotide should probably be comparable to the energy
of unpairing a single base so that energy liberated as the helix
opens in front could be used in closure at the rear and not be dis-
sipated as heat. It will also be necessary for these bonds to
"slide", that is be transferred sequentially from nucleotide to
nucleotide as the enzyme moves. Thus, the bonds must be equivalent
for the various bases. This is another reason to suspect that they
do not involve the base pairing sites on DNA. It will be interesting to see whether this slidable bond is similar to the one employed
by the DNA unwinding proteins discussed earlier in this Symposium
by Dr. Alberts, and whether any protuberance from the polymerase
protein is inserted in between the DNA strands.

As the enzyme moves laterally, there will be differences in
free energy depending on which base pairs are being opened at the
front relative to which are being closed at the rear. In addition
there may be stacking and folding energies to consider. All of
these will contribute to barriers to drift or "friction", which
could influence the efficiency of initiation of transcription and
provide potential sites for so-called promoter mutations.

Although many questions remain to be answered, the study of
transcription and its control will continue to benefit from the
parallel application of genetic and biochemical approaches. Bacteriophage λ, which has been thoroughly studied from both these points
of view, will therefore continue to be a very important tool in
this area. One thing I hope we can avoid in the future, however,
is the tendency to prematurely use genetic terms for biochemical
entities and vice versa. For example, the term "promoter" often
has been used interchangeably for the site of promoter mutations
and for the site of RNA polymerase binding and initiation. It now
appears that such interchangeable usage might not be justified.

ACKNOWLEDGMENT

The ideas and opinions presented in this review and in the
earlier paper by Blattner *et al.* (1972) were formulated in the
course of many spirited discussions with Jim Dahlberg and Waclaw
Szybalski; any of them which they disown are my responsibility.
The work was supported by NIH and NSF grants to W. Szybalski and
to J. E. Dahlberg.

REFERENCES

Adam, G. and M. Delbruck. 1967. Reduction of dimensionality in biological diffusion processes. In (A. Rich and N. Davidson, eds.) Structural Chemistry and Molecular Biology. p. 200. W. H. Freeman and Co., San Francisco.

Blattner, F. R. 1968. Interaction of RNA polymerase with T7 DNA molecules. Ph.D. Thesis. Johns Hopkins University.

Blattner, F. R. and J. E. Dahlberg. 1972. RNA synthesis startpoints in bacteriophage λ: Are the promoter and operator transcribed? Nature New Biol. 237: 227.

Blattner, F. R., J. E. Dahlberg, J. K. Boettiger, M. Fiandt and W. Szybalski. 1972. Distance from a promoter mutation to an RNA synthesis startpoint on bacteriophage λ DNA. Nature New Biol. 237: 232.

Haensel, V. and R. L. Burwell, Jr. 1971. Catalysis. Scientific American 12: 46.

Hayes, S. and W. Szybalski. 1973. Control of short leftward transcripts from the immunity and *ori* regions in induced coliphage lambda. Molec. Gen. Genetics, submitted.

Heyden, B., C. Nüsslein and H. Schaller. 1972. Single RNA polymearase binding site isolated. Nature New Biol. 240: 9.

Hinkle, D. C. and M. J. Chamberlin. 1972. Studies of the binding of *Escherichia coli* RNA polymerase to DNA. I. The role of sigma subunit in site selection. J. Mol. Biol. 70: 157.

Lozeron, H. A., M. L. Funderburgh, J. E. Dahlberg, B. P. Stark and W. Szybalski. 1972. Identity of *in vitro* and *in vivo* initiation of phage lambda mRNA: Analysis of *in vivo* cleavage products. Abstracts of the Ann. Meet. of the Amer. Soc. for Microbiol. p. 237.

Maniatis, T. and M. Ptashne. 1973. Multiple repressor binding at the operators of phage λ. Proc. Nat. Acad. Sci. in press.

Saucier, J. and J. C. Wang. 1972. Angular alteration of the DNA helix by E. *coli* RNA polymerase. Nature New Biol. 239: 167.

Tribel, H., K. E. Reimert and J. Strassburger. 1971. Persistence length of DNA from hydrodynamic measurements. Biopolymers 10: 2619.

NOTE ADDED IN PROOF

Since this manuscript was prepared we have isolated a new λ deletion strain which deletes almost all of the DNA between p_L and p_R without damaging either promoter. Electron microscopic examination showed its left endpoint to be about 300 nucleotides upstream of δ_L, placing a new upper limit on the size of the promoter-operator region.

With this deletion as marker, the position of $bio3$h-1 was remeasured with an increase in accuracy, and found to be in the neighborhood of 20-30 nucleotides upstream of the left end of $imm434$ (F. R. Blattner, M. Fiandt, K. Hass, and W. Szybalski, in preparation). This places the calculated position of the sex_1 mutation site 40 to 80 nucleotides upstream of δ_L. Thus, the size of the drift region might be considerably smaller than our earlier measurements indicated. Further analysis with this and similar deletions will enable us to ascertain more exactly whether its size exceeds that of a polymerase diameter.

25. STRUCTURE OF SIGMA-DEPENDENT BINDING SITES OF *E. COLI* RNA POLYMERASE TO PHAGES λ, T5 AND T7 DNA'S

Philippe Jeanteur* and Jean-Yves Le Talaër**

*Laboratoire de Biochimie-C.R.L.C., Hopital Saint-Eloi, 34000 Montpellier, France and **Unité de Biochimie, Institut Gustave Roussy, 94800 Villejuif, France

At variance with DNA replication, which is basically unselective insofar as it must yield an accurate and complete copy of the entire genome at each generation, the transcription process is highly restrictive. Indeed, at any given time, only a limited number of specific operons is actually transcribed. During early development of a phage, which depends entirely on the host transcription machinery, RNA polymerase initiates the synthesis of RNA chains at a very small number of discrete sites recognized by its cognate sigma factor (Bautz and Bautz, 1970). The very high degree of specificity involved in the initiation of transcription calls for the existence of some unique features of these DNA sequences involved in the recognition process. The structure of these sites is obviously of great interest since a number of regulatory factors act either positively (sigma-type factors, cyclic AMP-cyclic AMP recepor-protein system) or negatively (repressors) in their close vicinity.

During the past few years, our group has been intereted in finding some common peculiarities of the DNA sequences from different coliphages that are specifically recognized by *E. coli* RNA polymerase in the presence of sigma factor. We have found these sequences to be very rich in (A+T) pairs (67%) in the three phages (λ, T5 and T7, we have studied (Le Talaër and Jeanteur, 1971a,b and 1972; Le Talaër *et al.*, 1973).

ISOLATION OF RNA POLYMERASE BINDING SITES AS PROTECTED DNA

It was first observed independently by Novak (1967) and Blattner (1968) that the binding of bacterial RNA polymerase to DNA provided protection towards nucleolytic digestion of those DNA sequences

covered by the polymerase (referred to as pDNA) and therefore representing the binding sites. This protection phenomenon does not
depend upon the presence of nucleoside triphosphates (Blattner,
1968). All the experiments described in this paper have been performed in the absence of such substrates.

Methodology for RNA polymerase purification, DNA labeling and
extraction from $\lambda C_I 857$, T5 and T7 phages as well as the binding and
digestion conditions have been already described in detail (Le
Talaër and Jeanteur, 1971b; Le Talaër et al., 1973). These conditions, unless otherwise states, are as follows: varying amounts
of [^{32}P]DNA and RNA polymerase were mixed and incubated at 37°C for
15 minutes in 40 mM Tris-HCL (pH 8.0), 10 mM $MgCl_2$, and 1 mM $CaCl_2$.
Digestion was carried out in all cases by further incubation for
30 minutes at 37°C in the presence of both pancreatic DNase (200 µg/
ml) and venom phosphodiesterase (200 µg or 7.5 U/ml). When specified, tRNA was added to 1 mg/ml during this step. The resulting
mixture was then either directly filtered on Millipore filters or
treated with Pronase, extracted with sodium dodecyl sulfate phenol,
and ethanol-precipitated with or without added calf thymus carrier
DNA.

DISCRIMINATING AGAINST NON-SPECIFIC BINDING SITES

It is well established that the number of binding sites for
RNA polymerase exceeds by far the number of genuine promoters
(Pettijohn and Kamiya, 1967). It is therefore likely that pDNA
would contain an excess of non-specific over specific sites, unless
some action is taken to select against the former. This explains
the failure of earlier works on T7 (Blattner, 1968) and λ (Nakano
and Sakaguchi, 1969) to detect any differences in the base composition of pDNA as compared to total DNA.

However, it was observed that RNA polymerase binds with a much
higher affinity to a limited number of sites on λ (Stead and Jones,
1967) or on T7 DNA (Hinkle and Chamberlin, 1970, 1972). In this
latter case, it was shown that the sites of highest affinity were
for holoenzyme and should thus be considered as specific. Eliminat-
ing non-specific binding sites was then a matter of selection for
sites of highest affinity. This was achieved by different means.
First, as shown in Table 1, the use of tRNA as a competitor allowed
the selection of sites on λDNA that require both sigma and an ele-
vated temperature during binding in order to form a stable complex
(Le Talaër and Jeanteur, 1972). These results are in full agreement
with the findings of Hinkle and Chamberlin (1970) on T7. Our second
approach, which proved to be the most successful, was to reason that
only sites of lower affinity (non-specific) could dissociate during
the digestion step and eventually be degraded to a smaller size

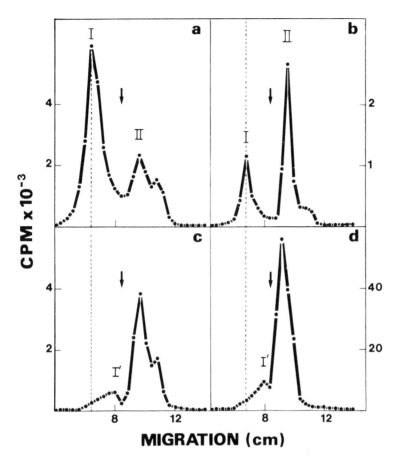

Figure 1. Radioactivity profiles on acrylamide gels of protected
DNA fragments from phage T5 DNA. Fragments obtained in the presence
(a,b) or absence (c,d) of sigma factor were prepared and analyzed
as described in methods. The binding mixtures contained per ml:
a) 40 µg DNA and 20 µg holenzyme; b) 40 µg DNA and 80 µg holoenzyme; c) 50 µg DNA and 25 µg core enzyme; d) 50 µg DNA and 250 µg
core enzyme. Arrows indicate the marker dye (Bromophenol Blue)
position.

although still be able to rebind polymerase and end up as pDNA. To
remove these non-specific sites, we fractionated pDNA on acrylamide
gels. In the case of T5, two populations could be separated according to size, as shown in Fig. 1. The first type of fragments, referred to as Peak I, was observed only when sigma was present during
the binding step whereas Peak II fragments of smaller size were always observed. Similar results were obtained with λ (Le Talaёr and

Jeanteur, 1971b) and T7 (Le Talaër and Jeanteur, 1973). However,
a very small peak of intermediate size (referred to as Peak I') was
detectable in the absence of sigma, especially with T5 and T7 as
can be seen in Fig. 1c and d. Except for this small contamination
by Peak I', Peak I fragments can be operationally defined as "promoter" on the basis of their sigma dependence. This definition is
discussed below in view of the recent work by Blattner *et al.* (1972
and this volume).

Table 1. Discrimination by tRNA and composition of two types of
RNA polymerase binding sites on λDNA.

Binding Conditions	Digestion Conditions	pDNA (% of input)	(A+T) content of DNA
No polymerase	−tRNA	0	(50.0)
	+tRNA	0	−
0°C, + σ	−tRNA	1.24	−
	+tRNA	0	−
37°C, + σ	−tRNA	1.21	−
	+tRNA	0.17	58.0
0°C, − σ	−tRNA	0.99	−
	+tRNA	0.02	−
37°C, − σ	−tRNA	1.07	50.2
	+tRNA	0.01	−

     Methods for pDNA preparation, retention and elution from
Millipore filters, and base composition analysis were as previously
reported (Le Talaër and Jeanteur, 1972).

          COMPOSITION AND STRUCTURE OF SIGMA-DEPENDENT BINDING SITES

     The results presented in Table 1 show that the base composition
of pDNA fragments not displaced by tRNA and therefore engaged in the
most stable complexes with RNA polymerase are significantly enriched
in (A+T) (58%) even under the unfavourable conditions of excess polymerase used in this experiment (Le Talaër and Jeanteur, 1972). Base
composition analyses of the different populations of pDNA resolved
by gel electrophoresis as in Fig. 1 are shown in Table 2. In all
cases, only the sigma-dependent Peak I fragments are enriched in
(A+T) whereas the composition of Peaks I' and II strictly reflects
that of total DNA. When the polymerase/DNA ratio was decreased to
favor the dissociation of the most weakly bound sites, the (A+T)
content of Peak I increased up to a maximum (about 67%) which was
strikingly similar for all three phages (Le Talaër and Jeanteur,

Table 2. Percent (A+T) of RNA polymerase binding sites to λ, T5
and T7 DNA's.

	λ	T5	T7
Total DNA	50.5	59.7	50.9
Peak I	66.8 (0.23) 65.4 (1.2) 59.8 (9.6)	66.4 (0.5) 65.3 (1.0) 60.1 (2.0)	67.5 (0.15) 55.2 (0.5) 55.4 (0.15)
Peak I'		59.1 (0.5 to 5.0)	51.4 (0.15)
Peak II	49.6 (0.9 to 20.0)	59.2 (0.5 to 5.0)	49.9 (0.15 to 5.0)

Methods for pDNA preparation, gel electrophoresis and base
composition analysis were as previously reported (Le Talaër and
Jeanteur, 1971a,b; Le Talaër *et al.*, 1973). The numbers in paren-
theses refer to the weight ratio between polymerase and DNA.

1971; Le Talaër *et al.*, 1973). These sigma-dependent sites were
shown to be double-stranded on the basis of their resistance before
and sensitivity after heat denaturation to the single-strand specific *Neurospora crassa* endonuclease (Le Talaër *et al.*, 1973).

ENTRY, DRIFT OR START SITES

From the above data, we conclude that DNA sequences of very
high (A+T) content are very similar for λ, T5 and T7 and recognized
by sigma. Similar results have been reported for the composition
of RNA polymerase binding sites on the replicative form of phage
fd DNA (Okamoto, Sugiura and Takanami, 1972; Heyden, Nüsslein and
Schaller, 1972) so it appears that the specific binding of *E. coli*
polymerase to (A+T)-rich sequences might be a general phenomenon.
Insofar as sigma mediates promoter recognition (Bautz and Bautz,
1970), these sequences can be operationally identified to promoters.
However, the promoter concept has been recently questioned by the
findings of Blattner *et al.* (1972 and this volume) which show that
polymerase actually initiates RNA synthesis on λDNA some 200 nucleotides away from the initial binding site (entry site). Whether
the sites dealt with here can be equated to the start site, the
entry site or any sequence between these two (drift region) remains
an open question. However, the observation by Wu *et al.* (1972)
that λ repressor can still inhibit transcription by a prebound polymerase would rather suggest we have been dealing with the entry
sites of λ. More work is obviously needed to select among these
possibilities.

ACKNOWLEDGMENTS

    This work has been supported by the Délégation Générale à la
Recherche Scientifique et Technique (contrats n° 72-7-0491 and 72-
7-0389), the Institut National de la Santé et de la Recherche Médi-
cale and the Ligue Nationale Francaise contre le Cancer. We are
indebted for the interest and support of Dr. C. Paoletti in whose
laboratory this work was achieved. Thanks are due to Miss S. Colin
for her expert technical assistance.

REFERENCES

Bautz, E. and F. Bautz. 1970. Initiation of RNA synthesis: the
function of σ in the binding of RNA polymerase to promoter sites.
Nature 226: 1219.

Blattner, F. 1968. Ph.D. Thesis. Johns Hopkins University.

Blattner, F., J. Dahlberg, J. Boettiger, M. Fiandt and W. Szybalski.
1972. Distance from a promoter mutation to an RNA synthesis startpoint on bacteriophage lambda DNA. Nature New Biol. 237: 232.

Heyden, B., C. Nüsslein and H. Schaller. 1972. Single RNA-polymerase binding site isolated. Nature New Biol. 240: 9.

Hinkle, D. and M. Chamberlin. 1970. The role of sigma subunit in
template site selection by E. coli RNA polymerase. Cold Spring
Harbor Symp. Quant. Biol. 35: 65.

Hinkle, D. and M. Chamberlin. 1972. Studies of the binding of E.
coli RNA polymerase to DNA. I. The role of sigma subunit in site
selection. J. Mol. Biol. 70: 157.

Le Talaër, J.-Y. and Ph. Jeanteur. 1971a. Preferential binding
of E. coli RNA polymerase to A-T rich sequences of bacteriophage
lambda DNA. FEBS Lett. 12: 253.

Le Talaër, J.-Y. and Ph. Jeanteur. 1971b. Purification and base
composition analysis of phage lambda early promoters. Proc. Nat.
Acad. Sci. 68: 3211.

Le Talaër, J.-Y. and Ph. Jeanteur. 1972. Discrimination by tRNA
of two types of isolated binding sites for E. coli RNA polymerase
on phage lambda DNA. FEBS Lett. 28: 305.

Le Talaër, J.-Y., M. Kermici and Ph. Jeanteur. 1973. Isolation
of E. coli RNA polymerase binding sites on T5 and T7 DNA: further
evidence for sigma-dependent recognition of A-T rich DNA sequences.
Proc. Nat. Acad. Sci. in press.

Nakano, E. and K. Sakaguchi. 1969. Isolation and base composition of sites on λ phage DNA which bind with RNA polymerase of *E. coli*. J. Biochem. <u>65</u>: 147.

Novak, R. 1967. Deoxyribonuclease resistance of DNA·RNA polymerase complexes. Biochem. Biophys. Acta 149: 593.

Okamoto, T., M. Sugiura and M. Takanami. 1972. RNA polymerase binding sites of phage fd replicative form DNA. Nature New Biol. <u>237</u>: 108.

Pettijohn, D. and T. Kamiya. 1967. Interaction of RNA polymerase with polyoma DNA. J. Mol. Biol. <u>29</u>: 275.

Stead, N. and O. Jones. 1967. Stability of RNA polymerase complexes. J. Mol. Biol. <u>26</u>: 131.

Wu, A., S. Ghosh and H. Echols. 1972. Repression of the cI protein of phage λ: interaction with RNA polymerase. J. Mol. Biol. <u>67</u>: 423.

26. GENETIC REGULATION OF QUINATE-SHIKIMATE CATABOLISM IN

*NEUROSPORA CRASSA**

Norman H. Giles, Mary E. Case and James W. Jacobson

Department of Zoology, University of Georgia, Athens, Georgia

In recent years genetic mechanisms responsible for regulating several metabolic pathways have been elucidated in considerable detail in certain prokaryotes. By contrast, much less is known concerning regulatory mechanisms in eukaryotes. However, certain eukaryotic microorganisms, particularly various fungi, provide especially favorable material for combined genetical and biochemical investigations of specific regulatory systems. This paper summarizes briefly the present status of studies on one such system in *Neurospora crassa*.

This system involves an inducible metabolic pathway that includes the first three reactions in the catabolism of quinic acid (QA) and shikimic acid (SA) (Fig. 1). This part of the pathway (prior to protocatechuic acid) is controlled by a tightly linked cluster of four genes - the *qa* cluster - located in linkage group VII very close to the methionine-7 (*me*-7) locus. In contrast to wild type, mutants in these genes cannot utilize quinate (or shikimate) as a sole carbon source for growth. In addition, when grown on minimal sucrose medium in the presence of quinate they are also non-inducible for one or more of the enzymes involved in quinate-shikimate catabolism. Three of these four genes are apparently the structural genes for individual enzymes (Rines, 1968; Chaleff, 1971). The *qa*-3 gene encodes quinate dehydrogenase (QHDase) which also acts as shikimate dehydrogenase (SDHase). This latter conclusion is based on the evidence that the two activities co-purify

---

* This paper is dedicated to Professor Karl Sax on the occasion of his eightieth birthday.

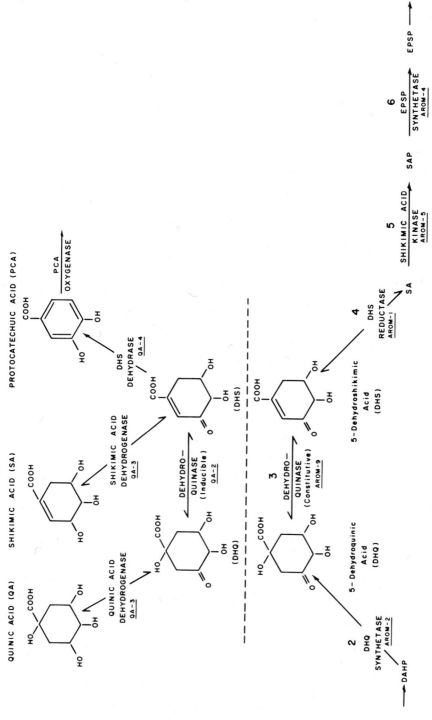

Figure 1. Diagram of the reactions in the quinate-shikimate catabolic (inducible) and the poly-aromatic (constitutive) pathways, indicating the metabolic interrelationships in *Neurospora crassa*.

(Rines, 1969) and that both are lost as a result of single mutations at the qa-3 locus (Chaleff, 1971). The qa-2 gene encodes catabolic dehydroquinase (C-DHQase). *Neurospora crassa* also has a constitutive, biosynthetic dehydroquinase (Fig. 1), which is part of the *arom* multienzyme complex encoded in the *arom* gene cluster (Giles *et al.*, 1967). The qa-4 gene encodes dehydroshikimate dehydrase (DHSDase). In contrast to the five *arom* activities, the three qa proteins are not physically associated, at least *in vitro*.

Mutants in the fourth gene in the cluster (qa-1) are of particular interest. These mutants are pleiotropic negative types, being non-inducible for all the enzyme activities encoded in the three adjacent qa genes. In general, qa-1 mutants are recessive and complement in heterocaryons with mutants in each of the three other genes (*i.e.*, such heterocaryons are able to grow on quinate as a carbon source). These results led to the hypothesis that the qa-1$^+$ (wild type-W.T.) gene produces a regulatory protein that exerts positive control over the synthesis of the enzymes encoded in the three adjacent structural genes in the qa cluster (Rines, 1969).

Additional evidence for positive control has been obtained as a result of the isolation of constitutive mutants (qa-1^C) in the qa-1 gene. These mutants produce high levels of all the qa enzymes when grown in the absence of an inducer. The initial qa-1^C strains were selected as revertants able to utilize quinate as a carbon source following ultraviolet treatment of certain qa-1 mutants (Valone *et al.*, 1971). Subsequently, a technique was developed for the direct detection of qa-1^C mutants induced in wild type conidia (Partridge *et al.*, 1972). In addition, a reexamination of the original qa-1 mutants isolated by Rines has led to the detection of two temperature-sensitive qa-1 mutants that are constitutive at 35°C but not at 25°C (Case, 1972). All these qa-1^C mutants map very close to, presumably within, the qa-1 locus. Tests with heterocaryons between qa-1^C mutants and qa-1$^+$ (W.T.) have indicated that certain qa-1^C mutants are dominant (or semi-dominant) to W.T. (Valone *et al.*, 1971). These results are interpreted as indicating a system of positive control only, rather than one, such as the arabinose system in *E. coli* (Englesberg, 1971), that combines both positive and negative control.

A number of features of the induction process have been examined in the qa system. Rines (1969) concluded that protein synthesis is involved since cycloheximide inhibits induction. Quinate, dehydroquinate, and/or dehydroshikimate are potent inducers, shikimate being much less, if at all, effective (Chaleff, 1972). Evidence that quinate can act as a "gratuitous" inducer comes from induction studies with qa-3 mutants since these mutants lack quinate dehydrogenase and hence cannot metabolize quinate. To date, no true gratuitous inducers have been detected although numerous quinate analogues have been tested (Partridge and Giles, unpublished). Uti-

lizing a qa-3 mutant, Chaleff (1972) demonstrated coordinate induction by quinate of catabolic dehydroquinase and dehydroshikimate
dehydrase activities. In addition, he also obtained evidence for
coordinate induction of quinate dehydrogenase and catabolic dehydroquinase. Prior results with qa-1^C mutants suggesting a possible
lack of coordinancy for the qa enzymes (Valone et $al.$, 1971) appear
to be attributable to the marked instability of the dehydroshikimate
dehydrase activity under the growth and extraction conditions used
(Chaleff, 1972). The evidence that all qa enzyme activities are
coordinately induced supports (but does not prove) the hypothesis
that there is a single initiator (promoter) region between the qa-1
locus and the adjacent three qa structural genes, and that polarized
transcription involves a single polycistronic mRNA. However, there
is as yet, no unequivocal evidence for either initiator or polar
mutants in the qa region. Present genetic evidence suggests that
the order of genes (from left to right in the right segment of linkage group VII) is qa-1 qa-3 qa-4 qa-2 (me-7, me-9) (Chaleff, 1972).
However, fine structure mapping has proved difficult because of the
leakiness of qa mutants as well as infertility problems, and the
order qa-4 qa-2, in particular, must be regarded as tentative. Initial attempts to detect polar mutants employed complementation tests,
which have been utilized so successfully in the $arom$ gene cluster.
However, it now appears that polarity may be much less pronounced
in the qa cluster and that quantitative enzyme assays may be required to detect polar mutants if they exist. Since an efficient technique for selecting double qa-2 qa-4 mutants is now available (Case
et $al.$, 1972), tests for possible polar (nonsense) mutants in either
the qa-2 or qa-4 genes (depending upon their order) can now be made.

A considerable amount of evidence is now available concerning
the nature of the qa-1 regulatory product. The detection of temperature-sensitive qa-1 mutants and of inter-allelic complementation
between various pairs of qa-1 mutants (Case, 1972) provides indirect
evidence that this product is a multimeric protein. To date, attempts to obtain nonsense mutants within the qa-1 locus have been
unsuccessful. Rines (1969), Case (1972), and Chaleff (1972) have
shown that qa-1 mutants can be divided into two groups - qa-1^S (slow)
and qa-1^F (fast) - on the basis of their complementation responses
with other qa mutants. The qa-1^S types are considered to exhibit
negative complementation to varying degrees and may be analogous to
the i^{-d} mutants of the lac operon in $E.$ $coli$. Genetic mapping data
localize these two groups into two discrete, non-overlapping regions
of the qa-1 locus. In studies to date, only qa-1^S and no qa-1^F types
have reverted to constitutivity (qa-1^C). One of the qa enzymes -
catabolic dehydroquinase - has been purified from an induced wild
type, from an induced qa-3 mutant, and from a qa-1^C mutant. Present
evidence indicates that catabolic dehydroquinase is a multimer (M.
W. $\sim$160,000) composed of a single type of monomer (M.W. probably
less than 14,000). The three preparations appear to be indistinguishable on the basis of preliminary amino-acid analyses and other

comparative data (Jacobson *et al.*, 1973), a result which supports the hypothesis that the only function of the qa-1^+ (W.T.) regulatory protein is to initiate the synthesis of the enzymes encoded in the qa gene cluster.

In summary, the overall results discussed in this brief paper appear best interpreted on the hypothesis that the qa-1^+ gene produces a multimeric protein that acts in a positive fashion to regulate the coordinate synthesis of three enzymes involved in quinate-shikimate catabolism in *N. crassa*. Furthermore, the genetic characteristics of the two types of qa-1 mutants suggest that qa-1^+ protein may have two discrete functional regions – one, an amino acid sequence that interacts with the inducer, and second, a sequence that interacts directly or indirectly to initiate transcription at an initiator (promoter) site proximal to the three qa structural genes. Additional evidence will be required to determine whether the qa gene cluster is equivalent in its organization and function to a prokaryote operon – as appears possible.

ACKNOWLEDGMENT

This research has been supported by Atomic Energy Commision Contracts AT (30-1)-872 and AT (38-1)-735.

REFERENCES

Case, M. E. 1972. Genetical and biochemical characteristics of qa-1 mutants in *Neurospora crassa*. Genetics <u>71</u>: 510A.

Case, M. E., N. H. Giles and C. H. Doy. 1972. Genetical and biochemical evidence for further interrelationships between the polyaromatic and the quinate-shikimate catabolic pathways in *Neurospora crassa*. Genetics <u>71</u>: 337.

Chaleff, R. S. 1971. Evidence for a gene cluster controlling the inducible quinate catabolic pathway in *Neurospora crassa*. Genetics <u>68</u>: 510A.

Chaleff, R. S. 1972. Studies on the genetic control of the inducible quinate-shikimate catabolic pathway in *Neurospora crassa*. Unpublished Ph.D. thesis, Yale University.

Englesberg, E. 1971. Regulation in the l-arabinose system. In (H. J. Vogel, ed.) Metabolic Regulation V. p. 257. Academic Press, New York.

Giles, N. H., M. E. Case, C. W. H. Partridge and S. I. Ahmed. 1967.

A gene cluster in *Neurospora crassa* coding for an aggregate of five aromatic synthetic enzymes. Proc. Nat. Acad. Sci. 58: 1453.

Jacobson, J. W., M. E. Case and N. H. Giles. 1973. Purification and properties of catabolic dehydroquinase produced by wild type and various mutants in the *qa* gene cluster of *Neurospora crassa*. Proc. XIII Internat. Cong. Genetics A. in press.

Partridge, C. W. H., M. E. Case and N. H. Giles. 1972. Direct induction in wild-type *Neurospora crassa* of mutants ($qa-1^C$) constitutive for the catabolism of quinate and shikimate. Genetics 72: 411.

Rines, H. W. 1968. The recovery of mutants in the inducible quinic acid catabolic pathway in *Neurospora crassa*. Genetics 60: 215A.

Rines, H. W. 1969. Genetical and biochemical studies on the inducible quinic acid catabolic pathway in *Neurospora crassa*. Unpublished Ph.D. thesis, Yale University.

Valone, J. A., Jr., M. E. Case and N. H. Giles. 1971. Constitutive mutants in a regulatory gene exerting positive control of quinic acid catabolism in *Neurospora crassa*. Proc. Nat. Acad. Sci. 68: 1555.

Barbara A. Hamkalo[*][1], O. L. Miller, Jr.[*][2] and
Aimée H. Bakken[†][3]

*Biology Division, Oak Ridge National Laboratory, Oak
Ridge, Tennessee and †Department of Biology, Yale
University, New Haven, Connecticut

Electron microscopic analysis of the material released by
gentle lysis of prokaryotic and eukaryotic cells has provided information on the in vivo structure of transcription complexes. We
have identified active nonribosomal and ribosomal RNA genes in both
cell types (for reviews see Miller and Hamkalo, 1972; Hamkalo and
Miller, 1973). This paper summarizes the comparative structural
features of these two types of transcription in three eukaryotic
cells (HeLa, Drosophila, and yeast).

Favorable electron microscopic preparations require rapid but
gently lysis of cells and nuclei; this is achieved by different
procedures for each system and these methods will be described below. The basic electron microscopic preparative procedure utilized
in all experiments was developed by Miller and Beatty (1969a) and
is detailed in Miller and Bakken (1972) and Hamkalo and Miller
(1973).

Present Addresses:

[1] Department of Molecular Biology and Biochemistry and Cell and
Developmental Biology, University of California, Irvine, California.

[2] Department of Biology, University of Virginia, Charlottes-
ville, Virginia.

[3] Department of Zoology, University of Washington, Seattle,
Washington.

HeLa CELLS

Miller and Bakken (1972) reported that treatment of rapidly growing HeLa cell cultures with 0.3% Joy (Proctor and Gamble) at pH 8 for 30 sec at 4°C results in lysis of both cells and nuclei. When the lysate is deposited on an electron microscope grid, stained, and studied in the electron microscope, one can identify both cytoplasmic and nucleoplasmic compoenents.

Although much of the deoxyribonucleoprotein (DNP) extruded from a HeLa nucleus appears to be inactive in transcription, as defined by the absence of attached nascent ribonucleoprotein (RNP) fibrils, some regions are seen that were being transcribed at the time of preparation (Fig. 1, a and b). Protein granules of various sizes are bound to the DNA at both active and inactive sites.

Fig. 1 illustrates the two major structural arrangements at RNA synthesis sites, initially distinguishable by differences in transcription initiation frequency. In Fig. 1a, nascent RNP fibrils are both free in the nucleoplasm and attached to the DNP fiber at widely spaced intervals. The long stretches of DNP between adjacent attached RNP's is probably a result of infrequent initiation of transcription. Such a low level of initiation is markedly different from the high frequency seen on ribosomal precursor RNA (rpRNA) genes (Miller and Beatty, 1969a,b, and below) and on lateral loops of amphibian oocyte lampbrush chromosomes (Miller *et al.*, 1970). In both these cases, adjacent RNP fibrils are very closely spaced, composing easily discernable short-to-long fibril gradients. A comparison of the length of DNP transcribed to a given RNP fibril on a lateral loop vs. the length of the RNP permitted Miller *et al.*, (1970) to estimate that the RNA within an RNP fibril is foreshortened about fivefold. Since the RNP fibrils in HeLa shown in Fig. 1a do not generate a short-to-long fibril gradient, we cannot deduce the foreshortening ratio of these RNA's. However, these regions presumably represent transcription of the rapidly metabolized, high molecular weight heterogeneous nuclear RNA (HnRNA) that comprises about 95% of the RNA synthesized in HeLa cells (Darnell, 1968).

Fig. 1b illustrates regions of HeLa DNP that are frequently read. That is, adjacent RNP's are very closely spaced, making up short-to-long fibril gradients. These RNP fibril matrices show structural similarities to the active rpRNA genes of amphibian oocytes as described by Miller and Beatty (1969a,b), as detailed below.

Based on a molecular weight of approximately 4.5×10^6 for the mammalian precursor (Loening, 1970), each rpRNA gene should measure about 4.5μ, assuming that there is no alteration of the B-conformation state of the DNA. A typical fibril gradient in Fig. 1b measures about 3.5μ, somewhat shorter than anticipated;

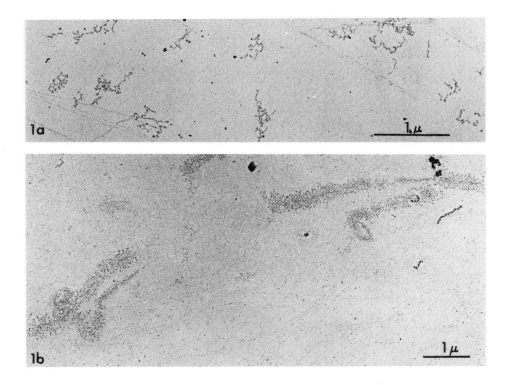

Figure 1. Portions of active chromatin from HeLa cells lysed by
30 sec treatment at 4°C with 0.3% Joy. Material was prepared for
electron microscopy by a brief, low-speed centrifugation (2350 X g;
5 min) through a 0.1M sucrose-10% formalin cushion onto a hydrophobic carbon support film. The electron microscope grid was
rinsed in 0.4% Kodak Photoflo, air-dried, stained in a 1% alcoholic
solution of phosphotungstic acid, rinsed in 95% ethanol and air-
dried. (a) HnRNA transcription; (b) putative active rpRNA genes.

it is possible, however, that the additive effect of local denatura-
tions at each active RNA polymerase along the gene might foreshorten
the DNA somewhat. Measurement of the length of fibrils at the
distal end of the fibril gradient permits an estimate of the amount
of foreshortening of the precursor molecule within the RNP fibril;
for HeLa, the longest RNP fibrils on these loci are only one-
thirtieth the contour length of a precursor molecule.

     Beginning about halfway along each locus, dense granules are
seen at the free ends of nascent RNP's. Although the composition
and function of these granules is presently unknown, they do appear
to be a consistent feature of nascent rpRNA's (Miller *et al.*, 1970,
see below).

The putative rpRNA genes tend to appear in clusters, although we have not yet achieved sufficient spreading to assess the number of units per cluster. *In situ* hybridization of rRNA to human chromosomes shows at least five nucleolus organizers on five chromosomes Henderson *et al.*, 1972). In regions where there is little DNP obscuring the background, it has been possible to follow the DNP strand between adjacent fibril gradients; these segments show no attached fibrils and are about the same length as the active loci. Such intermatrix DNP is presumably analagous to the untranscribed spacer between adjacent rpRNA genes of amphibian oocytes (Miller and Beatty, 1969a,b). This observation, then, provides the first evidence for the existence of spacer segments in mammalian ribosomal DNA.

DROSOPHILA EMBRYOS

Embryogenesis in *Drosophila melanogaster* provides an excellent system for the study of the eukaryotic replication apparatus (discussed by Hogness in the Symposium) and analysis of transcription during differentiation. Our initial observations on *Drosophila* embryonic nuclear material utilized embryos collected 4-6 hours after egg-laying. At this time the syncytial nuclei have migrated to the periphery, cell membranes have formed, and nucleoli are identifiable (Sonnenblick, 1965).

Following egg-laying on paper wetted with a solution containing 15% sucrose, 2% 95%-ethanol and 2% acetic acid embryos were gathered and placed in ice-cold 0.1% solution of Joy at pH 8. Chorions were removed manually with a needle and tweezers under a dissecting microscope and the embryo was disrupted. During chorion removal, material was in this solution for 10 min, permitting some dispersal. Released contents were mixed with a pipet and deposited on an electron microscope grid as described in the legend to Fig. 1. Fig. 2 illustrates several active regions of *Drosophila* chromatin. Polyribosomes and endoplasmic reticulum also are seen in these micrographs because the preparative procedure does not include a nuclear isolation step.

As in the other cells studied, two basic structural arrangements of transcribing regions are seen. Comparable to the bulk of HeLa chromatin, there are long stretches of DNP that are not being transcribed; however, compared to HeLa, active sites in general have a somewhat higher initiation frequency in these differentiating cells. Figs. 2a and b undoubtedly illustrate nonribosomal transcription. Nascent RNP fibrils are attached with apparent random spacing to the DNP axis. The region at the arrow in Fig. 2a is presumably a locus with very active transcription initiation, since nascent RNP's are closely spaced.

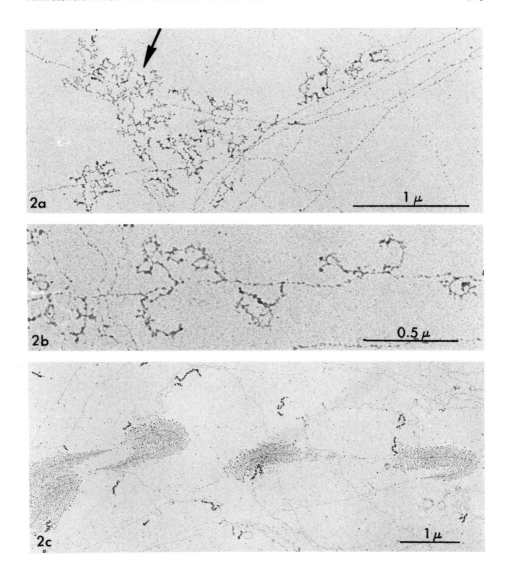

Figure 2. Portions of material extruded from 4- to 6-hr *Drosophila melanogaster* embryos after manual disruption and dispersal followed by preparation for electron microscopy as in Fig. 1. (a) Region showing both relatively inactive DNP and a site of high synthetic activity (arrow); (b) chromatin segment exhibiting a short-to-long fibril gradient of nonribosomal transcripts; (c) putative active rpRNA genes.

Fig. 2b shows a length of *Drosophila* chromatin along which the
nascent RNP's make up a short-to-long fibril gradient. The length
of DNP between the shortest and longest attached chains is about
1.75μ. Since the initiation site certainly is some distance proximal to the shortest fibril, we can estimate that this region codes
for an RNA molecule greater than 1.75 X 10^6 daltons. Since we cannot accurately extrapolate back to the approximate initiation site,
we cannot estimate the amount of DNP transcribed at the longest
RNP fibril and, hence, cannot arrive at a foreshortening ratio of
the RNA molecule within the RNP fiber.

Fig. 2c shows a portion of active *Drosophila* DNP that possesses
structural features common to all active eukaryotic rpRNA genes
studied. Each 2.65μ unit, composed of many closely spaced RNP fibrils making up a short-to-long fibril gradient, is only slightly
shorter than the length of the *Drosophila* precursor gene estimated
from a molecular weight of 2.85 X 10^6 for the precursor (Perry *et
al.*, 1970). Dense granules appear at the free ends of nascent
RNP's, and adjacent matrix units have the same short-to-long fibril
gradient polarity and are separated by variable lengths of DNP that
are inactive at the time of isolation. As with the putative HeLa
rpRNA genes, the intermatrix segments undoubtedly are analagous to
the untranscribed spacer between amphibian oocyte nucleolar genes.
Although the spacer lengths appear to be quite variable in *Drosophila*, the shortest measures about 0.4μ, or one-seventh a gene length.
Typical amphibian spacers measure about one-third the length of a
gene. Although the role of spacer DNA is still unknown, its apparent universal occurrence suggests some significant function in
ribosome biogenesis in most if not all eukaryotes.

                                   YEAST

Osmotically shocked spheroplasts produced by Glusalase-treat-
ment (Endo Labs) of logarithmically growing yeast cells, according to Shahin (1971), provide suitable material for ultrastructural
studies of transcription in a lower eukaryote. From a comparative
standpoint, it can be said that active yeast DNP (Fig. 3) is virtually indistinguishable from that of higher eukaryotes. Inactive
chromatin has a diameter of about 100 Å and possesses bound granules
of varying sizes. At sites of RNA synthesis, short, irregularly
spaced RNP fibrils are attached to the DNP (Fig. 3a). Once again,
since fibril gradients are not apparent, initiation of transcription
must occur at a low frequency, similar to that of the nonribosomal
transcription of HeLa chromatin (Fig. 1a).

Fig. 3b shows several regions in the nuclear contents from
Schizosaccharomyces pombe, a haploid fission yeast, that are sug-
gestive of partially unwound nucleoli (sites of rpRNA synthesis).

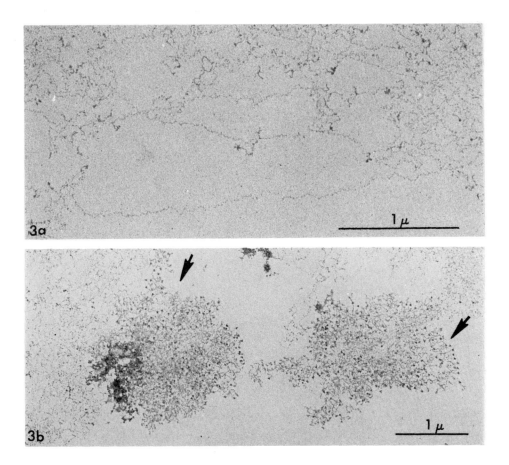

Figure 3. Material extruded from a yeast nucleus after osmotic shock. Log phase cells of *Schizosaccharomyces pombe* were converted into protoplasts according to Shahin (1971). Protoplasts were pelleted, resuspended in growth medium with 0.1M sorbitol and incubated for 2 hr at 30°C to allow macromolecular synthesis to resume. Osmotically shocked protoplasts were prepared for electron microscopy as in Fig. 1. (a) Portion of chromatin with attached RNP fibrils at sites of RNA synthesis; (b) low-magnification photograph of extruded contents showing two presumptive nucleolus organizers (arrow).

Further dispersal of this material should provide information on the arrangement of the redundant rpRNA genes of yeast as compared to other eukaryotes. In addition, visualization of *Saccharomyces cerevisiae* rpRNA genes might offer supporting evidence for the suggestion by Cramer *et al.* (1972) of the existence of clusters of rpRNA genes (10-32 cistrons per cluster) separated from other clusters by long stretches of nonribosomal DNA.

CONCLUSIONS

Comparisons of nonribosomal and ribosomal transcription in several eukaryotes provides a general picture of the structure of each type of active material. Nonribosomal activity is identified by RNP fibrils attached to the chromatin at highly variable intervals, with the exception of the closely spaced nascent transcripts of amphibian oocyte lampbrush chromosomes. In addition, nascent RNP's may grow to several times the length of mature rpRNP's because of the existence of transcription units that are longer than individual rpRNA genes. On the other hand, active rpRNA genes are composed of closely spaced RNP fibrils that form short-to-long gradients; each gradient is separated from its neighbor by untranscribed DNP. Differences between organisms are reflected in the length of each fibril gradient (related to precursor size) and the length of the spacer material.

With this information as a background, some of the questions that can be approached include the potential interaction between transcription and replication complexes and the identification of active genes coding for specific proteins. During this Symposium we have heard of systems that produce sufficiently high amounts of a specific messenger RNA so that the molecular species is easily isolatable (e.g. silk fibroin and histone messengers). The genes coding for these RNA's should be highly active in transcription, possibly with an initiation frequency approaching that of rpRNA genes. It should be possible to identify such active sites by electron microscopy using the techniques we have employed in these studies. Such experiments may provide significant information on the regulation of transcription that may not be obtained as easily by other less direct approaches.

ACKNOWLEDGMENT

Oak Ridge National Laboratory is operated by the Union Carbide Corporation for the U.S. Atomic Energy Commission.

REFERENCES

Cramer, J. H., M. M. Bhargava and H. O. Halvorson. 1972. Isolation and characterization of γDNA of *Saccharomyces cerevisiae*. J. Mol. Biol. 71: 11.

Darnell, J. E. 1968. Ribonucleic acids from animal cells. Bacteriol. Rev. 32: 262.

Hamkalo, B. A. and O. L. Miller, Jr. 1973. Electronmicroscopy of genetic activity. Ann. Rev. Biochem. 42: 379.

Henderson, A. S., D. Warburton and K. C. Atwood. 1972. Location of ribosomal DNA in the human chromosome complement. Proc. Nat. Acad. Sci. 69: 3394.

Loening, U. E. 1970. The mechanism of synthesis of ribosomal RNA. Symp. Soc. Gen. Microbiol. 20: 77.

Miller, O. L. and A. H. Bakken. 1972. Morphological studies of transcription. Acta Endocrinol. 168: 155.

Miller, O. L., Jr. and B. R. Beatty. 1969a. Visualization of nucleolar genes. Science 164: 955.

Miller, O. L., Jr. and B. R. Beatty. 1969b. Extrachromosomal nucleolar genes in amphibian oocytes. Genetics 61: 1.

Miller, O. L., Jr., B. R. Beatty, B. A. Hamkalo and C. A. Thomas, Jr. 1970. Electron microscopic visualization of transcription. Cold Spring Harbor Symp. Quant. Biol. 35: 505.

Miller, O. L. and B. A. Hamkalo. 1972. Visualization of RNA synthesis on chromosomes. Int. Rev. Cytol. 33: 1.

Perry, R. P., T.-Y. Cheng, J. J. Freed, J. R. Greenberg, D. E. Kelley and K. D. Tartof. 1970. Evolution of the transcriptional unit of ribosomal RNA. Proc. Nat. Acad. Sci. 65: 609.

Shahin, M. M. 1971. Preparation of protoplasts from stationary phase cells of *Schizosaccharomyces pombe*. Can. J. Genet. Cytol. 13: 714.

Sonnenblick, B. P. 1965. The early embryology of *Drosophia melanogaster*. In (M. Demerec, ed.) Biology of *Drosophila*. p. 62. Hafner Publishing Co., New York.

28. MOLECULAR CYTOGENETICS: A SYMPOSIUM SUMMARY

Hewson Swift

Department of Biology, University of Chicago, Chicago, Illinois

INTRODUCTION

I have been instructed by our chairman to keep my comments uncomplicated, remembering we have a broad audience, some of whom have never been distracted by the beauty of a chromosome let alone a whole live salamander, and others who might think that ethidium bromide was something you took for a headache, and hydroxyapatite for acid indigestion. I have taken notes on 32 different talks, considering genome sizes 1.5μ to 10 meters in length, more than 6 orders of magnitude in size, from *Polyoma* to *Triturus*. We have gone from replicating mechanisms in T4 which, though highly complex, can now be discussed in great detail, to replication mechanisms in higher eukaryote cells, which will scarcely be unraveled, except in a much more superficial way, within our lifetime. Yet I feel that there has been a certain coherence to this meeting, which I will try my best to impart.

These remarks have been divided into four rather obvious areas: 1) the nature of the genome, 2) DNA synthesis and its control, 3) transcription, and 4) post transcriptional control. We have considered these with decreasing emphasis--most on the genome, and least on translational control. So, not to end in an anticlimax, I would like to consider these topics reversed from the usual order, translation first, then transcription, then DNA synthesis, and finally working our way back to the genome.

POLY (A) AND TRANSLATIONAL CONTROL

We have really considered only one aspect of translational control, and that is presently enigmatic; in fact it may not in-

volve translational control at all. Darnell, in discussing an extensive series of studies on HeLa cells (e.g. Darnell et al., 1971;
Molloy and Darnell, 1973), brought up the problem of the role of
polyadenylic acid. Poly (A) as you know, was found by Kates (1970)
and Edmonds et al. (1971), attached to the 3'-OH end of vaccinia
message, and also to both HnRNA and mRNA of uninfected mammalian
cells. In HeLa it was found to be 200 nucleotides long. It was
present in both nucleus and cytoplasm, but after a 45 second pulse
with [3H]adenosine virtually all the label was nuclear (except for
a small mitochondrial fraction). This is unlike the situation during early cleavage of sea urchin eggs, where substantial cytoplasmic
poly (A) synthesis has been described, the polymers being covalently
attached to pre-existing high molecular weight RNA which serves as
primer (Slater et al., 1973). At first many people suspected that
one should find regions of poly (T) isostiches in the DNA to act as
transcription sites, but now one knows that poly (A) sequences increase with time, apparently built up with poly (A) synthetase on
the 3'-OH end of HnRNA molecules.

With the exception of histone (9S) message, most, if not all,
cytoplasmic message released from polysomes by EDTA had poly (A)
attached. Perry (with L cells) (see also Greenberg and Perry, 1972)
showed it was put on late, just before nuclear RNA was transported
to the cytoplasm. Once in the cytoplasm, poly (A) got shorter.
This suggested the ingenious mechanism that the HnRNA singled out
for translation was adenylated, which specified its transfer to the
cytoplasm. Once there, its poly (A) tail might gradually decrease,
and when it did so, possibly it was marked for destruction, like a
candle burning to the end.

However, histone message gets to the cytoplasm without poly
(A); and it is relatively stable, with a half-life of 11.5 hours
(shorter in G2 or mitotic cells), as compared to approximately 15
hours for adenylated message. Thus poly (A) *does not* impart stability. Length of the poly (A) tail cannot specify messenger life,
since young and old messages decay at the same rate, as Brown described for the silk message, where about 30% of the molecules were
found to have poly (A) tails of about 100 nucleotides long (Suzuki
and Brown, 1972). Also, some poly (A) breaks down in the nucleus,
since nuclear and cytoplasmic poly (A) do not show a simple precursor-product relationship. Thus some addition must be to HnRNA that
never makes it to the cytoplasm. Also, if poly (A) is needed to get
some RNA through the nuclear envelope, what is it doing on mitochondrial RNA, as recently found by Perlman et al. (1973)? Thus we
know a lot about poly (A), except its function. Could it specify
which messages go on membrane bound polysomes? This is unlikely
since it is on the wrong end of the molecule and besides the com-
partmentalization of protein synthesis is one problem we did not
discuss.

In closing Darnell pointed out an obvious point, but one that needs stressing. If there is translational control, and many believe there is, then this probably requires that an excess of potential message be made, to warm the bench so to speak, waiting to be called. This could be one reason for the seemingly wastefulness of nuclear RNA synthesis, where most HnRNA is destroyed soon after it is made in apparent profligacy. But in HeLa and most other cell types, less than 10% of the HnRNA ever gets to the cytoplasm; biological systems seldom seem so wasteful.

TRANSCRIPTION

Phage and Bacterial Systems

The traffic signals built into the DNA, whereby the RNA polymerase molecules are made to initiate or terminate RNA chains, were discussed by Chamberlin. There scarcely seems a better way to frustrate students of eukaryote transcription than to impress them with the complexities of such "simple systems" as T7. Six different classes of RNA transcription products are produced, varying in size from 0.2 to 5.5 X 10^6 daltons, from six different regions of the chromosome. Each region possesses its own promoter and terminator sites where *E. coli* RNA polymerase is bound and released. The promoter for region I can exist in an active or inactive state, where chain initiation is either extremely rapid or extremely slow. It has several separate binding sites for RNA polymerase molecules, producing r-strand transcripts with an ATP terminus. Another class I site produces l-strand transcripts initiating with GTP. There are innumerable details whereby the transcription of 12.6μ of DNA produces about three dozen proteins.

Zubay has studied simple lysates of λ or ϕ80-infected *E. coli* cells in which the viral genomes contained the *lac* operon. This produced an *in vitro* soup in which the enzyme was manufactured and an inducer like the classical IPTG was shown to stimulate enzyme synthesis. In addition the system required cyclic AMP; this requirement has been neatly analyzed to show that cyclic AMP binds to a specific protein (CAP) which then binds to the *lac* operon DNA to initiate the synthesis of β-galactosidase message. The rate of synthesis was doubled by addition of a penta- or hexanucleotide, called "magic spot" from the days when it was known only as a spot on a 2-dimensional chromatograph associated with enzyme activation. In a beautiful experiment β-galactosidase formation was made sensitive to the tryptophan repressor when a viral genome was used that carried fused portions of the *tryp* and *lac* operons. These are the kind of experiments eukaryote cell biologists dream of doing--but we need similar cell lysates containing only a tiny piece of the eukaryote genome--one which possibly Hogness and collaborators are

going to supply us if their attempts to insert a portion of the
Drosophila genome into the λ chromosome are successful.

Mitochondrial Protein Synthesis

Yeast mitochondrial genomes have their own complexities, as
discussed by Mahler. There are still some preparational hurdles to
cross, but with a little more time, the ρ^+ genome may become as well
known as that of T4. It has already been mapped by Casey *et al.*
(1973) and has at least one interesting property. The yeast cell
does not really need oxidative metabolism to survive, and so the
battered parasitic remnants of mitochondrial DNA, totally lacking
the translational system, can still replicate, ostensibly in a non-
functional state, the cell surviving on anaerobic glycolysis.

Like phage-bacterial interrelationships, mitochondria-nucleus
interactions are intricate, and the result of millions of generations of evolution (see Mahler, 1973 for review). Because of the
close integration-coupling, it has only recently been apparent
which proteins were coded on the yeast mitochondrial genome, which
probably consists of a circle of DNA 25μ in circumference. By using
labeled formate, it has been nicely shown which proteins are made
in situ, since mitochondrial proteins are initiated by formyl-
methionine as in prokaryotes. Pieces of 3 enzyme systems (cytochrome
oxidase, cytochrome c reductase, and ATPase), relatively-small hydrophobic proteins of the inner membrane comprising only a few percent of its mass, are apparently made *in situ*. All the rest, more
than 100 protein species, are imported from the cytoplasm. Mitochondrial RNA synthesis has been studied in a temperature sensitive
mutant in which cytoplasmic RNA is unstable at 36°C. At the restrictive temperature mitochondrial RNA synthesis continues, demonstrating that all mitochondrial RNA is transcribed from mitochondrial DNA.

Mahler also described a series of experiments in which wild
type yeast cells were "rescued" from the effects of ethidium bromide
by antimycin A, which, strangely, binds to the inner mitochondrial
membrane a long way from the DNA. The system is complex, and its
implications for the analysis of ethidium bromide mutagenesis are
not yet clear.

Silk Glands

Some 20 years ago, Butenandt and Karlson (1954) bought up all
the silk worms in southern France, several hundred kilos, with
which to determine the structure of ecdysone. It is too bad that
Brown was not around then, since it would have made a fine collaboration. I presume that most of the mulberry groves have by now been

replaced by nylon factories, but silk worms are still useful. Silk
fibroin is largely a glycine-alanine polymer with occasional residues of serine and tyrosine. Larvae in the fifth day of the fifth
instar were found to have a high molecular weight (50-64S) RNA in
its silk glands, which when isolated was 59% (G+C), and was broken
by T1 RNase into mono-, di-, tri-, and hexanucleotides with base
sequences exactly as predicted from the protein structure. This
analysis also indicated that only certain amino acid codons were
utilized in the mRNA molecule, other alternative codons for the
same amino acids being absent. The mRNA was purified by sucrose
gradient and acrylamide gel electrophoresis, and by passing it
through a poly C-cellulose column; the DNA sequences were purified
by equilibrium density gradient sedimentation in Ag^+-Cs_2SO_4. The
purified fibroin message was 10,000 nucleotides long (2.4×10^6
daltons). It hybridized to the DNA with a saturation level of
0.002%. Since the genome is small (0.5 pg) there can only be at
most 3 (probably 1 or 2) cistrons for fibroin per genome, thus there
was no specific amplification in these highly polyploid nuclei.
One can compute that each gene must make 10^4 mRNA molecules. These
are stable over 24 hours or more. During the final 2 to 3 days of
the last larval instar, each mRNA molecule would have to make about
10^{10} fibroin molecules. Since the mRNA was 59% (G+C), its DNA should
have high (G+C). Use of polylysine precipitation may help to isolate the specific gene. With purified gene and gene product it
seems likely that both the control mechanisms, as well as mRNA processing can be studied with this system. Its future seems to offer
considerable promise (Suzuki *et al.*, 1972).

Salivary Glands

    Another insect larva has been the subject of intensive study.
The aquatic larvae of *Chironomus* possess a modest economic importance as a food for trout, and more recently as indicators of stream
pollution, but they form the basis of an important series of cytological and biochemical studies. Together with *Rynchosciara*, *Chironomus* has the largest chromosomes yet found. Puffs were described
by Balbiani in 1881, and in the 1940s from *Sciara* by Poulson and
Metz--but as Daneholt has said, it was Beermann, Mechelke, and Pavan
who first emphasized their importance as signs of chromosomal activity (see Beermann, 1962 for review).

    Balbiani ring 2 on chromosome IV of *Chironomus tentans* in the
fourth instar is filled with large 450-500 Å granules, which are
RNA containing, and which are evident in both the nuclear sap and
in small numbers in the cytoplasm. These granules are apparently
formed in the Balbiani ring from nascent RNA and preformed protein,
and pass through pores in the nuclear envelope to the cytoplasm,
when they must undergo a configurational change and disappear. A
75S RNA, and its possible lighter molecular weight presursors, are

present in the puff. The 75S RNA is also a prominent constituent
of the nucleoplasm, and in addition forms a detectable component
of the cytoplasm after 3 hours of labeling. The 75S RNA is stable.
It comprises about 1.5% of the total RNA of the cell. It has a high
C/U ratio, 3.8 as opposed to 2.0 for RNA from other chromosomes,
and in autoradiographic studies by Lambert *et al.* (1972) can be
shown to hybridize selectively with the site of Balbiani ring 2 on
chromosome IV. The hybridization is rapid enough to indicate that
the 75S RNA is probably repetitive, or at least contains an internal repeat unit in its structure.

RNA from chromosomes I, II, and III is in part equally large,
but these RNA's have lower C/U ratios and do not form recognizable
peak components on gels from nuclear sap and cytoplasm. Also,
when labeled total cytoplasmic RNA was hybridizaed to the chromosomes, only Balbiani ring 2 on chromosome IV and the nucleolus organizer showed a clear concentration of label. Thus other RNA components probably do not occur in as large amounts nor are as repetitive. Electron microscopy did not show these large 450 Å granules
at other sites along the chromosome. Many smaller puffs contain
less regular granules about 150 Å in diameter (as shown by Stevens
and Swift, 1966 for *Chironomus thummi*). These studies suggest that
the product of Balbiani ring 2, and possibly also of Balbiani ring
1, are special messengers, associated with mass production of salivary gland protein secretion, as proposed by Beermann (1961) and
Grossbach (1969). The conclusions reached in these fine studies
by Daneholt, Edström and collaborators, the product of many years
of development of ultramicro techniques, strongly support the theory
that structural genes for protein secretion reside in Balbiani ring
2, are transcribed in 75S message, where they pass virtually *uncut*
into cytoplasmic polysomes, to be translated into salivary protein.
Whether the message is itself repetitive, whether the genetic information is surrounded by transcribed but "non-genetic" repeats, or
whether the message and hence the protein itself possess internal
repeat units, has yet to be determined. By analogy with the fibroin
message, one might suspect the latter alternative. One might also
emphasize that this is one of the only cases (possibly the only one
yet described) where a true eukaryote message has been localized
in the nucleus (except for viral messages) and apparently it is
passed to the cytoplasm with no detectable processing. The study
of the proteins of salivary gland secretion, the putative product
of the 75S RNA, poses several severe problems related to their
large size and the small quantities obtainable, but clearly needs
to be further studied.

Collagen

We obviously need other message systems before we have any
idea of what is typical and what is odd. The history of cell biolo-

gy was in a sense set back because Boveri drew general conclusions from *Ascaris*, and DeVries from *Oenothera*. Who knows whether these special secretions of silk worms and gnats are at all typical of protein synthesis in general? That is a major reason why one hopes the collagen synthesis system, briefly described by Brentani, fulfills its promise. Presently we need all the carefully studied examples we can obtain.

Puff Induction by RNA

We have talked little about experimental puff induction, but the report from Lara's laboratory, where 3rd or 4th instar larval RNA induced a DNA puff in late 4th instar *Rhynchosciara*, may afford a beginning for an interesting series of investigations. Presently there is a long list of unnatural treatments including anoxia, dinitrophenol, abnormally high or low salt concentrations, ribonuclease, etc. that nonetheless produce rather specific puffing patterns. Far fewer agents have been shown to be active at physiological concentrations, such as with Clever's careful studies with ecdysone (1962). Hopefully we can include these RNA fractions also in the category of natural inducers.

Chromosome Proteins

Histone message is markedly different from either fibroin or Balbiani ring mRNA's. It was first localized as a 7-9S component occurring just prior to the S phase in synchronized HeLa cells (Borun *et al.*, 1967). It was thereafter described as a 9S fraction in sea urchin, occurring in early cleavage at a time when most RNA synthesis was suppressed. As shown by Birnstiel and collaborators, it is a heterogenous collection of five fractions, probably each with a 1:1 correspondence to one of the five different major histones. Each RNA has a molecular weight of about 140,000. Hybridization studies have demonstrated that histone messages are made on repetitive sites, about 1,200 in all, clustered into one or several regions with the linkages unknown. During cleavage they have a rapid exit time from the nucleus, and a short half-life, being produced right before and during the rapid S period of egg cleavage. Histone message was found to be (G+C)-rich, and possesses no poly (A). The specificity of the 9S fraction in making histone-like proteins has also been shown *in vitro*.

The remarkable similarity between pea and beef histone IV, shown by DeLange *et al.* (1969), differing by only a couple of amino acids, is one of the most remarkable findings in evolutionary biology. Similar stability for histone III has also recently been reported (see DeLange *et al.*, 1971 for review). As mentioned by Birnstiel, this is one amino acid substitution, per site, per 100 billion

years. As shown by Easton and Chalkley (1972) and others, histone
I is much more variable. But even if the protein structure itself
remains virtually unchanged in evolution, the particular codons
within the message can still be altered. Cross hybridization
studies between different sea urchin species, and with *Drosophila,*
showed a surprising degree of divergence, much of it attributed to
shifts to alternate codons, but the exact sequences of the proteins
themselves have yet to be determined.

Gels of 9S RNA from the sea urchin *Lytechinus* presented by Kedes
showed 8 bands arranged in 3 clusters. Two dimensional slab gels
of a Tl digest showed a complex pattern, totally unlike that for
ribosomal RNA. It was suggested that the 9S RNA may perhaps be a
bit too big to be entirely translated.

Non-histone proteins, from amphibian lampbrush chromosomes,
as solubilized in guanidine HCl, were shown by Hill. On SDS gels
these showed 2 major bands, with molecular weights of 43,000 and
110,000. Several reports of HnRNA-associated nuclear proteins fall
in the 40,000 range (Georgiev and Samarina, 1971; Martin *et al.,*
1973). It is amazing how little we know of these components which
could easily play important roles in packaging, processing and
transporting messenger RNA's. Parenthetically, the fact, often
stressed by Callan (1963) and Gall (1958) for oocytes, or Hess and
Meyer (1963) for *Drosophila* spermatocytes, that different lampbrush loops have characteristic morphologies of their ribonucleoprotein granule components, poses an interesting problem. Is the
difference between a fusing loop and a large or a small granule
loop only in the *size* of the RNA transcript?

One has viewed the slow progress of *transcriptional control*
with some disappointment, since the interesting paper by Roeder and
Rutter three years ago (1970). Of particular disappointment was
the finding that the kosher nucleolar template, obtained in Brown's
laboratory, showed none of the hoped for specificity to nucleolar,
as opposed to nucleoplasmic, RNA polymerase (Roeder *et al.,* 1970).
Also, the postulated boon from a plethora of specific sigma factors
has not done so well either; but all that might have been too easy.
For this reason, the careful studies of Butterworth seem welcome.
We are obviously eventually going to have to consider using templates
resembling intact chromatin if the *in vivo* situation is to be understood, since the viral systems, or the sterilized "pure DNA" systems,
may obviously be too artificial. Real progress has been made on
understanding the heterogeneity of polymerases and their interaction
with α-amanitin. Studies on heparin, on nicked templates and on
the nature of the synthesized RNA products (as analyzed by DNA-RNA
hybridization kinetics); salt concentration effects; as well as
Hall's factor II, all seem important. But almost certainly there
are going to be other presumably elusive protein factors involved
in transcriptional control which are yet largely uncharacterized.

This is clearly a hard problem; possibly the detailed examination
of specific systems, like the silk gland, as well as temperature
sensitive mutants of specific polymerases mentioned by Hall, will
be of help.

DNA SYNTHESIS

Phage DNA Replication

It has been something of a pleasure for an outsider to see
the field of DNA synthesis grow from its early beginnings 16 years
ago. Now a couple of Nobel prizes later what is surely the most
complex series of biochemical events ever put together is, to say
the least, impressive, not only because of the sophistication of
the molecular biology, but also because of the beauty of the DNA
synthesis process itself. There is not time here to say much about
the replication process in phage, and after Albert's excellent presentation it would largely be superfluous. The T4 DNA synthesis
system requires the polymerase (the product of gene 43), and the
unwindase (from gene 32) which binds 150 molecules per replication
fork, as well as four other gene products now being characterized.
Synthesis may start with a displacement loop, with a small strand
separation at the site of the origin, which was nicely shown by
Mosig. Initiation probably involves the interaction of gene 32
protein plus a small piece of RNA made by the rifamycin-sensitive
host RNA polymerase. It can then proceed with addition of more
binding protein plus one polymerase on the leading side, and one
or more involved in short stretches of back synthesis on the lagging
side--producing 1000-base Okazaki fragments at the rate of 1 per
second, each of which begins with a short piece of RNA, and builds
on DNA at the 3' end. The structure of these primer RNA's, 81
nucleotides long for λ and 67 for ϕ80, was presented by Szybalski,
with interesting but unstated implications about the reasons for
their apparently similar secondary structure. Later the short
pieces of RNA are degraded, new DNA made with DNA polymerase, and
the gap sealed with ligase. The single stranded regions required
by T4 polymerase are provided by the unwindase protein. The advantage of an RNA primer was emphasized--since the initial match
to the template merely involves binding and does not have be be
perfect. The later replacement with DNA can involve a more careful
matching. Also, since as shown for *E. coli* polymerase I by Brutlag
and Kornberg (1972), the enzyme cuts a single-stranded 3' end until
it comes to a properly matched base pair, it may repair mis-repli-
cated bases during synthesis. A similar rectification mechanism
may be involved in T4, also requiring DNA synthesis in the 3' to
5' direction only. Implications for eukaryote systems are obvious,
and already evidence for DNA-binding proteins has been presented,

e.g., by Hotta and Stern for meiosis in lily (1971). Replication
forks of phage and *Drosophila* are also morphologically similar,
as discussed below.

The fact that there is still much to be learned about phage
DNA synthesis and its control in *E. coli* has been shown by Hausmann.
Results are complex, but the moral is clear. Many mutant strains
of *E. coli*, for presently unknown reasons, cannot support the
replication of T3 and T7. In two cases the lack of phage growth
could be attributed to restriction enzymes, but in five other cases
it could not. One must imagine changes in *E. coli* proteins which
have no detectable effect on growth of the uninfected host cell,
but which somehow are a matter of life or death to the virus. One
must assume, as in the case of the co-evolution of mitochondrial
with nuclear genomes, the replication of these phages is intimately
adapted to host cell function, in ways as yet unspecified.

Phage Evolution

Concerning the evolution of genetic systems, the studies of
Summers and collaborators (Summers *et al.*, 1973; Hyman *et al.*,
1973) should be a delight to old chromosome cytologists, who have
used the mismatch of homologous pairing in hybrids to map the
presence of chromosome alterations between species--a technique
dating back to Patau in 1935. The hybrids of phages T3, T7 and
their close relatives, seem exactly comparable on a molecular level,
and also perfectly fit the title of this symposium. An evolutionary
tree can be drawn for the relationships between DNA's of T3, T7,
QI, QII, W-31 (from *E. coli*) and H (from *Pasturella*). The more
closely related phages, which apparently can recombine in nature,
show regions of complete homology and of complete mismatch, while
less closely related phages show regions of partial homology.
Apparently, when recombination can occur, it helps to keep regions
of related genomes identical.

Eukaryote DNA Replication

We have heard several recent findings involving the timing of
DNA synthesis in eukaryotes. It has been obvious for many years
that the pattern of DNA synthesis was different in different nuclei
of the same organisms, but now with the precise measurements of
lengths of labeled DNA, by the Cairns (1966), and Huberman and
Riggs (1968) technique, presented by Callan, the evidence is very
clear.

Do chromomeres (or the probably comparable bands in salivary
gland chromosomes) represent single units of replication (replicons)?
The center to center spacing of labeled regions of stretched DNA

molecules, presumably a function of the spacing of initiation sites, averaged about 200 μ for tissue cultured cells of *Triturus cristatus*, was 43 μ for neurulae and approximately 2000 μ for early spermatocytes of the same species. Since the haploid genome contains 29 picograms of DNA, and there are an estimated 3,500 chromomeres, the average DNA-length per chromomere would be roughly 3,000 μ. Clearly the rapidly growing neurula cells have many more initiating sites than in the premeiotic S period. The *rate* of synthesis, in terms of chain elongation, between neurula and spermatocyte was 6 μ/per hour and 12 μ/per hour respectively. Thus *rates* of DNA synthesis per replication fork are roughly comparable. The 50 times more rapid S period in the embryonic tissue is largely due to the presence of many more simultaneously replicating sites along the chromosome.

A more extreme example, yet to be analyzed, is seen in the rapid cleavage nuclei of the *Drosophila* egg, where the S period is estimated to be 1 minute, as compared with the giant polytene nuclei of the salivary gland, with an S period of more than 12 hours. During the most rapid period of DNA synthesis in *Drosophila hydei* Wolstenholme (1973) found a replication fork on the average of every 0.5 μ. On the other hand, the average DNA length per salivary gland band (divided by the degree of polyteny) is some 30 times larger (Rasch *et al.*, 1971). Although each band in a polytene chromosome may contain a single initiation site for DNA synthesis, clearly there must be many initiation sites in the cleaving egg for a comparable length of DNA. These studies clearly indicate that one way an organism regulates the rate of DNA synthesis is through control of the number of replication forks present at one time.

The electron microscopy of *Drosophila* replication forks has been discussed by Hogness. The configurations of single and double stranded regions, and the presence of single stranded "whiskers," match closely those reported for the replication forks of phage λ by Inman and Schnös (1971). Clearly the replication processes of *Drosophila* and phage have much in common.

DNA Amplification

A major problem of DNA synthesis in eukaryotes concerns the question of DNA amplification, where one relatively small chromosome region, that of the nucleolus organizer, containing the genes for rRNA and their spacers, is differentially replicated many thousand times. The evidence of Hourcade and Bird for amplification via a rolling circle is to me one of the major new observations presented at this meeting. In 1970, in a speculative review, Thomas postulated a galaxy of rolling circles, one per gene, as one theory to explain the non-divergence in evolution of tandem

repeats. I always thought it was silly to imagine that floating
DNA molecules could be involved in the replication of such relatively large and stable entities as chromosomes. But at least for
the amplification of ribosomal cistrons in the amphibian ovary,
the postulate has been proven. The obvious question now is: where
else? Although unmeasured circles have been seen in spread boar
sperm DNA (Hotta and Bassel, 1965) and in yeast nuclei (Sinclair
et al., 1968) and yeast main band DNA (Guerineau *et al.*, 1971),
they are not evident in normal untreated somatic DNA, for example
in the *Drosophila* or *Chironomus* DNA studied by Wolstenholme *et al.*
(1968). In Hourcade's experiments DNA from *Xenopus* ovaries taken
during the period of amplification shortly after metamorphosis
was centrifuged in cesium chloride and the rDNA region on the heavy
side of the main band was collected. A small percent of the DNA
was circular in form, with circumferences of the expected length
of 4.5, 9, 13.5 μ, etc. up to 15 units long. Many of the circles
had tails attached, *i.e.*, were "sigma figures" or "lariats". No
circles of any kind were found in the main band region of the
gradient. The circles showed the expected blistering pattern,
when partially denatured by high pH or formamide. That these circles represented sites of rDNA synthesis was shown by Bird, when
labeled rDNA was spread for EM autoradiography, a high percentage
of silver grains was located over sigma figures.

THE STRUCTURE OF THE GENOME

Strandedness

     This brings us, lastly, to the problems of chromosome struc-
ture. We are, many of us, a bit tired of the problem of stranded-
ness. It was mentioned by Callan, who said that Taylor's [^{3}H]thy-
midine segregation experiments of 1957 and 1958 were best explained
by the unineme hypothesis--one DNA strand per chromosome. This is
very true, but, as Taylor pointed out, they did not rule out a
multiple stranded structure. I would merely like to emphasize that
Suzuki *et al.* (1972) have supplied strong evidence for a not-more-
than 2-stranded chromosome, with the hybridization saturation
studies on the fibroin message, where 1 or 2 (3 at most) copies per
haploid genome were indicated. Other studies by Bishop and Rosbash
(1973) with the duck hemoglobin message show much the same thing.
The unineme hypothesis has also been supported by the studies of
Laird (1971), where that fraction of the genome slowest to renature,
the so-called "unique" DNA, was shown to do so with kinetics indicating the presence of only a single copy of each nucleotide sequence per haploid genome. The proportion of unique DNA in various
plant and animal genomes varies from all but 1 or 2 percent to
less than half, but most evidence indicates the unique DNA contains

most of the structural genes of the organism, and comprises the major portion of the euchromatin. If these assumptions are correct, this clearly indicates that chromosomes are single stranded, but the conclusion has been questioned by Thomas (1970), as discussed below.

Repetitive DNA

In addition to the unique DNA, we have spent much time in discussing the characteristics of the repetitive DNA components of the genome. Most of us recognize two categories of repetitive DNA, the moderately repetitive and highly repetitive fractions, the latter usually equated with satellite or simple sequence DNA.

The moderately repetitive DNA's may comprise roughly between 5 and 30% of the genome, although the limit between moderately and highly repetitive fractions in some cases is an arbitrary one. The fact that nucleolus organizer DNA contains tandem repeats (500 per haploid chromosome set in *Xenopus*) is magnificently shown for several species by Hamkalo, Miller and Bakken, in their graphic and justifiably famous electron micrographs. The ribosomal cistrons in *Xenopus*, HeLa cells, *Drosophila* and yeast, with the nascent RNA and protein attached, are all strikingly similar in morphology, indicative of an underlying molecular homology. The extension of these methods to other genomes, *e.g.*, of mitochondria and chloroplasts, is in progress, and one awaits the results with interest.

The location of repetitive loci within the karyotype has been clearly determined by cytological hybridization and light microscope autoradiography. In *Xenopus*, as studied by Pardue, repetitive DNA's are clustered in certain specific regions of the genome. These beautiful preparations show that the 27,000 cistrons for 5S RNA are divided almost equally among all or nearly all the 18 chromosomes of *Xenopus laevis*, occurring at the end, or telomere, of each long arm. The localization in *X. mulleri* was identical, but this is not a universal distribution. In the newt *Triturus*, 5S sites were at numerous internal positions in the karyotype, and in *Drosophila melanogaster* Wimber and Steffensen (1970) have shown that 5S sites are all clustered at a single locus, in region 56 EF on the right arm of chromosome II. The position of the histone locus was also studied by cytological hybridization, using labeled 9S sea urchin histone message and salivary gland chromosomes of *Drosophila melanogaster*. Although the 9S message can be resolved on gels into 5 components, all label was localized on two adjacent bands, the 39 D-E region in the left arm of chromosome II. When the region was stretched, however, hybridization was also apparent between the bands. It is likely that the expected 5 histone loci are all clustered in this region, but it is also possible that at least one histone, most likely histone I, might not possess enough homology between sea urchin and *Drosophila* to form a stable hybrid.

Cytological hybridization is an exceedingly valuable method for the localization of specific chromosome regions. It has worked well where extremely hot RNA's have been obtained, and where the cistrons studied contained clusters of repetitive DNA, such as for the 5S, ribosomal, and histone regions. The method is presently not sensitive enough to indicate sites of single loci, for example that for globin or for SV-40 integration in the mammalian karyotype. Cytological hybridization is, of course, also aided by the use of polytene chromosomes, where each locus is laterally amplified several thousand times. Doubtless because of this, and possibly also because the locus itself is repetitive, or possesses an internal repeat structure, Lambert *et al.* (1972) were able to show by cytological hybridization that the 75S RNA of *Chironomus* is a product of Balbiani ring 2, as discussed above.

Cytological hybridization has also been exceedingly valuable in localizing the position of the highly repetitive simple sequence DNA. Most evidence suggests that these DNA's are not transcribed (*e.g.*, see Greenberg and Perry, 1971), but the DNA is, of course readily isolated on hydroxyapatite columns, or by cesium chloride gradients, and thus purified simple sequence DNA can be used as a template, together with bacterial RNA polymerase, to synthesize labeled complementary RNA *in vitro* (Pardue and Gall, 1970). This method has demonstrated that simple sequence DNA is primarily localized in areas of constitutive heterochromatin, *i.e.*, at centromeres or terminal knobs. Apparently one specific DNA, such as the (A+T)-rich satellite of the house mouse, may be localized at the centromere of each chromosome except the Y. In other cases, such as with satellite III in the human genome, it may primarily be localized on a single chromosome, *i.e.*, in the centromere region of chromosome 9 (Jones *et al.*, 1973).

The simple sequence DNA's of *Drosophila virilis* have been studied by Gall and collaborators. They comprise 41% of the *virilis* genome, more than half of it being in satellite I (comprising 25% of the genome), and the remainder in satellites II and III (8% each). These simple sequence DNA's are all lighter [more (A+T-rich)] than the main band, and are localized in the centric heterochromatin of all chromosomes except the Y (Gall *et al.*, 1971). Like other simple sequence DNA's, these components are highly variable between species, *i.e.*, they have not been conserved in evolution. The closely related *D. americana* possesses satellite I, but not II or III, and also a new satellite absent in *virilis*. The distantly related *D. melanogaster*, with only one obvious satellite comprising 8% of the total genome, shows no homology whatever of simple sequence DNA's. Clearly, these components are readily gained or lost in the evolutionary process. Some satellites form relatively minor components, but some organisms such as *D. certiloma*, possess a single massive satellite comprising 60% of the total DNA.

The three satellites of *D. virilis* have been sequenced by Gall. In spite of their markedly different buoyant densities and strand separation properties, all three are polymers of closely related heptanucleotides. Satellite I, which occurs in 10^7 copies per haploid genome, varies from satellite II by a single T for C substitute and I differs from III by a similar substitution at another site. Because of their close similarities, cRNA's made from different satellites should show appreciable cross hybridization, as shown by Blumenfeld (1973); thus it has not yet been possible to determine which satellites are located on which chromosomes. The structure of these highly repetitive DNA's also poses an important question. Although satellites II and III clearly seem to be derived from I, or vice versa, how does one obtain precisely the same base substitution in 3 million copies of a simple heptanucleotide? As discussed by Gall, it seems more than likely that the initial mutation occurred in a single heptamer, which was somehow "amplified" to produce several million copies within the genome. A comparable situation occurs in *Xenopus* (Brown *et al.*, 1972), where the spacer DNA between ribosomal cistrons is markedly different in X. *laevis* and X. *mulleri*, yet <u>within</u> one species, all spacer sequences appear to be the same. It is likely that base changes were readily accumulated during evolution in spacer DNA, since these appear to be non-transcribed regions where base sequence may be of little consequence. [These are the regions in the Miller and Beatty (1969) electron micrographs that lie between the feathers of attached RNA.] But by what mechanism are all the 400 spacers in the organizer of one species allowed to change with evolution yet be kept in an identical series? This is the process Brown *et al.* (1972) have termed "horizontal evolution," namely the spread of a mutation to multiple sites within one genome. The ability to keep tandem repeats identical should clearly be of value to the organism if it can prevent random accumulation of mutations within the transcribed loci of the moderately repetitive DNA, *e.g.*, within ribosomal and 5S cistrons, and the loci for tRNA's and histones. We now know, from the studies of Gall and Brown, that such a rectification mechanism, long ago postulated by Callan (1967), actually exists. But at present we have only hypotheses as to the nature of the process itself.

Several possible mechanisms have been suggested for the maintenance of identical sequences in tandem repeats. The "master-slave" theory of Callan (1967) proposed that the DNA strands comprising the master gene should somehow separate into H and L strands, and each be matched in turn with slave repeats, the L strand of the slave pairing with the H strand of the master and vice versa. Specific enzymes, similar to the correction property shown for polymerase I by Brutlag and Kornberg (1972) as mentioned above, would then seek out and excise any regions of mismatch in slave DNA. Excised regions would then be repaired, and the rectified slave looped out of the way so that another slave could take its place. Other theories include the rolling circle model, where the master

gene is located on a circle which rolls down the series of slaves
(Thomas, 1970). One could also imagine synthesis of DNA copies
away from the chromosome by a rolling circle process, similar to
that shown for rDNA amplification by Hourcade and Bird, and then
the reinsertion of amplified DNA within the genome. A process of
this kind has been postulated for *Drosophila* magnification by
Ritossa (1973). DNA could similarly be amplified by reverse transcriptase, as postulated by Tocchini-Valentini *et al.* (1973). Also,
a single mutation could spread along a series of repeats provided
that extensive unequal exchanges occurred between sister strands
of the newly replicated chromosome, as suggested by Smith (1973).

We are thus confronted with two major problems concerning
repetitive DNA's: first the nature of the rectification process,
which apparently provides the mechanism for horizontal evolution,
and second the function of simple sequence DNA. Although these
nonsense polymers are apparently not transcribed, are highly variable among related species and thus constantly changing in evolution,
they must be of some functional importance to the organism. They
are too widespread to be considered mere vagaries of evolution.
These two problems are closely related, so that the solution of one
may well lead to the clarification of the other.

Sequence Arrangement

Although many repetitive DNA's are clustered at specific sites
in the genome, such as at centromeres, telomeres, the nucleolus
organizer, etc., other repetitive DNA's are interspersed along the
chromosome arms. Much of this interspersed multiple copy DNA probably falls in the moderately repetitive class. This has been clearly
demonstrated by Gall *et al.* (1971) for the polytene chromosomes of
Drosophila virilis. When main band DNA, excluding satellites I, II
and III, was used as a template for synthesis of cRNA, cytological
hybridization was distributed along all the chromosome arms, but
as expected was light in the regions of the heterochromatin occupied
by the satellites. Under these conditions the sites of moderately
repetitive DNA were indicated, dispersed over all the regions of
euchromatin, but with some clustering in specific regions, being
particularly heavy over the X chromosome. The labeled cRNA would
not be expected to hybridize appreciably to the unique DNA during
the 15 hour incubation period used.

The detailed analysis of *Xenopus* DNA reported by Davidson (see
also Davidson *et al.*, 1973) has led to similar conclusions, based
on a completely different approach. *Xenopus* DNA has been shown to
possess a major repetitive component comprising about 30% of the
total (Hough and Davidson, 1972). Labeled DNA was sheared to pieces
of varying length from 250 to 3700 nucleotides, was denatured, and
then its binding to an excess of small (450 nucleotide) segments of

DNA studied by hydroxyapatite retention. Renaturation conditions (up to C_0t 50) were such that most associations were between sequences of the major repetitive component. Roughly 50% of the labeled pieces 450 nucleotides in length possessed a binding site for a single repetitive fragment, and as the length of the labeled DNA strands was increased, more of the 450 nucleotide pieces were bound, reaching a value of 80% for pieces 3700 nucleotides long. These data are consistent with the concept that the basic arrangement of DNA sequences in more than half the genome consists of interspersed repetitive and unique sequences. The unique sequences were estimated to be about 800 nucleotides (0.25 μ) in length. Much of the remaining DNA presumably contained longer stretches of unique DNA, also with the insertion of occasional repetitive sequences. It was suggested that in this model of the chromosome interspersed repetitive components could serve as binding sites for molecules engaged in the regulation of specific genes (Britten and Davidson, 1969, 1971). Evidence that at least some of the repetitive sequences were transcribed during *Xenopus* oogenesis was obtained by hybridization studies between repetitive DNA and oocyte RNA (Hough and Davidson, 1972). Evidence for a similar alternation of unique and repetitive regions was also found for sea urchin DNA. Davidson has concluded that this interspersion of base sequences is a highly regular and basic feature of eukaryote genomes. Similar findings were reported by Wu and Bonner (1972) for *Drosophila* DNA. Large denatured pieces were reannealed to an excess of short fragments, and the position of bound fragments was studied by electron microscopy. It was concluded that short repetitive sequences, roughly 150 nucleotides long, alternated with longer 750 nucleotide stretches of unique sequence DNA.

An alternate model for the arrangement of gene sequences within the chromosome has been proposed by Thomas and collaborators (Thomas *et al.*, 1970; Lee and Thomas, 1973) based on the ability of eukaryote DNA to form rings. *Drosophila* DNA was fragmented, and single-stranded ends were formed on the fragments by treatment with exonuclease III from *E. coli*. The preparations were then incubated at 60 to 65°C in 2XSSC for 2 hours, and then studied by electron microscopy. Under these conditions 15-20% of the DNA was present in the form of rings and lariats. (Rings could also be formed from the annealing of single-stranded pieces, but these preparations tended to aggregate, so the ring frequency became indeterminate.) Since the rings were stable and showed thermal denaturation characteristics not unlike native DNA it was concluded that they were formed by association of complementary sequences several hundred nucleotides long in the single stranded ends. The frequency of rings produced was a function of segment length. The largest percentage of circles was formed from fragments about 2 μ long. Smaller and larger pieces were less efficient. Further, the mode of breakage of the DNA, whether by mechanical shear, or by endonucleases from *E. coli* or *H. influenzae* had no effect upon ring frequency. It was concluded that breakage did not occur at special points, *e.g.*, regions of interspersed repetitive DNA, and thus rings were produced by association of randomly produced single stranded ends. Both salivary gland and adult *Drosophila* DNA produced rings at about the same frequency, thus the simple sequence DNA's, which are underreplicated in the salivary gland, apparently did not contribute to the cyclization process. Also no ring formation was obtained with prokaryote (phage or *E. coli*) DNA.

These experiments, as well as similar studies on mouse and salamander (*Necturus*) DNA, have been extensively analyzed by Thomas and collaborators (Lee and Thomas, 1973; Pyeritz and Thomas, 1973; Bick *et al.*, 1973; Thomas *et al.*, 1973). The subject was only briefly considered in our symposium, and these complex details cannot be given the attention here that they deserve. The fact that ring frequency decreased as segment length increased is interpreted to mean that similar adjacent sequences are clustered into relatively short regions of repetitive DNA's. The size of the regions, computed from the slope of the frequency-length curve, has been estimated at about 5 μ for *Drosophila*, roughly half the average amount of DNA per chromomere (or the number of visible bands) divided by the estimated number of polytene strands in the chromosome. If the efficiency of ring formation is considered as about 50%, then the data agree with the concept that each chromomere (on the average, 10 μ of DNA) consists of a collection of tandem repeats of an identical gene seqeunce. This *tandem repetition model* is favored over the *interspersed* (unique and repetitive DNA) *model* proposed by Davidson for two main reasons. First, as segments decrease in size, below 2 μ, they are progressively less efficient at ring formation, which would not be predicted from clusters of short repetitive sequences. Second, no evidence was found for unique regions among the repetitive sequences. It was argued that if indeed such unique sequences existed, then the structure of ring closures would be complex, *i.e.*, would show regions of mismatching between two matched regions, evidenced by single strand "blisters" in formamide-treated DNA; such structures were not found by Bick *et al.* (1973). It was concluded that if such unique regions were present they must be too short (less than 50 nucleotides) to be visible or too long to be contained within the closure region. It was also argued that, since the satellite DNA's were essentially absent from the salivary gland DNA that was studied, and the moderately repetitive DNA amount was negligible [estimated to be only 5% of salivary gland DNA in *D. hydei* (Dickson *et al.*, 1971)] the interspersion of a rare cluster of repetitive DNA's could not possibly account for the 20% circles obtained.

The process of ring formation in *Drosophila* embryo DNA has also been studied by Schachet and Hogness, as reported here by Hogness. Single-stranded ends were made by λ exonuclease, and the DNA was cyclized by incubation at 65°C. Closed circles were then made by addition of DNA polymerase and ligase, and the circular molecules were isolated in large numbers by differential centrifugation. The circles were then labeled by DNA polymerase in the presence of labeled nucleotide triphosphates, after nuclease treatment. Under these conditions some of the old DNA is replaced by newly synthesized radioactive DNA. The labeled DNA from the circles was then mixed with an excess of cold embryo DNA, heat denatured, and the renaturation kinetics studied. About 70% of the labeled (circular) DNA was in the rapidly renaturing category, probably simple sequence DNA, and the remaining 30% was in the moderately repetitive category. No labeled DNA was found in the slowest (unique) class. It was concluded that all rings were formed from repetitive DNA--in either the highly or moderately repetitive category. These results are inconsistent with the tandem repetition model, but are to be expected on the basis of interspersed moderately repetitive and unique sequences. At least under the conditions used, the unique DNA contributed not at all to ring formation.

Additional refutation of the Thomas tandem repeat model has come from Bonner and Wu (1973) and Laird *et al.* (1973) both of whom have demonstrated on theoretical grounds, ways in which the relation between fragment length and ring frequency, considered by Thomas to be evidence for tandem repeats, could also be explained on the basis of an interspersion model. Bonner proposed a model in which several unique sequences each about 750 nucleotides long, were considered to exist within one chromomere each interspersed by short repetitive sequences, 100 to 150 nucleotides long. All repetitive sequences within one chromomere would belong to a single family. Laird (see also Laird *et al.*, 1973) considered several other models. It was pointed out that high frequencies of ring formation could be produced even by relatively low percentages of moderately repetitive DNA, if these sequences were alternating and regularly spaced. Proposals of this kind could be tested by the production of fragments with specific terminal sequences. The bacterial restriction enzymes would be useful in such a study, but also, as reported by Bernardi, other deoxyribonucleases have some sequence specificity.

The Reality of Unique Sequences

In the evaluation of these conflicting models of chromosome structure it is important to inquire about the evidence for "unique" DNA. Does a substantial portion of the genome exist in the form of single copies per haploid chromosome set, as proposed originally by Britten and Kohne (1968) and supported by Laird, Davidson, and Hogness, or are nearly all structural genes composed of tandem repeats of a few to many copies, as proposed by Thomas? That fraction of the DNA that renatures most slowly clearly contains, as mentioned above, the majority of all structural genes of the organism. It is difficult to study because of its extreme slow renaturation rate.

Nevertheless, it has been concluded by Britten, Laird and others
that this slowest fraction, does indeed represent a unique class of
base sequences, represented only once per haploid chromosome set.
Evidence comes from the fact that a linear relationship apparently
holds between the amount of DNA in this unique class and the rate
of renaturation, as indicated by the $C_0t_{1/2}$ value over a 280-fold
range from T4, *E. coli, B. Subtilis, D. melanogaster,* the ascidian
Ciona and the mouse. The three prokaryotes on this list are well
known to possess uninemic chromosomes, with essentially all, or
nearly all, of their DNA falling in the unique category. Since the
same ratio of $C_0t_{1/2}$ value to DNA amount holds for the eukaryote
DNA's, this is seemingly convincing evidence that *one copy* and only
one of each gene is present in the haploid genome. This evidence
refutes the idea that all genes exist as multiple copies, either as
tandem repeats or in multiple stranded chromosomes. It supports a
unineme chromosome, containing unique gene loci. On the other hand,
Lee and Thomas (1973) have pointed out that the expected $C_0t_{1/2}$
values for a unique DNA, as compared to a DNA in which all loci are
represented 10 times, is only a factor of 3. Although a difference
of this magnitude should be clearly recognizable, the cumulative
uncertainties in determination of genome sizes and inaccuracies
in the estimation of C_0t values makes the 35-fold extrapolation
from *E. coli* to *Drosophila* somewhat uncertain.

The controversy is not yet solvable, but it might be pointed
out that whatever the outcome, the brilliant exposition of the
tandem repeat hypothesis by Thomas (1970) has provided a powerful
stimulus to students of chromosome structure. Much of the current
wide interest in the subject is due to his efforts.

Even the least initiated participant in this symposium must
come away with the realization that the eukaryote genome possesses
a highly complex organization. Like many controversies in biology,
I expect we will find that one single concept of the arrangement of
genetic material is insufficient. Although there is much evidence
that unique seqeunces exist in the genome, certain loci, such as
those for the 5 major histone fractions, (as well as for the rRNA,
5S and tRNA cistrons), are certainly all moderately repetitive.
Other loci, as yet undiscovered, will doubtless fall into this
category. And somewhere lost among the thousands of microns of
DNA that direct the formation of a eukaryote organism are the as
yet unfathomed mechanisms for rectification of tandem loci, the
role of the seemingly pointless simple sequence DNA, and the as
yet elusive answers to the problems of replication and transcription
control.

REFERENCES

Beermann, W. 1961. Chromosoma 12: 1.

Beermann, W. 1962. Protoplasmatologia 6D. 1.

Bick, M. D., H. L. Huang and C. A. Thomas, Jr. 1973. J. Mol. Biol. 77: 75.

Bishop, J. O. and M. Rosbash. 1973. Nature New Biol. 241: 204.

Blumenfeld, M. 1973. Cold Spring Harbor Symp. Quant. Biol. in press.

Britten, R. J. and E. H. Davidson. 1969. Science 165: 349.

Britten, R. J. and E. H. Davidson. 1971. Quart. Rev. Biol. 46: 111.

Britten, R. J. and D. Kohne. 1968. Science 161: 529.

Bonner, J. and J. R. Wu. 1973. Proc. Nat. Acad. Sci. 70: 535.

Borun, T. W., M. D. Scharff and E. Robbins. 1967. Proc. Nat. Acad. Sci. 58: 1977.

Brown, D. D., P. C. Wensink and E. Jordan. 1972. J. Mol. Biol. 63: 57.

Brutlag, D. and A. Kornberg. 1972. J. Biol. Chem. 247: 241.

Butenandt, A. and P. Karlson. 1954. Zeit. Naturforsch. 9b: 389.

Cairns, J. 1966. J. Mol. Biol. 15: 372.

Callan, H. G. 1963. Int. Rev. Cytol. 15: 1.

Callan, H. G. 1967. J. Cell Sci. 2: 1.

Casey, J., H.-J. Hsu, G. Getz, M. Rabinowitz and H. Fukuhara. 1973. J. Mol. Biol. submitted.

Clever, U. 1962. Chromosoma 13: 385.

Darnell, J. E., R. Wall and R. Tushinski. 1971. Proc. Nat. Acad. Sci. 68: 1321.

Davidson, E. H., B. R. Hough, C. S. Amenson and R. J. Britten. 1973. J. Mol. Biol. 77: 1.

DeLange, R. J., D. M. Fambrough, E. L. Smith and J. Bonner. 1969. J. Biol. Chem. 244: 5669.

DeLange, R. J. and E. L. Smith. 1971. Ann. Rev. Biochem. 40: 279.

Dickson, E., J. B. Boyd and C. Laird. 1971. J. Mol. Biol. 61: 615.

Easton, D. and R. Chalkley. 1972. Exp. Cell Res. 72: 502.

Edmonds, M., M. H. Vaughan and H. Nakazato. 1971. Proc. Nat. Acad. Sci. 68: 1136.

Gall, J. G. 1958. Symp. Chemical Basis of Heredity. (W. D. McElroy and B. Glass, eds.) Baltimore, The Johns Hopkins Press. p. 103.

Gall, J. G., E. H. Cohen and M. L. Polan. 1971. Chromosoma 33: 319.

Georgiev, G. P. and P. Samarina. 1971. In (D. Prescott, L. Goldstein, E. McConkey, eds.) Advance in Cell Biology. Vol. 2, p. 47. New York, Appleton-Century Crofts.

Greenberg, J. R. and R. P. Perry. 1971. J. Cell Biol. 50: 774.

Greenberg, J. and R. P. Perry. 1972. Biochim. Biophys. Acta 287: 361.

Grossbach, U. 1969. Chromosoma 28: 136.

Guerineau, M., C. Grandchamp, C. Paoletti and P. Slonimski. 1971. Biochem. Biophys. Res. Comm. 42: 550.

Henning, W. and B. Meer. 1971. Nature New Biol. 233: 70.

Hess, O. and G. F. Meyer. 1963. J. Cell Biol. 16: 527.

Hotta, Y. and A. Bassel. 1965. Proc. Nat. Acad. Sci. 53: 356.

Hotta, Y. and H. Stern. 1971. Devel. Biol. 26: 87.

Hough, B. and E. Davidson. 1972. J. Mol. Biol. 70: 491.

Huberman, J. A. and A. D. Riggs. 1968. J. Mol. Biol. 32: 327.

Hyman, R. W., I. Brunovskis and W. C. Summers. 1973. J. Mol. Biol. 77: 189.

Inman, R. B. and M. Schnös. 1971. J. Mol. Biol. 56: 319.

Jones, K. W., J. Prosser, U. Corneo and E. Ginelli. 1973. Chromosoma 42: 445.

Kates, J. 1970. Cold Spring Harbor Symp. Quant. Biol. 35: 743.

Laird, C. D. 1971. Chromosoma 32: 378.

Laird, C. D., W. Y. Chooi, E. Cohen, E. Dickson, N. Hutchison, M. Lamb, D. Nash, S. Olson and S. Turner. 1973. Cold Spring Harbor Symp. Quant. Biol. in press.

Lambert, B., L. Wieslander, B. Daneholt, E. Egyhazi and U. Ringborg. 1972. J. Cell Biol. 53: 407.

Lee, C. S. and C. A. Thomas, Jr. 1973. J. Mol. Biol. 77: 25.

Mahler, H. 1973. Ann. Rev. Biochem. 42, in press.

Martin, T., P. Billings, A. Levy, S. Ozarslan, T. Quinlan, H. Swift and L. Urbas. 1973. Cold Spring Harbor Symp. Quant. Biol. in press.

Miller, O. L. and B. R. Beatty. 1969. Science 164: 955.

Molloy, C. R. and J. E. Darnell. 1973. Biochemistry 12: 2324.

Pardue, M. L. and J. G. Gall. 1970. Science 168: 1356.

Patau, K. 1935. Naturwiss. 23: 537.

Perlman, S., H. T. Abelson and S. Penman. 1973. Proc. Nat. Acad. Sci. 70: 350.

Poulson, D. F. and C. W. Metz. 1938. J. Morphol. 63: 363.

Pyeritz, R. E. and C. A. Thomas, Jr. 1973. J. Mol. Biol. 77: 57.

Rasch, E. M., H. J. Barr and R. W. Rasch. 1971. Chromosoma 33: 1.

Ritossa, F., F. Scalenghe, N. DiTuri and A. M. Contini. 1973. Cold Spring Harbor Symp. Quant. Biol. in press.

Roeder, R., R. Reeder and D. Brown. 1970. Cold Spring Harbor Symp. Quant. Biol. 35: 727.

Roeder, R. and W. Rutter. 1970. Proc. Nat. Acad. Sci. 65: 675.

Slater, I., D. Gillespie and D. W. Slater. 1973. Proc. Nat. Acad. Sci. 70: 406.

Smith, G. P. 1973. Cold Spring Harbor Symp. Quant. Biol. in press.

Stevens, B. J. and H. Swift. 1966. J. Cell Biol. <u>31</u>: 55.

Summers, W. C., I. Brunovskis and R. W. Hyman. 1973. J. Mol. Biol. <u>74</u>: 291.

Suzuki, Y. and D. D. Brown. 1972. J. Mol. Biol. <u>63</u>: 409.

Suzuki, Y., L. P. Gage and D. D. Brown. 1972. J. Mol. Biol. <u>70</u>: 637.

Thomas, C. A., Jr. 1970. The Neurosciences: A Second Study Program. (F. O. Schmitt, ed.). Rockefeller Univ. Press, New York. p. 973.

Thomas, C. A., Jr., B. H. Zimm and B. M. Dancis. 1973. J. Mol. Biol. <u>77</u>: 85.

Thomas, C. A., Jr., B. A. Hamkalo, D. N. Misra and C. S. Lee. 1970. J. Mol. Biol. <u>51</u>: 621.

Tocchini-Valentini, G. P., V. Mahdavi, R. Brown and M. Crippa. 1973. Cold Spring Harbor Symp. Quant. Biol. in press.

Wimber, D. E. and D. M. Steffensen. 1970. Science <u>170</u>: 639.

Wolstenholme, D., I. Dawid and H. Ristow. 1968. Genetics <u>60</u>: 759.

Wolstenholme, D. 1973. Chromosoma <u>43</u>: 1.

Wu, J.-R., J. Hurn and J. Bonner. 1972. J. Mol. Biol. <u>64</u>: 211.

295446